MODELS OF
BRIEF PSYCHODYNAMIC THERAPY:
A COMPARATIVE APPROACH

Models of
Brief Psychodynamic
Therapy
A Comparative Approach

Stanley B. Messer
C. Seth Warren

The Guilford Press
New York London

Permission to reprint the following copyrighted material is gratefully ac-
knowledged:
Portions of Chapter 3 contain excerpts from: *Handbook of Short-Term Dynamic
Psychotherapy*, edited by Paul Crits-Christoph and Jacques P. Barber. Copyright
© 1991 by Basic Books, Inc.; *Principles of Psychoanalytic Psychotherapy*, by Lester
Luborsky. Copyright © 1984 by Basic Books, Inc.; and *Psychotherapy in a New
Key*, by Hans H. Strupp and Jeffrey L. Binder. Copyright © 1984 by Basic Books,
Inc. Reprinted by permission of Basic Books, a division of HarperCollins Pub-
lishers, Inc., New York, NY.
Portions of Chapter 4 contain excerpts from: *Time Limited Psychotherapy*, by James
Mann. Copyright © 1973 by the President and Fellows of Harvard College.
Reprinted by permission of Harvard University Press, Cambridge, MA.
Portions of Chapter 5 contain excerpts from: *American Journal of Psychiatry*, 141,
935–944, 1984. Copyright © 1984, the American Psychiatric Association.
Reprinted by permission.

©1995 The Guilford Press
A Division of Guilford Publications, Inc.
72 Spring Street, New York, NY 10012

Printed in the United States of America

This book is printed on acid-free paper.

Last digit is print number: 9   8   7   6   5   4   3   2

Library of Congress Cataloging-in-Publication Data

Messer, Stanley B.
   Models of brief psychodynamic therapy: a comparative approach /
Stanley B. Messer, C. Seth Warren.
      p.   cm.
   Includes bibliographical references and indexes.
   ISBN 1-57230-024-8 (hardcover).—ISBN 1-57230-340-9 (pbk).
   1. Brief psychotherapy.   2. Psychodynamic psychotherapy.
I. Warren, C. Seth.   II. Title.
   [DNLM: 1. Psychotherapy, Brief.   WM 420.5.P5 M584m 1995]
RC480.55.M47   1995
616.89'14—dc20
DNLM/DLC
   for Library of Congress   95-23628
                                                              CIP

To
Donna Evin Messer and Mary Kay Risi

Preface

We hope that this volume will be of special interest to graduate students in the fields of clinical and counseling psychology and clinical social work, and to residents in psychiatry. The book is also intended for psychodynamically and eclectically oriented clinicians who have been trained in long-term psychotherapy models but who, out of necessity or preference, are practicing or are about to practice brief forms of therapy in outpatient clinics, counseling centers, and private practice. Our aim has been to provide a volume that is both practical and scholarly, one that introduces psychotherapists and students to a variety of models. This will allow practitioners to choose among the models according to their evaluation of the theoretical power of the model, the evidence it offers, the one which seems best suited to the case at hand, and their own personality dispositions. The presentation of a variety of models can also more readily lead to an effort to integrate concepts from within or from outside the different models in a judicious and informed way.

How does this book differ from all other books on brief therapy? Prospective readers may be inclined to ask themselves this question before investing the time to read it and the money to buy it. We, too, posed a version of this question to ourselves before launching this project. There are four major answers that we can offer. The first is that this book, unlike others, organizes the panoply of brief psychodynamic therapies (BPT) and integrative therapies according to a conceptual scheme that reflects trends in both psychoanalytic and general psychotherapeutic theory. For example, whereas other texts typically present approaches to BPT — such as Davanloo's short-term dynamic psychotherapy, Sifneos's short-term anxiety-provoking psychotherapy or Malan's brief intensive psychotherapy — separately, this text will describe all three in one chapter under the heading of the drive/structural model of psychoanalytic theory and therapy. Similarly, the object relational/interpersonal approaches to brief therapy are clustered in one chapter, and the integrative and eclectic therapies in another. In this way the links connecting the therapies in each model can be highlighted, including (1) the *theory* underlying the model's view of personality and psychopathology, (2) its formulation of the psychodynamic *focus*, (3) the *theory of change it endorses*, and (4) the *techniques* of the therapy. Such a scheme also allows a comparison of similarities and differences across the different models of therapy.

Second, this volume takes research studies into account. It reviews the general outcome findings on brief treatments as well as the research on both process and outcome for each therapy covered. This permits one important kind of yardstick to be held up to these therapies, taking us beyond claims and speculations based on clinical experience alone.

Third, we try to stand back from the models — and the brief therapy movement itself — in order to provide a critical evaluation. What are the strengths and weaknesses, advantages and disadvantages, of each approach? Is it supported by research? Is it too narrow in its conception of psychopathology? Too confrontative in technique to be readily learned? Too restrictive in applicability? What are the limitations of brief therapy (and of managed care), especially in the treatment of the more severely disturbed patient?

Fourth, the volume tries to aid the teaching and learning of BPT, especially in the university classroom or field setting. It sets out the elements of a course in BPT and explores the intellectual and emotional concerns and resistances to be expected from novice and experienced psychotherapists as they try to adopt brief therapy models. It also offers copious case vignettes to allow the reader to get a firsthand view of the clinical application of each treatment approach. As with any applied skill, however, there is no substitute for doing BPT under supervision.

There are other, perhaps less central features that differentiate this volume from others. For one, it takes postmodern thinking into consideration by questioning the epistemological underpinnings of the models. For example, the question is raised as to whether good psychotherapy entails the discernment and working through of the correct and accurate underlying focus or conflict — which derives from a modernist, logical positivist perspective — or whether it is more like story construction or meaning making — an idea more wedded to a postmodern outlook. Can one model of brief therapy eventually prevail, or are there several equally valid ways to understand and treat mental problems? Is brief psychotherapy a scientific enterprise only, or, in assessing its value, does one have to consider the visions of reality that its practice entails?

For another, the book includes a chapter dealing with the thorny question of how to treat in short-term therapy the patient who really may need long-term treatment. That is, what are practitioners to do if necessity dictates a brief approach when they would advocate open-ended therapy? There is also a chapter on treating children, adolescents, and the elderly by viewing their problems in the context of lifespan development.

A sketch of the plan of the book will give the readers an overview of what is included. In Part I, Chapter 1, we describe the context of practice of BPT, which includes such topics as the typical length of outpatient therapy, therapists' preferences regarding long- or short-term therapy, and the role of brief therapy within the changing context of the mental health care delivery system. We give the history of BPT, starting with Freud and proceeding through Rank, Ferenczi, Reich, and Alexander and French, following the threads that lead from their ideas to current modes of practice.

We then review the research of brief therapy, including comparative studies, meta-analyses, studies correlating length of therapy to outcome, follow-up studies, and dose–effect relationships. We also view BPT in light of Northrup Frye's (1957) "visions" of reality, including the romantic, ironic, tragic, and comic. Finally, we take up the topic of learning and teaching BPT.

Part II describes two basic models of BPT, the first of which is the drive/structural model, which includes the therapies of Malan, Davanloo, and Sifneos (Chapter 2). The second is the relational model, examples of which include the therapies of Luborsky, Horowitz, Weiss and Sampson, and Strupp and Binder (Chapter 3). The therapies covered in Chapters 2–4 are described under the following headings:

1. The theory of personality and psychopathology
2. The formulation of a focus (or central issue)
3. The selection criteria: Indications and contraindications
4. The theory of change
5. The techniques of the therapy
6. A case (or case vignettes; cases may be subsumed under one of the preceding headings)
7. Review of research
8. A critical evaluation

Part III presents two types of integrative or eclectic approaches. One (that of James Mann) falls within the psychoanalytic mainstream but incorporates features from each of four basic psychoanalytic viewpoints—drive, ego, object, and self (Chapter 4). The second examines brief therapies that combine psychoanalytic understanding or approaches with concepts or techniques from other, nonpsychodynamic therapies (Chapter 5). One of these integrative approaches extracts common factors from a number of therapies (Garfield), another is technically eclectic (Bellak), and a third is theoretically integrative (Gustafson).

Part IV addresses three special topics that cut across the models: Assessing and treating the difficult patient (Chapter 6); treating children, adolescents, and the elderly: A developmental lifespan approach (Chapter 7); and epilogue: whither (wither?) psychotherapy? (Chapter 8). The first of the three chapters discusses the treatment of patients considered unsuitable for BPT, but whose therapy is frequently brief and for whom some models of treatment have been formulated. This includes, among others, problems such as narcissistic disturbances, the borderline personality, the presence of physical loss or illness, cultural differences, somatic complaints, and adults with traumatic histories. The second chapter adopts a lifespan or developmental perspective as it relates to the issues of assessment, selection, and therapeutic technique with different age groups. The final chapter raises broader, societal issues regarding the practice of short-term and long-term psychotherapy in the era of managed care.

We alternate the terms "client" and "patient" in accordance with their usage within different contexts. In using the term "psychodynamic therapy," we refer to the broad and somewhat nebulous tradition of psychotherapy which has at its core certain basic psychoanalytic theoretical and technical assumptions. These assumptions include the concept of transference as a central psychological structure arising in the course of development, which organizes and thematizes an individual's experience of self and others. We would also include the idea of psychic conflict as intrinsic to human experience, the use of defense mechanisms to mediate painful affects such as anxiety and depression, and the comprehensibility of psychological symptoms in such terms. We regard the attainment of insight in the context of a new relational experience as a central goal of psychodynamic therapy.

Although the term harkens back to Freud's theory of drives, we understand "psychodynamic" to include psychological configurations of self, other, and self-with-other, consistent with object relations and self psychological theories. We frequently use the term "psychodynamic" and not "psychoanalytic" to acknowledge a broader range of clinical techniques, such as the crucial ones of time limitation, once-weekly sessions, and the inclusion of supportive and nonpsychoanalytic techniques.

The central features of brief psychodynamic therapy include a range of 1 to 40, but more typically 12 to 25, sessions; a time limit; a psychodynamically informed focus; use of the major concepts and techniques of psychoanalytic psychotherapy; a relatively active therapist; and goal-setting.

Although we start with the drive therapies because they were developed first, didactically they are probably the hardest for the neophyte therapist to accept and to learn. Mann's therapy is easier to grasp and its techniques are gentler to employ. Next in user friendliness come the relational therapies and the eclectic approaches. An instructor using this volume may want to bear this in mind in accordance with the level of students' previous knowledge and experience.

ACKNOWLEDGMENTS

There are many people who have influenced our thinking and who have, in one fashion or another, been most helpful to us in bringing this volume to completion. We owe a special debt of gratitude to our colleague Bertram Cohen, who carefully read and commented on each page of each chapter. He challenged us to clarify our thinking, to consider alternative possibilities, and to fill in gaps where they existed. The reader assigned by The Guilford Press, Jeffrey Binder, the coauthor of an important volume in this field, also has been very supportive and helpful from the time of his reading of the initial proposal to his comments on the full draft.

Seymour Weingarten, Editor-in-Chief of The Guilford Press, knew well how to be encouraging without exerting undue pressure. It has been a pleasure working with him. The staff of The Guilford Press, including Rubina Yeh, Rowena Howells, Jeanne Ford, Jeannie Jhun, and especially Tom Penketh have been most helpful.

In addition to these acknowledgements, which we share, each of us speaking individually would like to make mention of the following:

S.B.M.: My colleagues and students at the Graduate School of Applied and Professional Psychology at Rutgers University have been a source of intellectual stimulation and friendship over the years. Sandra Harris, Dean, and Ruth Schulman, Associate Dean, have supported my endeavors through their democratic and benign leadership styles, creating conditions that gave me the time and psychic energy to pursue this project. Their friendship also mattered greatly. Louis Sass and Daniel Fishman have contributed to my knowledge base in the area of philosophical psychology. Arnold Lazarus and Cyril Franks, coming from a behavioral standpoint, have challenged me to think carefully about the strengths and weaknesses of the psychodynamic outlook. Nancy McWilliams has been a font of information and wisdom in all matters psychoanalytic. Sue Wright, secretary to the Department of Clinical Psychology, has made my duties as Chairperson much more manageable, freeing up my time to devote to this book.

William Hamovitch, Ph.D., (a. k. a. Uncle Bill), has been a staunch supporter of my academic career through the best and worst of times. I deeply appreciate his wise counsel over the years on matters both professional and personal. Seth Warren, former student and now colleague and co-author, has been an absolute delight to work with. The intellectual stimulation he provided made this volume possible.

My family has been very understanding of my work schedule and has taken in stride the deprivations of a sometimes absent husband and father. I thank my children, Elana, Leora, and Tova, just for being there, and my loving wife, Donna, to whom I dedicate this book.

C.S.W.: I would like to thank my friends and colleagues Whitney Collins, Mark Konecky, and Laura McCann, co-participants in the Rutgers Psychotherapy Research Project back when this book was just a gleam in my eye. My teacher and supervisor Nancy McWilliams has been a long-time source of encouragement and wisdom throughout the evolution of my career as a psychotherapist, for which I am deeply appreciative. I thank Art Robbins and the members of my supervision group, Al Shire, Helene Schwartzbach, the members of my peer groups, and Mike Eigen, all of whom have influenced, supported and encouraged me in important ways over the years and during the course of this project. My students and supervisees at the Graduate School of Applied and Professional Psychology at Rutgers have challenged, affirmed, and inspired me, and I am grateful for all I have received from them during the past five years.

I wish to thank my coauthor, Stanley Messer, who introduced me to brief psychotherapy more than a decade ago and has since fostered a long and fruitful collaboration of which this book is the culmination. As teacher and colleague his consistent encouragement, openness, and deep commitment to scholarly work have greatly shaped and enriched my intellectual and professional life.

Most of all, I wish to thank my wife, Mary Kay Risi, to whom I dedicate this book, and my children, Sam, Andrew, and Joanna, for sharing so generously in the sacrifices that this work entailed.

STANLEY B. MESSER
C. SETH WARREN

Contents

PART I

Introduction

CHAPTER 1

The Advent of Brief Psychodynamic Therapy

THE CONTEXT OF PRACTICE

The advent of brief psychotherapy probably owes more to changes in the social, political, and economic environment in the late part of the 20th century than to progress achieved in theory or research. In the public sphere, for example, the Community Mental Health Centers Act of 1963, and its refinement, the Mental Health Systems Act of 1980, led to the democratization of the mental health movement. Whereas previously it was largely the upper middle class who availed themselves of outpatient psychotherapy, this form of help now became available to people from all social strata. The press for service increased, leading to long waiting lists and the necessity for efficient modes of treatment, such as short-term and group therapies.

At the same time, the popularization of psychotherapy by the media through newspaper articles and features, television shows, and movies improved public awareness of, and interest in, psychological treatments for emotional and interpersonal disorders. For example, the advice columnist Ann Landers, after offering solutions to her anguished letter writers, often recommends that they seek professional counseling for their problems. On television, *The Bob Newhart Show* depicted a nonthreatening, congenial clinical psychologist who was seen conducting group therapy. In the movies, the actors Judd Hirsch and Barbara Streisand each portrayed a psychotherapist treating a troubled adolescent or adult, helping them to deal with traumatic memories and dysfunctional families.

This kind of publicity has decreased the stigma attached to psychologically based treatment, thereby increasing the demand for service. In the private sphere, the advent of health maintenance organizations, employee assistance programs, and preferred provider organizations has also changed the face of practice. These organizations typically limit the number of sessions covered or the dollar amount allowed, which has effectively increased the practice of brief therapy. In an effort to control costs, many private insurers have followed suit and have instituted peer review of long-term cases, increasing pressure on therapists to be efficient in their use of time.

Three other factors have enhanced the use of brief modalities. First, at the same time that the revolution in biologically based treatment decreased the need for lengthy hospitalization, it concomitantly increased the need for outpatient psychotherapy, including brief approaches. Second, the documented success of behavioral and family modes of treatment, which tend to be relatively brief, has presented a challenge to the time-unlimited orientation of psychoanalytic psychotherapy. To compete in the marketplace and remain viable, psychoanalytically oriented practitioners have had to adapt their techniques to a shorter time frame. Third, the advent of the dual-career family and the associated decrease in leisure time has probably affected the preference of consumers for brief therapy.

In our view, however, political, social, and economic factors are not sufficient to warrant the use of short-term therapy. There must be more clinically based reasons that are grounded in the theoretical sophistication of the brief dynamic therapy models and in the results of empirical research. A major thrust of this volume is to assess short-term therapy in light of these standards.

The changing face of practice causes many questions to arise: How much therapy are patients actually receiving and is it as much as they want? What are the attitudes of therapists—especially those who are psychodynamically oriented—toward time-limited versus time-unlimited psychotherapy, and have these changed over time? How is the medical care delivery system changing in the United States, and how is this affecting the role of brief therapy within it? We turn now to a consideration of the context of practice in the evolution of brief therapy as it relates to patients, therapists, and the health care delivery system in which they function.

The Patient's Perspective

How much therapy do patients seeking it actually get? Upon surveying the relevant literature, Garfield (1986) concluded that public clinic patients typically remain in therapy between five and eight sessions only. About 70% drop out before the tenth session. The modal number of interviews is one, the median is about three to five, and the mean varies from five to eight (Phillips, 1985). DeLeon, VandenBos, and Bulatao (1991) reported that for health maintenance organization participants utilizing outpatient mental health services, "63% were treated in fewer than 10 sessions; 26% were seen for between 11 and 20 sessions; and 11% had more than 20 sessions" (p. 22). They estimated that the average length of treatment was about 10.5 sessions. As it turns out, then, most treatment in public clinics is rather brief.

In the National Medical Expenditures Survey, over 38,000 individuals were sampled about their use of psychotherapy (Olfson & Pincus, 1994). Thirty-four percent had 1 to 2 visits, 37% had 3 to 10, 13% had 11 to 20, and only 16% had over 20 visits.

These figures may surprise practitioners whose time is largely spent with relatively few patients who are seen long term. They come to believe that most patients actually receive long-term treatment, a phenomenon known as the "clinician's illusion" (Cohen & Cohen, 1984). For example, in a study of 405 patients selected for psychodynamically oriented outpatient psychotherapy, those who attended one to four sessions (about 24%) accounted for only 2% of the 10,749 sessions utilized (Howard, Davidson, O'Mahoney, Orlinsky, & Brown, 1991). By contrast, those who attended more than 26 sessions (32%) accounted for 76% of the sessions used, and those who attended more than 52 sessions (16%) utilized 56% of the sessions. In another study, Taube, Kessler, and Feuerberg (1984) found that even fewer patients (16%) used more than 24 sessions, a finding similar to the National Survey results. It appears that a relatively small number of patients consume most of the therapy resources available. It is not surprising, then, for clinicians to think that most therapy is long term since they spend much of their time treating the relatively small percentage of patients who continue on to long-term treatment.

Phillips (1985) studied the length of treatment to learn whether such findings were restricted to particular settings and patients. He gathered data from counseling centers, health maintenance organizations, time-limited or time-unlimited settings, and community mental health clinics, in some cases repeating the measures in succeeding years. When he plotted the number of sessions in relation to the number of cases remaining after each session for each of these settings, he found a negatively accelerating, declining curve, which he referred to as the "attrition curve" (see Figure 1.1 for the general shape of the distribution, which, again, is quite similar to the National Medical Expenditures Survey results reported above). It existed across diagnosis, age, sex, presenting complaints, ethnic features, and time-limited or unlimited treatment. It even held for individuals followed from one clinic to another. Furthermore, Phillips did not view the results as suggesting

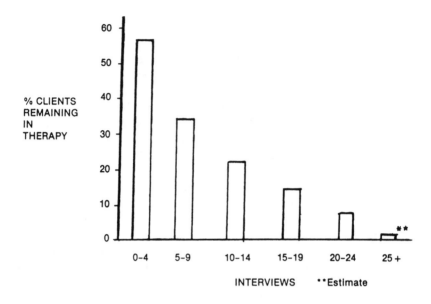

FIGURE 1.1. Phillips's "attrition curve." From Phillips (1985, p. 8). Copyright 1985 by Lawrence Erlbaum Associates. Reprinted by permission.

that the "dropouts" were necessarily therapeutic failures, but rather that many were satisfied with the help they received.

Because the preceding results emanated from public clinics of different sorts or from all sources, we may ask whether psychotherapy offered in private practice is more likely to be long term than that in public settings? Koss (1979) conducted a study in a private psychological clinic where the therapists were eclectic but always included verbal insight techniques in their treatment. Most of them favored long term psychotherapy. Based on 100 different patients seen over the period of 1 year, 80% received short-term therapy, with patients attending a median of only eight sessions. Similarly, Langsley (1978) set out to determine if there were differences in the length of treatment by private and clinic-based psychiatrists in California based on a total of 4,072 cases. The median for private psychiatrists across all diagnostic groups was 12.8, whereas for clinic psychiatrists it was 10.3. He then compared the cases of the private psychiatrists in California to a national sample of 14,381 cases treated by private psychiatrists. The length of treatment for the national sample was similar to the California group.

Regarding patient preferences, Cummings (1988) described a private, managed mental health delivery system called the Biodyne Model, in which specific interventions were developed for specific psychological conditions. When psychotherapists are trained in this model, Cummings states that "85% of patients will opt for fewer than 15 sessions, with an average of 6.2 sessions, whereas 10–15% will require long-term treatment and do receive it" (p. 312). In contrast, a study of counseling center clients by Gelso, Spiegel, and Mills (1983) found that when queried 18 months after termination of therapy, both therapists' and clients' evaluations favored time-unlimited therapy over an eight-session, time-limited therapy. However, it should be noted that the average length of the time-unlimited therapy was only 20 sessions, which still falls within the range of brief therapy.

Another study (Pekarik & Wierzbicki, 1986) demonstrated a positive relationship between clients' expected and actual treatment duration. That is, when queried at their initial appointment, the more sessions that clients expected to attend, the more visits they attended. Interestingly, 65% of the therapists in this private, nonprofit mental health clinic preferred a therapy of over 15 sessions, but only 12% of the clients expected to stay for this many sessions.

The conclusion is clear: Most people receive brief treatment, whether in public or private settings. That the perception is otherwise may be attributed to the clinician's illusion, based on the fact that more clinician hours are spent with the longer-term patients. We know rather less about the preferences of patients for short- versus long-term therapy or the reasons for the brevity of treatment, suggesting the need for more research in this area.

The Therapist's Perspective

How do mental health clinicians view the practice of time-limited therapy compared with time-unlimited therapy? To explore this question, Burlingame and Behrman (1987) surveyed the attitudes of a stratified, random sample of psychiatrists, psychologists, and social workers. Although the clinicians rated the overall value of both treatments similarly, there was an interaction between diagnosis and treatment type: Not surprisingly, time-limited therapy was regarded as superior to time-unlimited therapy for adjustment reactions and time-unlimited therapy was viewed more positively for the four remaining diagnostic categories (neurotic depression, other neuroses, personality disorders, and psychosis). This reflects a similar, earlier finding by Ursano and Dressler (1977). Also, therapists working in agencies reported having greater skill in time-limited versus time-unlimited therapy, whereas private practitioners reported no difference between the two, probably due to the familiarity and frequency of use of the two modes by the two sets of practitioners.

Burlingame and Behrman hypothesized that therapists' attitude to brief therapy may be partly a function of their theoretical orientation. Bolter, Levenson, and Alvarez (1990) studied this question, as well as attitudinal differences between short- and long-term therapists. A questionnaire tapping such variables was sent to licensed psychologists practicing in private and institutional settings in California. In accordance with Burlingame and Behrman's speculations, they found that only 17% of the behavior therapists favored a long-term approach, whereas 91% of the psychodynamic therapists and 69% of the existential–humanistic therapists did so. The greatest split in attitudes about short-term therapy between short- and long-term therapists of the same orientation was within the psychodynamic group.

Psychologists who favored long-term work were also more likely to be practicing privately (87%) than in agencies (60%). In terms of attitudinal differences, short-term versus long-term therapists more typically believed that change could occur outside of therapy and that setting a time limit intensified the therapeutic work. The authors summarized their results by saying that long-term therapists value a timeless quality in therapy and are more likely to view personality as relatively static and immutable, whereas short-term therapists take more of an adult-developmental perspective, believing that "only those interventions aimed at resuming growth are necessary" (p. 289). One implication of their findings is that attitudinal differences may be sources of resistance by therapists in learning and practicing brief therapy, especially those whose orientation is psychodynamic or existential–humanistic. How to understand and deal with such resistances, and whether these can be changed by training programs in brief therapy, will be discussed in the final section of this chapter.

A random sample of 1,500 licensed psychologists in California and Massachusetts was surveyed to determine their brief therapy experience, training, and self-reported skills (Levenson, Speed, & Budman, 1995). Among the 850 respondents, 80% were presently conducting at least some brief therapy. Of the 17 private practice hours they conducted on average each week, one-third were brief; of the 6 hours of work in public agencies, over one-half were brief. The more experience the psychologists had with brief therapy, the more positive was their attitude regarding its effectiveness. Not surprisingly, greater self-rated skill in brief therapy was associated with more experience and training and a more positive attitude toward it. Psychodynamic therapists were less positive about brief therapy than cognitive-behavioral or systems therapists.

Mahoney and Craine (1991) assessed the current and early-career beliefs of the members of two prominent psychotherapy societies. One of the questions posed concerned the importance these psychotherapists now placed on the length of therapy as a factor in its success compared with what they believed at the beginning of their careers. Respondents reported a significant decrease in their belief that length of therapy was one of the most important factors determining the success of psychotherapy; this was true regardless of theoretical orientation. Furthermore, among ten variables they rated, only the therapist's theoretical orientation was rated as low in importance as the length of therapy.

In summary, the research literature indicates that most clinicians conduct brief therapy and that it makes up a substantial percentage of their practice. They tend to view brief therapy as best for situational disorders but as less applicable to other conditions. Those working in agencies report more skill in brief versus long-term therapy, whereas private practitioners feel themselves to be equally skilled in both. Psychodynamic and existential–humanistic practitioners in general prefer longer-term therapy, especially as compared to behavior therapists. However, length of therapy seems to be regarded as less important later in therapists' careers than earlier on, and it is not considered by therapists of any persuasiion to be a major factor in determining success in therapy. Regarding our special interest in psychodynamic therapy, the results emphasize the importance of examining the reasons behind psychodynamic therapists' preference for longer-term work, and we will do so below when discussing the visions underlying the different approaches and the kind of training that psychodynamic therapists need if they are to become more accepting of short-term approaches.

The Context of Mental Health Care Delivery

Health care costs in the United States have been rising rapidly. In 1973, for example, $90 billion was spent on health care, but by 1986, that figure had ballooned to $500 billion, which constituted 11% of the Gross National Product. Of that amount, $15 billion went to mental health care (Zimet, 1989). Chrysler Corporation estimated that health care benefits were adding $600 to the cost of producing each car, leading some analysts to speculate that health care costs were a threat to American competitiveness on the world market (Broskowski, 1991). Increased costs have been traced to increasing prices charged for health care and to increased health care usage.

Far from being immune to the phenomenon of cost inflation, expenditures for mental health care, including alcohol and drug abuse, have risen much faster than general medical costs due primarily to increased utilization, especially of inpatient facilities in both psychiatric and general hospitals. In general, the costs of hospitalization and residential treatment consume much more of the mental health dollar than outpatient therapy (Lowman, 1991; Pepe & Wu, 1988), and probably account for most of the rise. Factors leading to increased utilization of mental health services include (1) the lessened stigma of seeking treatment for mental illness, (2) an increase in drug and alcohol use, (3) the greater availability of providers, and (4) the influence of popular culture. In terms of the organizational structure of health care delivery, high costs and increased use has led the field toward managed care systems.

Managed care typically involves an organization's actively overseeing and administering a patient's treatment in such a way as to coordinate continuity of care and to control costs. The best known of these systems is the health maintenance organization (HMO), which is a prepaid plan with its own staff or a hired group practice. HMO enrollments have grown so rapidly that they had reached 45.2 million members by the end of 1993 (Belar, 1995). Another type of managed care is the preferred provider organization (PPO), in which the insurer gets a discounted rate from the provider (e.g., a physician, psychologist, or social worker) and the provider is ensured a flow of referrals. There are also variations on these models known as independent practice associations (IPAs), with greater accommodation to traditional fee-for-service practice, and case management organizations (CMOs) that combine various ways of providing care while containing costs.

As an example of how such a system may operate, consider the treatment of the seriously disturbed. As inpatient care for such patients has not shown superior results to outpatient alternatives, and long-term inpatient care has not been shown to be superior to short-term stays (Lowman, 1991), a managed mental health system typically will provide the less expensive alternatives — short-term hospitalization and/or outpatient psychotherapy, which also may be short term. Similarly, taking cognizance of the findings that the provision of short-term psychotherapy and other psychologically informed care reduces the use of medical inpatient utilization (Mumford, Schlesinger, Glass, Patrick, & Cuerdon, 1984), an HMO will include short-term psychotherapy as one of the services it provides.

As Kiesler and Morton (1988) pointed out, most current professional psychology students (and, we may add, other mental health professionals in training) are destined to work in HMOs, PPOs and other emergent health care settings such as employee assistance programs and nursing homes. As a national health plan or state health plans come into being, these organizations will be operating under new reimbursement and incentive policies. To meet the challenge of cost containment policies and the integration of services occasioned by the health care revolution, Kiesler and Morton and others (e.g., Broskowski, 1995) encourage psychologists and other providers to develop their skills in brief, planned psychotherapy.

There are at least three different ways in which short-term therapy has been proposed in an effort to meet patient needs while simultaneously containing costs. In one, short-term therapy is highly reimbursed, whereas long-term therapy carries a higher deductible. Thus, the first ten sessions are reimbursed 100%, the next ten, 75%, the following ten, 50%, and so on (Lowman, 1991). In a second—the Biodyne model referred to above—brief therapy is offered on a sporadic basis throughout the life cycle, especially when crises occur, much in the style of a family practitioner who is available as the need arises (Cummings, 1988). In this model, treatment is not viewed as a once-in-a-lifetime intervention, but is conceived of as responding to developmental issues and/or life crises. In a third, practitioners in a managed care system are hired on the basis of their knowledge of short-term therapy or are trained on the job to perform rapid assessments and to provide focused care within a time limit for most clients (Haas & Cummings, 1991; Richardson & Austad, 1991).

To summarize the nature of practice in managed health care settings, therapists

> generally set clearly defined treatment goals rapidly, provide for crisis intervention, schedule sessions flexibly so that their frequency and length are based on client need more than on traditional routine, engage in cooperative interdisciplinary collaboration in treatment planning, work with not only the client, and use a modified version of primary care. (Richardson & Austad, 1991, p. 57)

Our presentation of the current move to managed health care and its emphasis on brief therapy should not be construed as a blanket endorsement of it. Many aspects of managed care are problematic. There is the clear conflict of interest involved in third-party payers regulating their own reimbursement. There is the use of less skilled case reviewers to supervise the services of more skilled and better trained providers. There are significant intrusions into patient privacy, burdensome record keeping, and the dictation of services to providers who will feel compelled to conform more to cost factors than to the needs of the patient. Perhaps most important to acknowlege is that certain patients with chronic and severe dysfunctional conditions need long-term (even lifelong) mental health services, including supportive psychotherapy (see Chapter 6). In brief, we believe that short- and long-term therapy should be available as possible choices for patients according to professionally judged and documented need (see Chapter 8).

THE HISTORICAL CONTEXT OF BRIEF PSYCHODYNAMIC THERAPY

The history of brief psychodynamic therapy (BPT) is worth telling not only for its own sake but because the connection between the work of the early pioneers and current BPT models is quite strong.

Sigmund Freud

We know that Freud's treatments tended to be short by today's standards, rarely lasting more than a year. He also conducted some very brief therapy: For example, he treated the conductor Bruno Walter in only six sessions in 1906 for a partial paralysis of his right arm. This therapy, however, relied more on suggestion than interpretation. In 1908, he relieved the impotency problem of Gustav Mahler, the composer, in a single 4-hour session, apparently by exploring its psychodynamic roots (Jones, 1957, pp. 79–80).

More relevant than the specific cases were the way in which therapy was conceptualized and the kind of techniques advocated by Freud and Breuer in the early days of psychoanalysis. To effect a cure, they believed that the cause of the symptoms, repressed traumatic memories, had to be made conscious in conjunction with an abreaction of the related affects. Psychotherapy allows "strangulated affect . . . to find a way out through speech; and also subjects the idea to associative connection by introducing it into normal consciousness" (Breuer & Freud, 1895/1955, p. 17). Hysterical symptoms, for example, were considered to be caused by the motivated extrusion of upsetting ideas from consciousness. Catharsis was the method by which the cure was effected and remains an important part of the approach of brief dynamic therapists, especially those whose work derives from the drive/structural model (e.g., Davanloo, Malan, Sifneos; see Chapter 2).

The selection criteria that Freud set out for his new therapy included at least a moderate level of intelligence, the patient's confidence in the procedure, a positive attitude toward the therapist, and a high level of motivation. For their part, therapists had to have confidence in their technique and be prepared to attack the resistance which inevitably arose as the patient came closer to the disturbing ideas creating the symptoms. The therapist was not only forceful in insisting on the patient's ability to remember but was also supportive, as well as educative about the workings of the mind. Transference was recognized but not emphasized, and treatment was limited to focal areas related to the symptoms (Flegenheimer, 1982, 1985). Many of these elements of the cathartic method are recognizable in the drive/structural brief therapies practiced today, especially the frontal attack on the resistance in the therapies of Davanloo and Sifneos.

Freud eventually abandoned the cathartic method, replacing it with the method of free association. With this change, the therapist became less active, less challenging, and less supportive. The technique became one that was optimal for inducing a regressive transference neurosis in which the arena of interpretation was largely the way in which the patient experienced the analyst, and the connection of this experience to early figures in the patient's life. A sense of timelessness was fostered, without any specificity of focus being necessary or desirable. As a result, Freudian therapy was no longer brief. As we shall learn in Chapter 2, the drive/structural brief therapists clearly operate with Freud's theory in mind, but have tried to recapture some elements of the abandoned cathartic method. Even during Freud's lifetime, however, there were psychoanalysts who were impatient with Freud's turn to the passivity of the free associative method, and who introduced both theoretical ideas and techniques that have been resurrected in modern BPT. The most prominent of these theorists were Otto Rank and Sandor Ferenczi.

Otto Rank

Whereas the vicissitudes of the oedipal complex were the primary focus of Freud's therapies, issues of separation and union were central for Rank. He posited that in the course of human development, we constantly move between the pole of emotional attachment and dependency and that of separation and independence. At first he emphasized the trauma of biological birth as the core event requiring analysis, but then moved to viewing this event as a metaphor for the separation and individuation that all human beings must undergo throughout life, including the ultimate separation of death. Rank argued that anxiety is due, not to the failure of the defenses to contain sexual and aggressive impulses, as had Freud, but to "a primal fear, which manifests itself now as a fear of life, another time as a fear of death" (Rank, 1929/1978, p. 123).

Human beings, however, are not merely driven by fear of attachment and separation, but by the will to individuate, grow, and develop. Rank's notion of will is akin to Freud's ego—an organizing and integrating force of the personality (Novey, 1983). The neurotic is unable to make choices in a constructive way and becomes paralyzed by the fear of life and of death. What he or she must learn, according to Rank, is self-acceptance, and the capacity to accept and assert responsibility without guilt, thereby overcoming existential fear (O'Dowd, 1986). Rather than viewing resistance as the force arrayed against experiencing and understanding—as something to be overcome by the therapist's technique of confrontation or interpretation—Rank saw resistance in a positive light, as the patient's unwillingness to accept the assertion of the therapist's will against his or her own. The danger of Freudian therapy was that patients would merely come to accept a new explanation for their behavior but, in so doing, deny their own will. Rank's object was to free his patients by allowing them the experience of "willing" in the therapy, thereby becoming more accepting of themselves as separate individuals. Regarding the termination of therapy, patients have to learn to resolve and accept the limits of the relationship just as they must learn to perceive other relationships as necessarily limited.

To travel this route to healing, Rank advocated an emphasis on the present experience of the relationship rather than on past events, an emphasis on the transference as an effort to reestablish the biological tie to the mother rather than on the sexual manifestations of it, and the setting of an announced endpoint to therapy, as opposed to allowing an open-ended venture. He encouraged the expression of feelings in the interaction with the therapist, as well as an analysis of patients' wish to deny and avoid them.

When Rank sensed that the patient was struggling with the will to individuate, he insisted that a termination date be set. "I looked also for criteria in the patient's own expressions of will even if not always obvious, in order to discover when he himself should be ripe for the definite time of termination" (Rank, 1929/1978, p. 14). O'Dowd (1986) nicely sums up Rank's attitude to end setting as follows: It "provides an arena for working out issues of dependency, separation, and relatedness. The key aspect of this process is maintaining the connection, the sense of belonging and attachment, along with the new-found capacity to will and to create a separate individual" (p. 146).

There are important continuities as well as differences between Rank's innovative ideas and contemporary brief dynamic psychotherapies. The most obvious link is to James Mann's time-limited psychotherapy, the subject of Chapter 4. Like Rank, Mann emphasizes the process of engagement, attachment, and eventual loss, through which the patient learns to deal with separation from an ambivalently loved object. Oedipal issues are not at the forefront as they are for Sifneos, for example. To promote this focus, Mann, unlike Rank, sets a time limit from the start so that the necessity for separation serves continuously as a catalyzing background factor. Like Rank, he regards time-limited therapy, for at least some patients, as the treatment of choice insofar as it requires them to deal with the dread of time and its implications for loss. This is quite different from the advocacy of brief therapy as a response to long waiting lists, limited resources, and other exigencies of public practice.

Rank's model is not one of medical cure, but of growth and development, which he viewed as a lifelong task. As O'Dowd (1986) described it, the goal of Rank's therapy is to empower the person to will, to act, and ultimately to create. For this to occur, the individual must learn to separate. Whereas, according to Rank, other models of psychotherapy, such as the Freudian, Jungian, or Adlerian, tried to adjust individuals to a social, biological, or normal standard, his therapy tried to free their ability to construct and create their inner and outer reality. This lifespan developmental approach informs some models of brief therapy, as discussed in Chapter 7.

Rank's focus on the relationship and its corrective potential also resonates with the interpersonal and object relational therapies described in Chapter 3, and with the work of Alexander and French, considered below. But first we turn to the work of Sandor Ferenczi, whose approach bears a relationship to the spirit of brief therapies that integrate psychoanalytic understanding and technique with those of other therapies as described in Chapter 5.

Sandor Ferenczi

Ferenczi (1920/1950) objected to psychoanalysts' increasing passivity and their excessive reliance on intellectual explanations of associations, dreams, symptoms, and complexes. In a book he wrote with Rank (Ferenczi & Rank, 1925/1986), they expressed their complaints as follows:

> The theoretic analyst always runs the danger of looking, for example, for arguments to prove the correctness of a new statement, while he thinks that he is promoting the process of curing a neurosis. Important proofs for certain theories could be found in this way, but the process of healing the abnormal dynamics of mental life was scarcely promoted. (p. 52)

They suggested that analysts should "push their academic interests aside as much as possible in their practical applications" (p. 53). Bauer and Kobos (1987) and Novey (1983) have summarized some of Ferenczi's recommendations for promoting a more rapid and effective therapy:

1. He encouraged patients to face their phobic objects or situations in order to mobilize anxiety which could then be analyzed.
2. He prohibited some behavior patterns, such as rituals in obsessional patients. In this way, the feelings that were discharged through motoric channels would become conscious and available for analysis.
3. He encouraged patients to fantasize about those topics that appeared spontaneously in their associations, in order to more readily expose their unconscious conflicts—akin to maintaining a focus.
4. He advocated provoking affective experience in the transference, either through frustration or gratification, to aid the recovery of memory.

The purpose of these maneuvers was to enhance the emotional experience of psychoanalysis, leading to a briefer therapy. In response to the charge that such parameters negated analytic neutrality, he pointed out that neither were the interpretations of traditional psychoanalysts "neutral" but actually guided patient thoughts in particular directions.

Most modern brief dynamic psychotherapies can be viewed as continuing the work started by Ferenczi. The high level of emotional involvement through therapist activity and the guiding of patient associations along the lines of a focus clearly characterize current approaches. In addition, those therapies that introduce more active or even behavioral techniques can be seen as linked to the first and second recommendations in the preceding list, although their purpose and explanation differ. That Ferenczi and Rank (1925/1986) had in mind the potential utility of combining techniques from different psychotherapies is apparent in the following statement:

> The splendid isolation which was indispensable to the creation and development of psycho-analysis need then no longer be strictly adhered to: indeed, we should not wonder, if the point were finally reached when other psychotherapeutic methods which had proven themselves useful according to analytic understanding (as we tried to show, for example, in hypnosis) were legitimately combined with psycho-analysis. (pp. 63–64)

They then refer approvingly to Freud's dictum regarding the future mass application of psychoanalysis in which its "pure gold" would be alloyed with the "copper" of direct suggestion. The integrative and eclectic models of therapy described in Chapter 5 have taken this dictum seriously.

Franz Alexander

Alexander considered his approach a continuation of the work of Rank and Ferenczi. He introduced many new ideas into psychoanalysis which have found their way into currently practiced modes of BPT. His contributions emanated from the therapies and research that he and his collaborator, Thomas French, conducted at the Chicago Institute of Psychoanalysis in the 1940s.

Best known among his concepts is the "corrective emotional experience," which shifts the curative element of psychoanalysis (although not entirely) from insight based on interpretations to emotional change based on reexperiencing of old conflicts in a new context: the therapeutic relationship. Alexander and French (1946) wrote, "Because the therapist's attitude is different from that of the authoritative person of the past, he gives the patient an opportunity to face again and again, under more favorable circumstances, those emotional situations which were formerly unbearable and to deal with them in a manner different from the old" (p. 67). More important than the similarity between the old conflict and the transference situation, maintained Alexander, were their differences, in which lay the therapeutic value of the analytic procedure.

In expanding on this idea, Alexander and French proposed the "principle of flexibility." The therapist attempts to create an interpersonal climate that highlights the discrepancy between the patient's transference attitude and the actual situation between patient and therapist.

> For example, if the original childhood situation which the patient repeats in the transference was between a strict punitive father and a frightened son, the therapist should behave in a calculated permissive manner. If the father has a doting, all-forgiving attitude towards his son, the therapist should take a more impersonal and reserved attitude. (Alexander, 1965, p. 89)

In response to the critique that such a stance was artificial, he responded that it was less so than that of the emotionally nonparticipating attitude of the standard analytic approach. He also emphasized as corrective the fact that the standard analyst's reactions in the transference situation were more rational and more objective than those of early figures who had contributed to the neurosis (Marmor, 1986).

Alexander stressed the need to formulate a comprehensive dynamic understanding of the patient in the first few interviews and to use it to plan the treatment. Goals should be established from the outset and potential complications anticipated. Like Ferenczi and Rank, he believed in making therapy an emotionally intensive experience, observing that long analyses too often ran aground on the shoals of intellectualization. He also warned against promoting dependency in the patient by allowing regression beyond the point of origin of the problem. To prevent such undue dependency, and what he viewed as the unnecessarily long analyses of the time, he proposed that treatment be interrupted for time periods to allow the patient to actively work on life problems. His stated intention was to make therapy as brief as possible.

In this connection, Alexander encouraged patients to apply what was learned in therapy to their life situation. In fact, the therapy was to focus on current life problems more than on the past, which was considered useful only insofar as it shed light on present concerns. Therapy should be "a process of emotional reeducation" (Alexander & French, 1946, p. 95) and should help the patient resume and complete an interrupted learning process.

In retrospect, it is apparent that Alexander—and Ferenczi and Rank before him—presaged a shift from Freud's one-person psychology to the two-person psychology of modern psychoanalytic schools, especially object relations and interpersonal psychoanalysis (Aron, 1990). Although they did not articulate it as such, these pioneers were shifting from the intrapsychic, drive-oriented emphasis of Freudian psychoanalysis to the more relational, interpersonal psychology developed by Balint, Guntrip, Fairbairn, Winnicott, and Bowlby in England, and Sullivan, Thompson, Fromm, and Fromm-Reichmann in America (Aron, 1990; Mitchell, 1984).

Consider, in this connection, the concept of transference. In the Freudian view, it takes place in the mind of the analysand, uninfluenced by the unique personality of the analyst, who is technically neutral and anonymous. This is so even if it unfolds in the presence of the analyst: It is an intrapsychic phenomenon. In the relational view, transference unfolds in relation to the personality and behavior of the analyst, and the patient's associations are, in part, determined by them. It is an interpersonal phenomenon. Similarly, countertransference, which was once considered entirely intrapsychic and detrimental, a source of undue *interference* with therapy, is now recognized as a potentially valuable source of *information* about the patient's struggles as they impact on the therapist.

An examination of the time-limited dynamic psychotherapy of Strupp and Binder in Chapter 3 illustrates the way in which the patient reacts to all of the therapist's current behavior, even his or her silence or shadowy presence, which then becomes fodder for examination of the vicissitudes of their developing relationship and its problems. Also discussed in that chapter is the therapy proposed by Weiss and Sampson, in which the patient is said to test the therapist's willingness not to respond as the neurotogenic parent had in the past. It is this test passing by the therapist that is a corrective emotional and cognitive experience.

The commonality between Alexander and such modern relational therapies lies not in their "manipulation" of the transference but more in their emphasis on the importance of the real (actual, contemporary) experience of the patient in the therapeutic relationship. By highlighting the centrality of that relationship for the patient's improvement, Alexander was setting the stage for viewing the relationship as other than a projection screen for patients' fantasies of the therapist. Ferenczi's experiments in gratifying or frustrating his patients, and Rank's stress on patients' working out their separation–individuation problems with the therapist pointed in a similar direction.

In advocating the early formulation of the patient's problems and planning the route to be followed in therapy, Alexander and French were proposing what has become the *sine qua non* of all forms of BPT, namely, a focus. Not everything can be attended to in a brief therapy, and it is crucial that the therapist have a road map of the journey. There must be benign neglect of some aspects of the the patient's personality or even of subsidiary problems that are not central to the person's current adaptation.

There is also a link between the eclectic brief dynamic therapies described in Chapter 5 and Alexander's advocacy of therapy as an emotional reeducation and as a learning experience in the service of adaptation. Since the purpose of the therapy was to provide an intense, emotional, focused experience rather than the fullest insight and understanding possible, he, like Ferenczi before him, realized that there was more than one way to go about this task. There are ways to heighten the emotional intensity, focal point, and adaptive quality of therapy that are not purely interpretive. These included experimenting with the spacing of sessions and with end setting, as well as variations in the very way that therapists were to act in the relationship. These principles find their counterpart in the attention of some integrative therapies to the patient's family situation (e.g., Gustafson), to the incorporation of suggestive or behavioral techniques (e.g., Garfield), and to advice giving and support (e.g., Bellak and Small). Of course, the sense in which such therapies remain "psychodynamic" must be evaluated along with the trade-offs such deviations from the standard approach entail.

Wilhelm Reich

As Magnavita (1993) has pointed out, Reich was not a proponent of brief therapy, but his impact on the brief treatment of personality or character disturbances was important nevertheless. The prevailing approach to interpretation in Reich's time was "the principle of minimal doses" (Strachey, 1934, p. 144), in which interpretation was titrated to allow affect to emerge very gradually. In contrast, Reich (1933) wrote that "many neuroses are not accessible to mild measures" (p. 146), advocating instead a stronger attack on character resistances with the object of bringing about an emotional breakthrough. Once this occurred, he asserted, the treatment, energized by the affect, would proceed rapidly. "Reich's style of heavily confronting the character resistances had the effect of giving rise to strong transference feelings, particularly to aggressive impulses" (Magnavita, 1993, p. 361).

The penetration of character resistances as the route to unlocking underlying trauma has been adopted by Davanloo in his intensive short-term dynamic psychotherapy (ISTDP; see Chapter 2). By attacking the character defenses, Davanloo, like Reich before him, elicits patients' aggressive feelings in the transference. This is supposed to change the character pattern both by means of a corrective emotional experience (the lack of a punishing response by the therapist) and by insight based on interpretation. Both Reich and Davanloo acknowledge the need for the patient to possess good ego strength to withstand the relentless pressure of character analysis. In addition to Reich's influence on ISTDP, the treatment of personality disorders in brief therapy more generally (see Chapter 6) is indebted to his work.

The pioneers of brief treatment were not popular in their day. Freud objected to the work of Ferenczi and Rank, and Alexander's approach was so strongly attacked by the psychoanalytic establishment that from the mid-1940s until the mid-1960s brief therapy did not reemerge.

In the scientific climate of the recent past and foreseeable future, demonstrating the effectiveness of brief psychodynamic therapy will be critical for its wide acceptance. We turn to a consideration of the main research findings

THE CONTEXT OF RESEARCH IN BRIEF PSYCHODYNAMIC THERAPY

Does brief therapy in general, and BPT in particular, make a difference to the patients for whom it is intended? If, for example, the research revealed little gain for patients in brief therapy, or was a very poor cousin of long-term therapy, our assessment of its worth would be affected accordingly. Throughout this volume, we will take into consideration the empirical literature on psychotherapy process and outcome as it bears on each of the models or topics that we cover. In this section we will examine the question of the overall value of time-limited therapy in general, and BPT in particular. It should be mentioned at the outset that investigators were usually selective in the patient populations treated, recognizing that short-term treatment is not for everyone. In addition, one must keep in mind that the goals, and hence the outcome measures for brief therapy, may not be the same as those for long-term psychoanalytic therapy, as we will discuss below.

In reviewing the empirical literature on brief therapy, there are several questions which we will try to answer.

1. Is brief therapy helpful, and is it more or less helpful than long-term therapy?
2. Is one form of brief therapy more helpful than other forms and, in particular, is long-term psychdynamic therapy more helpful than BPT?
3. Do patients diagnosed as depressed or anxious improve faster than borderline patients?
4. Do general measures of well-being and symptoms record improvement sooner than measures of life functioning, such as the ability to work and to enjoy good interpersonal relationships?
5. Do the results of brief therapy depend on the source of the outcome measures (patient, therapist, or tests)?
6. Do patients in brief therapy maintain their gains on follow-up?
7. Are the measures employed for judging outcomes pertinent to psychoanalytic therapy?

Comparative Studies

Time-Limited versus Time-Unlimited Therapy

Luborsky, Singer, and Luborsky (1975) compared eight controlled studies of brief time-limited to time-unlimited therapy. Time-limited therapy was superior in two studies and time-unlimited in one; there were no differences in the other five. More recently, Orlinsky and Howard (1986) compared seven such studies: Three found time-limited therapy superior, three showed no difference, and one demonstrated time-unlimited therapy to be superior. The authors cautioned however, that time-unlimited therapy may not have been very long, due to high dropout rates. Koss and Butcher (1986) also reviewed the research on comparative studies of outcome in time-limited vs. time-unlimited therapy, and concluded that there was "little empirical evidence of differences in overall effectiveness" (p. 660). The most recent review of such studies came to the same conclusion (Koss & Shiang, 1994).

Brief Psychodynamic Therapy versus Alternative Therapies

Studies have compared brief therapies based on different theoretical orientations, such as psychodynamic, client-centered, behavioral, cognitive, and so forth (e.g., Cross, Sheehan, & Khan, 1982; Levene, Breger, & Patterson, 1972; Patterson, Levene, & Breger, 1971; Sloane, Staples, Cristol, Yorkston, & Whipple, 1975; Strupp & Hadley, 1979; Thompson, Gallagher, & Breckenridge, 1987). Few significant differences have been found among these therapies, which parallels similar findings in the general psychotherapy outcome literature (Smith, Glass, & Miller, 1980; Stiles, Shapiro, & Elliott, 1986).

To cite just just two of the most sophisticated of the comparative studies, the National Institute of Mental Health collaborative study of depression (Elkin et al., 1989) compared interpersonal psychotherapy (IPT), cognitive-behavioral therapy (CBT), imipramine hydrochloride (an antidepressant) combined with clinical management (IHCM), and placebo combined with clinical management (PCM). All patients improved in general functioning and depressive symptoms over the 16 weeks of treatment, with IPT and CBT showing similar results, and falling between IHCM (which was more effective) and PCM (which was less so).

In the most recent comparative study of brief psychodynamic–interpersonal therapy (PI) with cognitive-behavioral (CB) therapy, Shapiro et al. (1994) studied patients with different levels of severity of depression who were treated for either 8 or 16 weeks. Patients showed substantial improvement in both treatments, with six of seven outcome measures showing no difference between PI therapy and CB therapy, irrespective of patients' initial severity of depression or the length of therapy (that is, 8 or 16 weeks). The one measure that favored CB therapy was the Beck Depression Inventory which, as the authors point out, is grounded in a CB model of depression, thus predisposing it toward CB therapy. There was no overall advantage to the 16 versus 8 session therapy except for the most severely depressed patients, who improved much more in the 16-session therapy.

Meta-Analysis

Another way of comparing studies is through meta-analysis, in which the individual findings from a large number of studies are aggregated by extracting a common metric, such as an effect size. The latter expresses the differences between the means of the groups, compared in standard deviation units. In their classic study comparing 475 studies of treated and untreated groups, Smith and colleagues (1980) found that the average effect associated with psychotherapy was 0.85 standard deviation units. This means that the average treated person is better off than 80% of an untreated sample at the end of therapy. Since the therapies compared were usually short, averaging 15 sessions, these results can be viewed as supportive of the effects of brief therapy. In addition, on the basis of their analysis, the authors concluded that the major impact of treatment occurs in the first six to eight sessions.

More recently, Crits-Christoph (1992) and Svartberg and Stiles (1991) published meta-analyses of studies focusing on the effects of brief psychodynamic therapy. Of the two, the Crits-Christoph review was more exacting in the selection of studies for inclusion in the meta-analysis. The criteria were use of a specific form of BPT as represented in a manual-like guide; comparison of BPT and either a waiting list control condition, an alternative therapy, medication, or a nonpsychiatric treatment (such as a self-help group, drug counseling, or low-contact treatment); and the study's provision of the information necessary to calculate effect sizes. Two other important criteria were a minimum of 12 sessions and therapists who were experienced in conducting BPT. The outcome measures compared included target symptoms, general level of psychiatric symptoms, and social functioning. The results of the meta-analysis of the 11 studies reviewed were that BPT demonstrated large effects compared to the waiting list control, slight superiority to the nonpsychiatric treatments, and equal effects to other psychotherapies and medication. (See Svartberg & Stiles, 1993, and Crits-Christoph, 1993, for a critique and response.)

The Svartberg and Stiles review included 19 studies, only 2 of which overlapped those in Crits-Christoph's review. This was because the former included only studies appearing between 1978 and 1988, whereas most of the studies in the latter review appeared after 1988. Svartberg and Stiles defined their inclusion criteria as follows: group designs which included BPT and either a no-treatment control or an alternative group, or both, and two of the following conditions: The underlying theory of the approach was psychodynamic, the stated goal was the acquisition of insight or the achievement of personality change, and the techniques emphasized interpretation and transference. In addition, there had to be a conceptually planned brief duration of treatment of less than 40 sessions.

BPT showed a small but significant superiority to the no-treatment condition at termination of therapy, but this had disappeared by 1-year follow-up. However, those studies that included such a follow-up averaged only 6.8 sessions in duration, which the authors point out (and the dose–effect relationship described below confirms) may not have been enough time for BPT to show its benefits. Compared with alternative approaches such as behavioral or cognitive therapy, BPT was inferior at posttreatment, not so at 6-month follow-up, but considerably so at the 1-year follow-up. In comparing the results by diagnostic group, the only category that presumably showed clear superiority for an alternative therapy was major depression, and the alternative treatment that was more effective was cognitive-behavioral therapy. It should be noted, however, that this conclusion was based on a particularly strong result in only one of four studies. Another interesting finding was that fixed time limits were more effective than flexible time limits.

The difference in results between the two reviews prompted us to look more carefully at the individual studies in these reviews and our findings are instructive. The most consistent difference between the reviews was in the nature of what was considered BPT. Whereas the Crits-Christoph review included only well-specified, manual-driven examples of BPT (e.g., Mann, psychodynamic–interpersonal, etc.), the studies in the Svartberg and Stiles review were often quite vague as to the extent to which the therapies were truly psychodynamic or psychoanalytic. Phrases such as "patterned after Malan," or "use whatever verbal techniques are most helpful" were common, as were references to eclectic forms of BPT that included some unspecified mixture of other elements, such as offering advice or looking at precipitating factors. In other words, it seemed to us that use of the term BPT was stretched too far in describing these therapies, especially if one compares them to existing models.

In addition, the therapists most typically were either trainees with little or no experience conducting psychoanalytic therapy (long-term or short-term), or, at the other end of the spectrum of experience, psychoanalysts who had practiced long-term therapy only. As pointed out by Crits-Christoph (citing Budman, 1981), long-term psychodynamic therapists, including psychoanalysts, are often slow to adapt to the philosophy of brief therapy. Another limitation of several of the studies included in the meta-analysis was the nature of patient problems, some of which included psychosomatic difficulties, drug addiction, severe depression, and eating disorders, all commonly considered unsuitable for BPT, as discussed in the chapters to follow. Other frequent problems were small sample sizes and, hence, low statistical power, a small number of therapy sessions (e.g., six to eight); lack of a time limit, and lack of randomization of patients among the groups. Svartberg and Stiles did attempt to separate out some of the methodological and treatment-related moderators (e.g., therapist experience) of overall effectiveness of BPT, with largely negative findings.

To tease out variables one at a time and relate them to variation in outcome, however, is to neglect all the other problematic aspects of these studies, which in our view, render the results of this meta-analysis highly ambiguous. In this connection, Rachman and Wilson (1980) have criticized the practice of including methodologically flawed studies in meta-analyses, since this only serves to add questionable effect sizes to the larger pool. Finally, had the better, more recent studies been included in the Svartberg and Stiles review, their results would have been more favorable to BPT, at least with respect to waiting list controls.

Diguer et al. (1993) were also puzzled by the discrepancy between the two meta-analyses and undertook their own, insuring that each study met preselected criteria, including a quality rating that they used as a weight in calculating effect sizes. They came up with 13 studies, 8 overlapping those of Svartberg and Stiles, which allowed for 17 comparisons between BPT and other therapies. The overall effect sizes revealed no significant differences in efficacy between BPT and other forms of psychological therapy at termination. Diguer and colleagues, as well as other authors (e.g., Barber, 1994) make the important point that future studies should assess other outcome areas of special interest to psychodynamic clinicians, such as interpersonal relationship patterns and psychodynamic conflicts.

Meta-analysis is still a relatively new procedure and, in spite of its apparent exactness and objectivity, subjective judgment does enter into it. The major source of bias is the criteria used for inclusion of studies, which can vary considerably (Piper, 1988). Another problem involves averaging effect sizes of several outcome measures from the same study, where some might be positive and others negative, leading to a washout. A similar problem exists across studies: Taking mediating variables such as the nature of the outcome measures used into account could make a significant difference in the conclusions reached on such important issues as the effect of the therapy's theoretical orientation on outcome (Shadish, 1992; Shadish & Sweeney, 1991).

Short-Term versus Long-Term Psychoanalytic Therapy

A very relevant kind of comparative study for a volume emphasizing psychodynamic approaches to brief therapy would be one directly comparing the effects of long-term versus a planned short-term psychoanalytically oriented psychotherapy. There is only one such study that we are aware of, and we will report its method and results in some detail because of its importance to our topic and its methodological sophistication. Piper, Debbane, Bienvenu, and Garant (1984) compared four types of psychoanalytically oriented therapy: short-term individual (STI), long-term individual (LTI), short-term group (STG), and long-term group (LTG). The patients were suffering from neurotic or mild-to-moderate characterological problems, with complaints concerning anxiety, depression, low self-esteem, and difficulties with interpersonal relationships. The therapists were three male psychiatrists, experienced in the four treatment modalities, each of whom served as his own control across the four therapies. The short-term therapy followed Malan's technique, which derives from a drive/structural theoretical approach (described in Chapter 2). The two long-term forms of therapy averaged 76 sessions, and the short-term forms, 22 sessions, for a ratio of 3.5 to 1.

Patients were matched on the basis of age, sex, and the composite sum of five selection criteria, including verbal skill, chronicity of problems, psychological-mindedness, motivation for individual therapy, and motivation for group therapy (patients had to be willing to accept either individual or group therapy). Outcome measures included traditional psychiatric symptomatology, interpersonal functioning, and personal target objectives. For the latter, the patient formulated a written set of objectives with the assistance of an independent assessor. Outcome was rated from the point of view of patient, therapist, and an independent evaluator.

Seventy-five percent of the patients (79) remained in therapy, with no significant difference in dropout rate between therapy groups. There was a significant interaction found between type of therapy (individual vs. group) and duration of therapy (long vs. short). From the therapist's perspective (on the outcome measures of an average of all target objectives, the most important target objective, and overall usefulness of therapy), STI therapy was rated best, followed closely by LTI and LTG therapy, with STG therapy a distant fourth. From the patient's perspective (on the outcome measures of shyness/inhibition, severity of disturbance, and overall usefulness of therapy), LTG therapy was rated best, followed closely by STI. LTI therapy was third and STG a distant fourth. Patients in all four forms of therapy evidenced improvement over pretherapy status. To their credit, the authors also conducted a 6-month follow-up. Patients either maintained their gains or showed additional improvement in all four therapies. However, in comparing the therapies, "the worst outcome was associated with STG therapy and the best outcome with LTG therapy and STI therapy" (p. 274).

Piper and his colleagues then conducted a cost-benefit analysis. In terms of the patient, the time ratios were 1 (STI): 2 (STG): 4 (LTI): 7 (LTG); that is, patients spent twice as much time in STG as in STI, four times as much in LTI, and seven times as much in LTG. In terms of therapist time, the ratios were 1 (STG): 4 (LTG): 5 (STI): 20 (LTI). The authors concluded that "in terms of cost-effectiveness and the quality of therapy process as viewed by the therapists LTG therapy and STI therapy were regarded as superior" (p. 278).

Psychoanalytic Outcome Criteria

We view these findings, as did Piper and colleagues, as very supportive of the value of brief, individual psychoanalytic therapy even when compared to long-term psychoanalytic therapy. However, it should be noted that psychoanalytically oriented critics could complain that the outcome measures were slanted toward more overt, objective, readily measurable effects and did not include variables that they value, such as changes in patients' productivity, self-knowledge, underlying conflicts, quality of life, and personality (Barber, 1994). The implication is that the research as it stands does not do justice to the goals of long-term psychoanalytic therapy. Baker (1985) lists the following as the five basic goals of all forms of psychoanalytic treatment:

1. A decrease in the intensity of irrational impulses and the mature management of instinctual strivings by appropriate conscious ego controls;
2. an enhancement of the repertoire, maturity, effectiveness, and flexibility of ego defenses;
3. the development and support of those values, attitudes, and self expectations that are based on an appropriate assessment of reality and that facilitate adaptation;
4. the development of a capacity for mature intimacy and productive self-expression;
5. a lessening of the punitiveness of the superego and the associated perfectionism that is rooted in the demands and inhibitions of the conscience. (p. 37)

Although some of these features may have been captured by Piper and colleagues, especially in the interpersonal measures, most were not. Perhaps some of these goals are more appropriate for long-term psychoanalytic therapy or psychoanalysis proper, but not for brief therapy. The kind of measures needed to tap the variables outlined by Baker are hard to come by, but are not impossible to construct. In addition, the traditional psychoanalyst may be more inclined to rely on measures such as changes observed in the nature of transference or in the content of dreams, which are less subject to patient or therapist distortion. Of course, these are not as readily assessed in a psychometrically reliable way, which may explain why they are infrequently employed in empirical research.

Another way of thinking about BPT is to view it as an introduction to a process through which patients expand their conscious awareness of the nature of their problem, their role in creating it, and the potential to do something about it. They become more attuned to their feelings, more honest with themselves, and more able to be intimate. These are some of the ways in which Schafer (1973) has conceptualized brief dynamic therapy, and it differs from both Baker's and Piper and colleagues' perspective. In his view, BPT lies on a continuum with psychoanalysis and long-term psychoanalytic therapy, with no hard and fast distinction between them. The Rutgers Psychotherapy Research Group created a scale to measure, session by session, mini-outcomes based, in part, on Schafer's concept of BPT (Sogg & Messer, 1995). The items, a sample of which are presented in Table 1.1, are rated by the therapist or researcher on a 5-point Likert scale, defining the degree to which progress is being made. The scale takes account of the steps ("process-like" items) that form the foundation for more external change (traditional "outcome-like" items).

Correlational Studies on Length of Treatment and Outcome

While the foregoing studies compared the outcome of brief therapies with longer-term or other therapies, the correlational investigations seek an association between the number of sessions attended and therapy outcome. The trend in these studies is quite different from that in the comparative studies. For example, Luborsky, Chandler, Auerbach, Cohen, & Bachrach (1971) found that "in 20 of 22 studies of essentially time unlimited treatment, the length of treatment was positively related to outcome; the longer the duration of treatment or the more

TABLE 1.1. Some Items from the Rutgers Session Outcome Measure

Process-like items

What is the quality of the relationship between the client and the therapist?
Does the client believe that his or her problems are understandable, potentially manageable, and potentially resolvable?
Does the client recognize the relationship between session material and the main theme(s) of the therapy?
Does the client have a well-defined and comprehensive idea of the scope and complexity of his or her problems?

Outcome-like items

How has the client been feeling?
Has the client been initiating or maintaining action that positively affects his or her well-being?
What is the client's level of self-esteem?
Has the client been demonstrating a healthy level of autonomy—that is, a balance between feeling able to use the support of others and feeling able to act independently of support from others?

Note. From Sogg & Messer (1995).

sessions, the better the outcome!" (p. 154). Similar conclusions were reached by Johnson and Gelso (1980) and Orlinsky and Howard (1986).

There are several important points which should be kept in mind in interpreting these results. First, Johnson and Gelso found that the percentage of studies favoring longer-term therapy varied considerably with the source of the outcome measurement. For therapist-rated outcome, 89% of the studies favored long-term treatment, but for client-rated outcome, the figure dropped to 50%. When outcome was gauged by behavioral measures or psychological tests (the most unbiased measures), the percentage favoring time-unlimited therapy fell even further, to 25%. They suggested that therapists may be biased in attributing change in those patients whom they have seen over a longer period of time, either in accordance with their expectations or as a result of cognitive dissonance. That is, the greater amount of time invested would lead therapists to judge results as more satisfactory, thereby justifying the increased effort and expense. (In a later statement, Gelso, 1992, pointed out that there is too little recognition of the special expertise of the therapist in making judgments about clients' progress.) However, they also found in a small subset of studies using observer-rated outcome, where a therapist bias would not be operating, that the correlation between length of therapy and outcome held in 71% of them.

Another possibility for the superior showing of time-unlimited therapy is that the type of behavior change observable to a dispassionate rater may not be manifested early. The longer therapies may allow time for changes to occur that are a function of time. In fact, the two studies that used observer ratings and rated improvement at follow-up rather than posttherapy found no relationship between time in treatment and improvement.

A related hypothesis to explain these differences concerns the nature of the ratings themselves (Johnson & Gelso, 1980). Typically, there is no difference in global ratings between time-limited therapy and time-unlimited therapy, or time-limited therapy is found to be superior. A ceiling effect could begin to operate for the general ratings of discomfort relief, which would not be true for the more extensive ratings, resulting in a lack of variance and thereby reducing the significance of the relationship of time in treatment to outcome. Based on the findings of two studies, Johnson and Gelso (1980) reported that

> client ratings of specific problem relief were very high regardless of amount of treatment, while the more extensive areas of self-respect, interpersonal relationships, and suicidal inclinations required more therapy sessions to show greater improvement. . . . When global ratings are used, some clients

> may note vast improvement because they feel better, while counselors may
> believe improvement means deeper changes, requiring more time, and thus
> rate global improvement lower. (pp. 71–72)

They concluded that time-limited therapy helps clients, but that the extent of improvement depends on the type of measure considered — global versus specific.

There are now some data available which tend to confirm Johnson and Gelso's conjectures. Howard, Lueger, Maling, and Martinovich (1993) posited a phase theory of psychotherapy in which improvement would first take place in patients' subjectively experienced well-being ("remoralization"), followed by a reduction in symptomatology ("remediation"), and then by enhancement in life functioning (e. g., interpersonal relations, work functioning, self-management), which they referred to as the "rehabilitation" phase.

In a test of their model, patients with mild to moderate psychological disorders were treated in time-unlimited psychodynamic therapy, which the investigators monitored at intake and at sessions 2, 4, and 17. Large improvements in *well-being* occurred by session 2. *Symptomatic change* also changed fairly early and steadily, although less dramatically, through the 17 sessions. *Current life functioning* improved later and to a lesser extent than well-being or symptoms, but did improve significantly within the 17 sessions. Furthermore, the investigators demonstrated a causal temporal ordering of phases such that symptomatic improvement was not likely to occur if subject well-being enhancement had not occurred first, and improvement in life functioning was not likely to occur unless symptomatic reduction had been previously achieved. Similarly, in another study of brief dynamic therapy, symptomatic distress abated more rapidly than interpersonal problems (Horowitz, Rosenberg, Baer, Ureño, & Villaseñor, 1988).

A second methodological problem is the confounding of time in therapy versus the passage of time per se. Lorr, McNair, Michaux, and Raskin (1964), for example, studied patients seen twice weekly, weekly, or biweekly, and found that improvement was related to time duration of treatment but not to the number of treatment sessions. Johnson and Gelso (1980) suggest that "given at least some treatment, a client may require time per se rather than specifically time in therapy to make improvement" (p. 72).

Another important methodological issue is the timing of the outcome assessment. There is some evidence, reviewed by Steenbarger (1994), that the relationship between duration and outcome may be quite different in a very brief therapy (fewer than 10 sessions) than in a more typical BPT of 12 to 25 sessions. For example, Svartberg and

Stiles (1991) found that duration was related to outcome only for those psychodynamic therapies that were longer than 12 sessions.

Perhaps the most important point, one mentioned by Johnson and Gelso (1980), Koss and Butcher (1986), and Koss, Butcher, and Strupp (1986), is that many of the older studies referred to above did not employ a specifically planned brief therapy with therapists experienced in such a modality, where a focus was chosen, goals set, the time limit stated to the patient, and high activity maintained. Compared to studies where the patient dropped out of what started as a time-unlimited therapy, which was then considered time-limited, we would expect an even better showing by brief therapy, and it is more of these kind of comparative studies of planned brief therapy that are needed.

Follow-Up Studies

A frequent challenge addressed to brief therapy is that its effects may not be enduring. Although few studies have conducted follow-ups, Johnson and Gelso (1980) found six studies, yielding seven measures, that did. Seventy-one percent found no difference between time-limited and time-unlimited therapy, one found time-limited therapy superior and one found time-unlimited therapy superior. Two studies, however, found that a minimum frequency of sessions (once per week) or minimum total number of sessions is necessary for stable long-term improvement. Johnson and Gelso concluded that "a minimal amount of counseling may be needed to get improvement started; after this point, the actual duration of the counseling is not predictive of long-term improvement" (p. 73).

These results are reflected in the meta-analysis conducted by Nicholson and Berman (1983) on 67 follow-up studies of different kinds of therapy (most of which were brief) with patients suffering from a broad variety of neurotic problems. They found that differences among treatments apparent at termination were maintained at follow-up. The status of patients at termination correlated with follow-up status regardless of the length of time that had elapsed (see also Lambert, Shapiro, & Bergin, 1986). Landman and Dawes (1982) reported similar results. These studies offer no support for the criticism that the gains of brief therapy are ephemeral.

However, some studies have found that a reasonably high percentage of patients treated in brief therapy return for more therapy (e.g., Budman, Demby, & Randall, 1982; Patterson, Levene, & Breger, 1971). In this vein, Gelso and Johnson (1983) found that the return rates after 1 to 1 ½ years for clients seen at the University of Maryland counseling center were 48% for an 8-session time limit, 33% for a 12-session time limit, 25% for a 16-session time limit, and 23% for a time-unlimited therapy. These figures suggest that following the shorter brief therapies clients are more likely to return for more therapy, but at the same time they demonstrate that a 16-session therapy is as effective as a time-unlimited therapy as evaluated by return rate.

Two comments are in order regarding the latter results: First, except for the Gelso and Johnson (1983) study, we do not know in general what percentage of patients seek more therapy following longer treatments. Second, that patients return may say as much about their enthusiasm for therapy after a brief experience as it says about its limitations. A course of brief therapy may select and prepare some proportion of patients for further psychotherapy.

The Dose–Effect Relationship: Probit Analysis

Howard, Kopta, Krause, and Orlinsky (1986) set out to determine the form of the relationship between the dose of therapy, using the session as the unit of exposure to the active ingredients of therapy, and the effect of therapy expressed as a percentage of patients improved at any particular dosage. They analyzed two sets of data from a Chicago psychiatric outpatient clinic. The first set consisted of 151 patients whose closed charts were rated by researchers following termination of treatment. The second set, taken from 148 of these patients, was based on the session-by-session patients' subjective report of their emotional well-being. Figure 1.2, which presents the results of their studies, shows a rapid rise in the percentage of patients improved in the early sessions according to both the objective (researcher) and subjective (patient) reports. By 13 sessions, roughly 55 to 60% of patients were considered improved. We note, too, that with increased sessions, the percentage continues to rise, but at a slower rate than in the earlier sessions.

The authors also examined the percentage of patients improved in therapies of different lengths to control for the possibility that improvement was due to nonimprovers terminating earlier than improvers. They found that the percentage of patients improved was similar in therapies of different lengths, and concluded that the curves in Figure 1.2 were not caused by differential patient attrition. These findings are somewhat at variance with those of Smith and Glass, reported above, which indicated that the major benefit of therapy occurs in the first six to eight sessions. Regarding this apparent discrepancy, Howard and colleagues (1986) note that the Smith and Glass work "was based on a between-study analysis and has no necessary implication

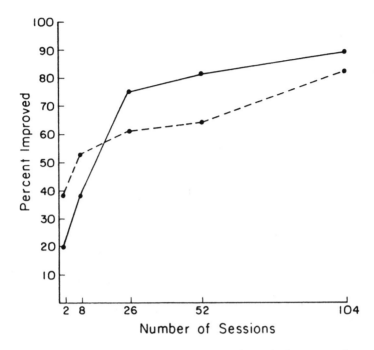

FIGURE 1.2. Relation of number of sessions of psychotherapy and percentage of patients improved. Objective ratings at termination are shown by the solid line; subjective ratings during therapy are shown by the broken line. From Howard et al. (1986, p. 160). Copyright 1986 by the American Psychological Association. Reprinted by permission.

for the relationship between duration and benefit within each study" (p. 159).

Upon scanning the literature for studies reporting improvement as a function of varying lengths of treatment, Howard and colleagues found 15 samples covering 30 years and 2,431 patients in individual outpatient psychotherapy. "These samples represented a variety of outpatients, therapists, therapeutic orientations, treatment settings, and outcome criteria" (pp. 160–161). Patients were typically diagnosed as depressive or anxiety neurotic. The therapists came from the usual mental health professions and their orientation was generally psychodynamic or interpersonal, making these data particularly instructive for our purposes. The outcome ratings were global and did not employ psychological tests.

The authors were able to estimate percentage of patients improved using best-fit lines produced by the probit analysis. Thus, the means, given in Table 1.2, are interpolated or extrapolated values of the expected percentage improved for the specific number of sessions indicated. Howard and colleagues (1986) summarized the findings as follows:

> [Table 1.2] indicates that 10% to 18% of patients could be expected to have shown some improvement before the first session of psychotherapy, simply as a function of initiating contact with the therapist or clinic, and that by eight sessions, 48% to 58% of patients would be expected to have measurably improved. About 75% of patients should have shown measurable improvements by the end of six months of once-weekly psychotherapy (26 sessions) and about 85% by the end of a year of treatment. (p. 162)

It can also be noted from the table that at 13 sessions, roughly the time limit set in some psychodynamic brief therapies, such as that of James Mann (see Chapter 4), 62% of patients should be expected to improve, according to these figures. Thus, it appears that brief therapy does a lot of good for many patients, at least as measured globally, while, at the same time, longer therapy increases the percentage of patients improved.

These authors then examined the percentage of different diagnostic groups improving at different dosages. As we might expect, those individuals diagnosed as borderline–psychotic lagged behind in rate of improvement (as judged both by researchers and patients) compared to the depressives and anxiety neurotics. For example, at *13 sessions,* while about 55% of the depressives and anxiety neurotics showed improvement on the *researcher* ratings of closed clinical charts, only 11% of the borderlines had done so. For the *patient ratings,* about 57% of the depressives and anxiety neurotics improved, compared to 42% of the borderlines.

By *26 sessions,* about 80% of the depressives and neurotics were improved compared to 38% of the borderlines, based on *researcher rat-*

TABLE 1.2. Interpolated and Extrapolated Estimates of Percentage of Patients Improved for Selected Amounts of Psychotherapy

	Number of sessions								
	0	1	2	4	8	13	26	52	104
Means	14	24	30	41	53	62	74	83	90
95% of confidence band (+/−) for estimate of mean	4	4	5	5	5	6	6	5	4

Note. Excerpted from Howard et al. (1986, p. 162). Copyright 1986 by the American Psychological Association. Excerpted by permission.

ings. According to *patients' self-reports,* about 66% of the depressives and anxiety patients had improved, as had 60% of the borderlines. It appears that researcher ratings generally lagged behind patient self-report ratings of improvement for sessions 13 to 26.

Howard and his colleagues have now extended the dosage model beyond significant improvement in global functioning. They examined symptom clusters (rather than global functioning) where the measure of change was return to normal range—that is, *clinically* significant change verus statistical improvement only (Kopta, Howard, Lowry, & Beutler, 1994). Using a symptom checklist (SCL-90-R), they grouped symptoms into three classes on the basis of the rate at which they responded to time-unlimited psychotherapy: acute distress (e.g., anxiety, depression, somatization, and compulsive symptoms), chronic distress (e.g., cognitive disturbances and interpersonal problems), and character problems (e.g., paranoid ideation and schizoid traits). For acute distress symptoms (e. g., feeling fearful, crying easily), it took five sessions on the average for 50% of the patients to recover normal functioning (a stiff criterion by which to gauge change). For chronic distress symptoms (e.g., feeling easily hurt, feelings of guilt, feeling blocked), it took 14 sessions on average. For character symptoms (e.g., can't trust others, urges to harm someone, feels something is wrong with his or her mind), it took more than 52 sessions, and quite a few symptoms in this category showed little change even after 100 sessions. For the most frequently occurring acute and chronic symptoms, it took a year of therapy to produce recovery among 75% of the patients. Similar dose-effect studies have been conducted for interpersonal problems (Maling, Gurtman, & Howard 1995) and work functioning (Lueger & Howard, 1994).

Of course, as the dose-effect studies are of open-ended therapy, the results may differ for planned, focused brief therapy with a set time limit, but these studies are probably suggestive of what areas of functioning are likely to be ameliorated within the parameters of brief dynamic therapy. In such a study, it was found that people with problems of hostility, dominance, or coldness were less likely to succeed in brief dynamic therapy than those with issues of submissiveness (Horowitz, Rosenberg, & Bartholomew, 1993). Taken together with the Kopta et al. (1994) findings, this suggests that it may be easier to help patients become more assertive in BPT if they are not too hostile (with urges to harm others), cold, or mistrustful to begin with.

Conclusions

Stated in the most general terms, time-limited therapy is helpful to a substantial proportion of patients and is often as helpful as time-unlimited therapy. Its effects seem to be as lasting as those of time-unlimited treatment. However, these global conclusions must be qualified in several ways. First, the dose-effect studies suggest that although time-limited therapy is helpful to a substantial percentage of patients, that percentage increases the longer that therapy continues. Similarly, the breadth of change may be greater for long-term therapy. In a sense, it can be said both that brief therapy is helpful but also that longer term therapy can be even more helpful.

Second, we cannot say that any one form of brief therapy is clearly superior to another form of brief therapy (with the possible exception of cognitive-behavioral therapy for major depression, but this conclusion is based on only one of the studies reported by Svartberg & Stiles, 1991), to medication, or to some forms of nonpsychiatric treatment. Nor can we say that longer-term psychoanalytic therapy is superior to brief psychoanalytic therapy.

Third, patients diagnosed as depressed or anxious improve faster than patients diagnosed as borderline. Reasonable proportions of the latter, however, also make gains in a relatively brief time period (2 to 6 months, depending on the source of measurement). Similarly, acute and chronic symptoms improve sooner than characterological features.

Fourth, measures of well-being and symptoms show earlier improvement than do general measures of life functioning, including interpersonal relationships.

Fifth, the results of time-limited versus time-unlimited therapy are dependent on the outcome measures employed. Therapist-measured outcome often yields superior results for time-unlimited therapy, especially compared to outcomes gauged by tests or behavioral measures.

Sixth, patients in time-limited psychotherapy tend to maintain their gains, although one study suggests that return rates for patients treated in fewer than 16 sessions is quite high.

Seventh, from a psychoanalytic perspective, the kind, or source, of outcome measures typically employed is not specifically targeted to the sort of change that psychoanalytic practitioners often look for. Clients, for example, may wish to please therapists in order to maintain their love, leading to an overly positive evaluation, or they may be angry or frustrated, resulting in an overly critical or disparaging evaluation (Messer & Warren, 1990). Therapists, too, have a stake in the outcome and can be influenced in their evaluation by their idiosyncratic reactions to clients based on their relationship to them. Outside observers may be less biased, but will be lacking the privileged information of the therapist. The choice of rating source involves trade-offs, and psychotherapy researchers must always ask themselves which individuals are in the best position to assess the particular constructs of interest to them.

THE CONTEXT OF VISIONS OF REALITY

While modes of psychotherapy differ from one another in both theory and technique, they diverge even more fundamentally in the view of human reality they encompass. Such an outlook is not peripheral to a psychotherapeutic approach, but is intrinsic to its very warp and woof, determining the basic stance taken by the therapist, wittingly or unwittingly. Because a therapy's unique vision embodies a way of regarding life's possibilities and limitations, it affects the kind of process fostered and the change that it is intended to bring about.

What concerns us here is the vision of reality encompassed by psychoanalytic therapy and what modifications in this vision BPT requires. Although there are different ways of conceptualizing the psychoanalytic vision, one particularly apposite scheme has been elaborated upon by the literary critic, Northrop Frye (1957, 1965) in connection with genres or mythic forms in literature; this framework was subsequently applied by Schafer (1970) to psychoanalysis. The "visions" are referred to as romantic, ironic, tragic, and comic. Messer and Winokur (1980, 1984, 1986) employed Frye's fourfold categorization to compare the visions of reality in psychoanalytic, behavioral, and humanistic therapy and to determine how the differences bear on the prospects for their integration. For present purposes, we will briefly present each vision and then discuss its application to long-term and short-term psychoanalytic therapy.

The Romantic Vision

From the romantic viewpoint, life is an adventure or quest in which the person as hero transcends the world of experience, achieves victory over it, and is liberated from it. "It is a drama of the triumph of good over evil, of virtue over vice, of light over darkness, and of the ultimate transcendence of man over the world in which he was imprisoned by the fall" (White, 1973, p. 9). The romantic vision emphasizes exploration and conquest of the unknown, the mysterious, the irrational. It is more the world as we would like it to be than the world as it often is. Romance, after all, flourishes in the dark, where blemishes are harder to spot.

The romantic vision idealizes individuality and what is "natural," since it views human nature as intrinsically good. To express oneself freely is prized. As Strenger (1989) described the romantic vision, "the fully developed individual is characterized by true spontaneity, by the richness of his subjective experience" (p. 595).

In stressing exploration of the unconscious, the irrational, and the unknown, psychoanalysis and long-term psychoanalytic therapy are influenced by the romantic vision. These therapies are often viewed as taking the patient on a journey, a quest for personal redemption. Schafer (1976) depicts the romantic quest as a "perilous, heroic, individualistic journey, an essentially lonely, drawn out, conflict ridden and difficult process . . . which ends after crucial struggles with exaltation" (p. 31). In our experience, and consonant with this vision, many patients in psychoanalytic therapy at some point dream of being on an airplane, train, or car with the therapist or themselves viewed as pilot, conductor, or driver. The therapeutic process itself encourages regression away from everyday reality and into the world of fantasy, free association, and dreams. Psychoanalytic therapists, in a romantic mode, hold an attitude of curiosity and openness to unexpected developments in the patient. They are interested in exploring and understanding the contradictory and uncertain aspects of human nature.

BPT also partakes of the romantic vision by stressing a tailor-made, dynamic formulation of the patient's problems: In doing so, it prizes individuality and the uniqueness of the patient's quest. It values dreams, fantasies, and spontaneity, encouraging patients to speak freely, to open up and explore the unknown, to face the dragons of their unconscious and to slay them. As in psychoanalysis, it expects the process to be conflict ridden, painful, and difficult. On the other hand, by emphasizing a rapid formulation of the patient's problems and the early setting of a focus, the open-endedness of the romantic quest is thereby curtailed. The therapist, by selecting interventions along the line of the focus, and specifying goals in advance, deliberately narrows the quest. Similarly, the extensity of the journey is foreshortened by virtue of the time limit, and the degree of "redemption" or change brought about is often circumscribed. Nevertheless, rapid termination — going on to face life on one's own — also lies in the spirit of the romantic vision.

The Ironic Vision

The ironic attitude is the enemy of romance. It is an attitude of detachment, of keeping things in perspective, of recognizing that there is more than one way to view any phenomenon. Ambiguity of meaning or intention is paramount. Each aspect of a person's behavior may represent something else, be it the manifest versus latent content of a dream, the distorted or displaced wish represented in a symptom, or the screen versus core memory. It is the essence of the ironic posture to take nothing for granted and to spot the antithesis to any thesis. Irony challenges our cherished beliefs, traditions and (romantic) illusions. Like the tragic vision, it emphasizes the inherent difficulties of life, the impossibility of mastering the world or even of truly knowing its mysteries.

Psychoanalytic therapists adopt the ironic attitude when they take a position of relative detachment (Stein, 1985) in order to detect the underside of the client's utterances and behavior—the hidden meanings, contradictions, and paradoxes. The ironic vision does not deny the patient's view of reality so much as it insists on the recognition of other significant realities that the patient may resist recognizing or acknowledging. The psychoanalyst is basically silent, adopting the technique of irony, which says "little, meaning as much as possible" (Frye, 1957, p. 40). In that no explanation is ever complete, psychoanalysis is inherently interminable.

Brief psychodynamic therapists incorporate an ironic posture insofar as they strive to discern hidden meanings, to uncover the impulse behind the defense. Like psychoanalysts, they adopt an attitude of suspicion toward the patient's statements, taking nothing for granted. They challenge the patient's illusions, although not in as thoroughgoing a way as in psychoanalysis. The greater activity and dialogic nature of brief dynamic therapy, however, may tend to obscure the recognition of irony on the therapist's part. Also, since brief dynamic therapy is not open-ended and inherently interminable, it deliberately limits the possibility of uncovering multiple meanings and the layers of impulse and defense.

In this connection, Kupers (1986) has discussed the loss in BPT of protracted self-reflection. It is this quality of psychoanalytic therapy that Habermas (1971) has referred to as emancipatory. It is the ability to get beyond superficial and mystifying appearances to the deeper levels of personal or social truth. The more that brief therapy is narrowly technical, adjustive, or purely clinical, the more conformist it becomes. To the extent that BPT limits self-reflection, the possibility for unfettered exploration leading to radical criticism of self and society is compromised.

The Tragic Vision

Tragedy and irony are connected in that both include a distrust of romantic illusions and happy endings in life. In addition, they are reflective in attitude, whereas the romantic and comic visions are more action oriented. Unlike irony, however, tragedy involves commitment. In tragic dramas, the heroes have acted with purpose and in so doing have committed an act causing shame or guilt, at least in their own minds. They suffer by virtue of the conflict between passion and duty and, after considerable inner struggle, arrive at a state of greater self-knowledge. In tragedy the flaw is present in the hero from the start, and thus is fated or destined, even if external circumstances contribute to it. It evokes fear and pity in the onlookers. What interests us in the work of the tragic poet "is the glimpse we get of certain profound moods or inner struggles. Now, this glimpse cannot be obtained from without" (Bergson, 1937/1956, p. 167). Such a mode may be contrasted with "the kind of observation from which comedy springs. It is directed outwards" (Bergson, 1937/1956, p. 169).

The limitations in life are accepted within a tragic vision: Not all is possible, redeemable, or realizable. Human nature cannot be radically perfected, the clock cannot be turned back, and death cannot be undone. Tragedy "requires one to recognize the elements of defeat in victory and of victory in defeat; the pain in pleasure and the pleasure in pain; the guilt in apparently justified action; the loss of opportunities entailed by every choice and by growth in any direction" (Schafer, 1976, p. 35). Thus, a good therapeutic outcome within a tragic view is a quiet acceptance of a certain degree of despair; it produces wisdom.

More than any other therapy, psychoanalysis falls within the tragic vision. People are viewed as trapped within early fixations which are then subject to repression and, thus, lie beyond their ken. The fixations result from our sexual and aggressive nature and the conflicts this nature gives rise to, from which we cannot be totally free. "Freud's vision resides in his emphasis that humankind cannot achieve fulfillment at a low price" (Strenger, 1989, p. 598). Only through suffering can our consciousness be illuminated (Mujeeb-ur-Rahman, 1990).

During psychoanalytic therapy, patients must be helped to recognize themselves as tragic heroes in the sense of coming to a full recognition of their internal dilemmas and the limitation placed upon them by their early experiences, rather than perceiving the source of their difficulties as essentially external. The kind of self-knowledge to be acquired from a tragic vantage point demands a thoroughgoing internal focus. The reconciliation that occurs at the end of a psychoanalytic therapy is not unmixed joy and pleasure. Rather, it is a fuller recognition of the nature of one's struggles and the conditions of life with which one has to cope. These conditions "set the limits on what may be aspired to and what may be legitimately aimed at in the quest for security and sanity in the world" (White, 1973, p. 9).

The tragic outlook is present in brief dynamic therapy as it is in most forms of psychoanalytic therapy (but see the discussion below, regarding the changes that revisions in psychoanalytic therapy have brought about). Its theoretical base is similar, as are some of its modes of intervention. Ironically, the time limit simultaneously renders it both more and less tragic. BPT is more tragic in that it often settles for circumscribed gain at the expense of fuller character analysis and broader structural change. It sets limits on what is possible by virtue of its brevity, focus, and goal setting. The practice of brief psychodynamic therapy recognizes the difficulty, if not impossibility, of transforming patients in the miraculous and thorough way they often hope for when seeking treatment. It accepts the limitations of both inner and outer resources for the task at hand.

At the same time, there is a decided hopefulness engendered in BPT, especially at its outset. The presentation of a focus emphasizes that problems are comprehensible and definable. The time limit conveys a message to patients that some problems are, after all, resolvable or ameliorable in a finite time period. It highlights the potential for human change and improvement. The need for separation, however, returns the person to the tragic vision at the end of therapy. Even at this point, however, the therapist conveys confidence that the patient can examine separation fears, go through with termination, and cope with these fears. This attitude actually falls more within the the comic vision, to which we turn next.

The Comic Vision

In contrast to the tragic vision, the comic vision emphasizes the familiar, predictable, and controllable aspects of life. Conflict is viewed as centered in situations that can be ameliorated by effective problem solving and action. If, in tragedy, things go from bad to worse, in comedy the direction is from bad to better. Obstacles and struggles are ultimately overcome, and a reconciliation takes place between hero and antagonist, between the person and his or her social world. Harmony and unity, progress and happiness are achieved. This is why comic operas and other dramatic comedies often end with festive celebrations.

The kind of knowledge attained by the comic hero "is not necessarily an introverted knowledge which is of little use to a comedy, but a sense of proportion and social reality" (Frye, 1965, p. 79). This kind of understanding cannot be regarded as self-knowledge in the tragic sense but rather is an increased capacity to perform social roles more adequately. The conflicts portrayed in a comedy are ones between people and the unfortunate situation in which they find themselves, and not the kind of inner struggles or implacable oppositions encountered in dramatic tragedy.

The comic vision is less evident in psychoanalysis than it is in behavioral and humanistic therapies. Behavior therapists, for example, are not so much interested in their patients' internal struggles as they are in the direct alleviation of suffering and a rapidly achieved positive outcome. Although behavior therapy increases self-knowledge, the term applies to an increased pragmatic capacity to fulfill social roles, not to attain the tragic hero's self-knowledge. Likewise, in humanistic therapy, the true self one comes to know is not one fraught with struggle, nor is it one seeking reduction of tension, but rather it is an authentic self, free of conditions of worth, in touch with its natural, organismic valuing, and satisfied with life's substantial possibilities for self-enhancement and growth. From the perspective of humanistic therapy, a freer, more joyful existence is decidedly attainable.

Despite its strongly tragic overtones, psychoanalysis does aim "to clear the way towards sustained hopefulness, the experience of security and pleasure" (Schafer, 1976, p. 28). It is only in a relative sense that psychoanalysis can be considered to fall more within tragic, romantic, and ironic visions than within the comic. Successful interpersonal relations and the capacity to cope with situational obstacles are also valued within psychoanalysis, even if insight is incomplete and patients have not attained full reconciliation with and self-knowledge of their condition (Messer & Winokur, 1984).

In fact, it is the drive/structural approach that is most guarded about the comic outlook, compared with the newer psychoanalytic therapies. In self psychology and object relations approaches, there is as much emphasis on the experience of the relationship as there is on offering interpretations leading to insight. The importance of the holding environment (Winnicott, 1965), empathy (Kohut, 1977), and the real relationship (Tuttman, 1982) are stressed in the belief that one can, in some measure, make up for or repair early deprivations through the healing power of the relationship. Similarly, the neo-Freudians and the ego-psychologists deemphasize the relentlessness of biologically given drives. The former stress the power of cultural and social forces or current life situations in distorting personality development and functioning, whereas the latter grant more ability to the ego (the individual as agent) to control the drives and to foster an adaptive, more conflict-free existence.

BPT is more comic in outlook than traditional psychoanalytic therapy. To formulate a focus is to regard patient problems as familiar and predictable. The brief therapist approaches therapy in a more optimistic spirit, believing that worthwhile change is achievable within the set time limit, even without the development and resolution of a transference neurosis. The therapist's heightened activity in BPT is also more consonant with the comic and romantic visions' stress on problem solving and action, in contrast to the more contemplative and reflective stance of the psychoanalyst within the ironic and tragic views. Insofar as brief therapies incorporate behaviorally based elements (see Chapter 5), they take on even more of the coloring of the comic vision. Insofar as specific goals are set and aimed for in brief therapy, it is more comic in thrust than tragic.

For the practitioner whose major mode of practice is long-term therapy, an adjustment in vision of reality is required to conduct BPT. There is enough similarity between long- and short-term modes that the shift is not a totally radical one, but it is a significant shift nevertheless. It means that BPT is not for every clinician, which can be said of any particular mode of practice. However, the mix of visions is somewhat different for each of the models we cover in this volume, and it can be expected that therapists, by virtue of their personalities, education, and training will resonate to them differently.

THE CONTEXT OF LEARNING AND TEACHING BRIEF PSYCHODYNAMIC THERAPY

A survey of practicing psychologists in California and Massachusetts (Levenson et al., 1995) found that psychodynamic therapists saw themselves as having less skill in brief therapy than did therapists of other orientations. The major factors positively predicting self-perceived skill were experience with brief therapy, attitude toward its effectiveness, and training. In this section we take up the issue of training in BPT and the many negative attitudes and forms of resistance that the educator, trainer, and both neophyte and experienced therapists must confront and resolve in order to become practitioners of effective short-term psychodynamic therapy. BPT engages the student of brief therapy, as it does the patient, in a learning process with both emotional and intellectual facets that are worth spelling out in advance so that they can be managed in an optimal way. (Some of the material below is drawn from Hoyt, 1985; McWilliams, 1987; Weddington & Cavenar, 1979; and Winokur & Dasberg, 1983.)

Emotional Challenges in Conducting Brief Psychodynamic Therapy

Guilt and Anger

Perhaps the most common feeling aroused in practicing BPT is guilt over shortchanging the patient. There is the nagging feeling that if only one had another five sessions, another 5 months, or even another year or two, the patient would be properly cured. The guilt can lead to anger at "the system"—be it the clinic, the insurance company limiting payment, or a society that does not provide sufficient resources for healing the mentally ill or for human growth and development to take place in those who feel stuck and in need of professional help. That is, if the prospect of an imminent or early ending of the treatment relationship is prone to induce transference issues in the client, it also can induce countertransference issues in the therapist. At such times it may be reassuring to recall the research that supports the value of BPT, especially that there is no conclusive evidence that it is inferior to long-term psychoanalytic therapy.

Perfectionism and Grandiosity

We may believe, in setting out to practice psychotherapy, that we will cure all comers and that we can do so categorically and completely. Such exaggerated hopes, secret or otherwise, may not be uncommon in the novice therapist practicing psychotherapy of any length and according to any orientation. We choose to practice therapy mainly because we want to help distressed individuals; the more thoroughly we are able to do so, the more satisfaction we are likely to experience. To recognize the limitations imposed by intractable human nature, by our own all-too-limited human capacities, and by the inevitable strictures of work settings or other circumstances can be experienced as a narcissistic blow. The practice of BPT can be an especially sobering experience in this regard. If such an attitude of therapeutic grandiosity, feelings of guilt and anger, or lowered self-esteem are sufficiently strong or uncontrolled, they will compromise brief therapy from the start. The therapist will convey dissatisfaction in one way or another to the patient, who will view the therapy as second rate at best, thereby fulfilling the therapist's ambivalent expectations regarding outcome.

To help mitigate these concerns, therapists need to recognize that the standard to which they may be comparing BPT is overly perfectionistic and hardly ever realized in practice. To take an extreme case, does it ever happen that we do not recognize the personality of people we know after they have been in psychoanalysis because structural change has been so complete? By our own seemingly admirable but too lofty standards, any outcome will be insufficient because life itself does not yield perfect or uncomplicated solutions. This is an aspect of the tragic vision which, far from being merely pessimistic as it may appear at first glance, allows us to proceed to do the best we can with the recognition of all that it means to be human.

Affects Concerning Separation and Termination

The many emotions aroused by the termination phase of BPT are frequently problematic for brief psychodynamic therapists, because leave taking comes about so quickly and, if one is conducting several brief therapies at once, so frequently. We may feel *guilty* for "rejecting" or "abandoning" the patient. We may feel *sad* at the prospect of losing an intense and satisfying relationship. In a sense, the more progress that the patient has made in therapy, the more acute the loss. As Goldberg (1975) has noted, the therapist may *mourn* because he or she is no longer a needed object for the patient. Therapists may also feel *disappointed* that there will not be time to explore other facets of patients' problems and personality and to contribute to their amelioration. At the other end of the emotional spectrum, therapists may feel *relieved* at ending therapy with patients who have been stormy, sullen, or otherwise resistant.

There are other emotional difficulties that may arise at termination of BPT. The therapist may have learned too late that the patient was not suitable for brief therapy. In this situation, therapists may feel that a Pandora's box has been opened by uncovering unconscious issues without sufficient time to see them through to resolution, leaving the therapists feeling that they have brought about more harm than good. On the other hand, they may feel that the real issues have not been addressed because they came to light too late. A further concern may be that the process was too intellectual, especially if therapists are too intent on interpreting everything according to some theoretically driven "focus."

In spite of these all-too-real difficulties, often some important issues have been addressed in therapy, immediate appearances notwithstanding. There may be a changed developmental trajectory, a partial internalization of a healthy therapist-patient relationship, and a degree of working through after termination. We should not put all our emotional eggs in the basket of outcome, neglecting the benefits of the *process* of therapy (Schafer, 1973). In place of externalizing, projecting, and perceiving themselves as passive victims, patients' awareness of internal conflicts can lead to an altered view of themselves as actively bringing about their dilemmas. This can result in decreased use of their psychic energy in the service of defense, and an increase in constructive action even after therapy has terminated. They can now see themselves, in part, as tragic heroes — sadder but wiser.

One frequent therapist reaction to the impending termination of therapy is an emotional withdrawal from patients, with too little exploration of the personal meaning that separation holds for them. As we will learn in Chapter 4, which describes the 12-session therapy of James Mann, termination presents important opportunities for affectively charged exploration and growth that can be lost if the therapist neglects interpreting the protective stance patients frequently adopt at this juncture. Another common reaction to termination is to try to do too much in the final stage of therapy, to engage in a "frenzy to cure," as if the number of interventions will make up for the lack of time to truly complete the therapy. This, too, will leave the patient, at the end of therapy, confused and regretful rather than reasonably satisfied. However, such foreknowledge can forearm brief therapists to be alert to their own reactions, whether based on the vicissitudes of the current therapy relationship or difficulties separating from others in their own past.

Power and Authority

BPT also elicits conflicts in the therapist over power and authority. Most forms of BPT require a more active stance by the therapist than does long-term psychoanalytic therapy, in order to channel the therapy in the area of the dynamic focus. The techniques employed by the drive/structural therapists, especially Davanloo and Sifneos, include direct confrontation of patients' defenses, which requires a rather bald show of therapist authority and assertiveness. For novice therapists there is bound to be anxiety over expressing what they may experience as their own aggressive impulses, thus possibly eliciting the patient's ire. Too great a need by therapists to express their power can lead either to more activity than the patient can comfortably tolerate or to excessive passivity as a way of guarding against the exertion of authority. Power needs can also result in therapists becoming irritated by patients who do not accept their authority or who resist doing the work of therapy. Awareness of either the potential abdication or misuse of their legitimate power and authority, and the ability to modulate them, are therapists' major assets in mitigating such negative effects.

Feelings of Inadequacy

In learning BPT, there are many points at which students may not feel equal to the task. They may be concerned at the outset about their diagnostic skill, both in selecting suitable candidates for BPT and in formulating a focus correctly. Therapists may wonder, for example, whether they are "pushing" a formulation of their own making that does not resonate to the patient's concerns. Then there is the threat from defining goals of therapy in advance, which more readily confronts the therapist with success or failure than typically would be true for a more open-ended, long-term therapy.

Carrying out a new kind of therapy brings inevitable anxiety over the adequacy of one's therapeutic skills. In this connection, there may be a fear that one is conducting a "wild analysis" or pursuing a personal agenda at the patient's expense. A related fear is of going too deep too quickly or, on the other hand, of keeping interventions at too superficial a level. If BPT is being learned in a group context, there is also the risk to therapists of being embarrassed about mistakes that they will make along the way. Among other ways of expressing this anxiety unproductively are therapists' efforts to prove themselves or the method as adequate by trying to persuade patients of its value through an overabundance of interventions that, as a result, are experienced by patients as an assault.

Aside from the value that accrues from recognizing these feelings, there are other ways to alleviate the anxiety over felt inadequacy. First, it is important for therapists to maintain a sense of themselves as "good enough" to borrow Winnicott's phrase, in spite of errors or not accomplishing it all. On a practical level, Malan (1963) recommended the use of the case conference for formulating patient problems and psychodynamics. Group discussion of the case diminishes the chances of a therapist's blind spots prevailing and can lend confidence to the therapist as to the correctness of the formulation. Along similar lines, psychological testing, which was employed in the Tavistock project led by Michael Balint and David Malan, can yield important information as to suitability of the dynamic focus, as well as alerting therapists to typical defenses the patient will employ. In fact, the advent of BPT could lead to a resurgence of psychological testing. It could also sharpen the focus of the diagnostician's task and the formulation of the referral for testing. The extra clinical time employed in such assessment may lead to more efficient and successful brief therapies.

Anxiety over Formulating the "Correct" Focus

Implied in this discussion, and undoubtedly contributing to the novice's discomfort regarding his or her adequacy, is that there exists only one correct dynamic formulation, so either the therapist has hit the target or is off base. This has been the prevailing point of view in psychoanalysis ever since Glover (1931) distinguished between accurate versus inaccurate and complete versus incomplete interpretations. In this outlook, an incomplete, inaccurate, or inexact interpretation constitutes "an ego-syntonic displacement system" such as a symptom, or a "substitution-product" (p. 410), but does not correctly identify the "true" source of the anxiety or impulses involved. That is, one has not tapped into the unconscious fantasy systems that lie ready to be unearthed. Such inaccurate or incomplete interpretations may make patients feel better, the argument continues, but cannot constitute a proper psychoanalytic cure in that they do not bring the patient closer to "psychological truth" (p. 419). Stated differently, such interventions are more in the realm of suggestion, allowing for the building up of defensive structures rather than penetrating to the unconscious core.

However, developments in psychoanalytic metapsychology (Edelson, 1975, 1977; Schafer, 1976, 1978; Spence, 1982) and in the experimental psychology of memory (Loftus & Ketcham, 1991; Palermo, 1978) lead to a different view of the accuracy of dynamic formulation and, hence, of therapeutic interventions. Palermo (1978) concludes that the evidence supports the view that memories are creative reconstructions rather than veridical recollections. Memories are not stored like photographs, but as abstracted essences of experience which can be used to construct a coherent memory. The important implication here is that there is no single correct reconstruction, but multiple and equally viable possibilities for such reconstruction, and, hence, of the dynamic formulation as well (Winokur, Messer, & Schacht, 1981). For Edelson, too, interpretations help to make sense of events, with the implication that it is not possible to label only one formulation as correct. As assessors and therapists, we help to create a life history for patients that organizes their experience in a way that allows it to become more intelligible to them (Schafer, 1981).

In a related vein, Howard (1991) views psychotherapy as an exercise in "life-story" repair. Psychotherapy usually begins by the therapist inviting clients to tell their story. In the telling, the therapist gets a rough idea of clients' orientation toward life, including their plans, ambitions, and the events involved in the presenting problem. "So, from this perspective, part of the work between client and therapist can be seen as life-story elaboration, adjustment or repair" (p. 194). Howard goes on to point out that a life becomes meaningful when clients see themselves as actors within the context of a story. There is always more than one story for clients to live by. "Nonrational constructions of reality are what one gets from stories. Stories slice the world up (or urge us to view the world) from a variety of different perspectives, points of view, and value positions, and thus construct noncomparable frames of reference through which reality might be grasped" (p. 191). Thinking about dynamic formulations or foci in this way should be reassuring to novice therapists who might otherwise feel that their formulations and interventions are either accurate or they are not, and, therefore, that they are competent or they are not.

We hasten to add that not that any kind of formulation or story line will do. There must be some resonance to the patient's feelings and life experience and to the ability of therapist and client to organize and extend that experience in a subjectively convincing way. It is also possible that the more a "story" is historically true, the more readily will interpretations that are consistent with it prove therapeutically mutative — although this statement can rarely, if ever, be empirically demonstrated (at least in the absence of historical data). But within these parameters, the formulation and reconstruction can fall along different story lines such as oedipal, separation guilt, separation anxiety, structures of knowing, and so on. In other words, we take a pluralistic stance regarding the truth value of dynamic formulations: More than one will fit.

Frustration of Curiosity

Since BPT is focused, there is less of a sense of adventure and timelessness in its conduct than is true in longer-term therapy. The romantic vision, as discussed above, views life as an open-ended quest emphasizing exploration and conquest of the unknown. For some therapists, to close down options and to limit exploration in brief therapy is too much of an abrogation of the romantic outlook. One should keep in mind, however, the appeal to patients (and many therapists) in the shift to a more comic vision of definable problems and reachable goals. There are trade-offs here, which anyone with a tragic perspective on life would readily acknowledge.

Intellectual Challenges to Brief Psychodynamic Therapy

In learning to conduct long-term psychoanalytically oriented psychotherapy, the student or practitioner also learns a set of beliefs or attitudes about what constitutes good therapy and about how to proceed in an optimal way. Brief dynamic psychotherapy challenges these beliefs and, in some cases, actually contradicts the values of long-term psychotherapy. In this section, we will try to spell out some of the more prominent beliefs espoused in long-term therapy and offer a different perspective on them, in keeping with the goals and values of BPT (Hoyt, 1985; Winokur & Dasberg, 1983).

1. *The need to work through takes time.* In long-term therapy, we learn that clients need time to assimilate new learning and that it is important to approach the same issue many times from different angles in order to bring about change. Also, given that personality is complex, there are many areas to address, and this takes time to accomplish. By

contrast, in BPT only one focus is chosen which, to begin with, means that not all problems or character facets will be explored. Within that focus, one keeps in mind the conflict area and addresses it through the triangle of impulse-anxiety-defense (described in more detail in Chapter 2). Furthermore, one explores the problem area as it manifests itself in the triangle of insight or persons (Menninger & Holzman, 1973), that is, in connection with (1) people toward whom the problem is manifested most strongly, (2) persons in the past, particularly parents or siblings, towards whom the problem was once or is presently exhibited, and (3) the therapist, or in the transference. This allows for some working through of the problem, even in the context of brief therapy.

The therapist working within a BPT mode also relies on some of that working through taking place outside of therapy sessions and after therapy terminates. The point of the therapy is to bring about enough change to equip clients to notice their maladaptive perspectives and behavior, and to alter them accordingly. BPT sets a process in motion which, if all goes well, leads to a trajectory of change, not all of which may be manifest at the outset. Findings such as those by Piper and colleagues (1984), which found no difference on 6-month follow-up between clients in brief (22 session) and longer-term (75 session) psychoanalytic therapy, lends credence to this outlook.

2. *Transference develops slowly and cannot be rushed.* The traditional outlook on transference is that it is subtle and that only through listening and waiting patiently in an atmosphere of stringent therapist neutrality and abstinence will it emerge in a convincing way. The alternate view, held by the brief therapist and by some psychoanalysts as well (e.g., Gill, 1982), is that transference is ubiquitous and present from the outset of therapy. We must make a distinction between a full-blown regressive transference neurosis as required by psychoanalysis, in which the major effort of therapy is directed toward fostering the enactment of the neurotic conflict and character structure in the therapist-patient relationship, and transference viewed more modestly as patients' experience of the therapist in ways akin to their view of other significant figures, especially from the past. Within this view, clients cannot help but relate to the therapist in accordance with their set patterns, templates, or schemas, and it is the therapists' job to discern the role relationships into which they are cast, bring them to light, and relate them to other such enactments in the present or past. A regressive transference neurosis, while holding out the promise of a more thoroughgoing change, also promotes dependency, which may not be resolved in a brief therapy.

3. *A good therapeutic relationship develops only slowly.* The accepted view is that client trust, comfort, and liking of the therapist take time to es-

tablish, and until they are firmed up, therapy will operate only on a superficial level. Whereas this belief holds for the more disturbed client, it often does not for the better adjusted client who comes to therapy with a more trusting attitude toward the therapist. For this reason, it is not surprising that selection criteria for BPT often include the ability of the client to engage in a meaningful interpersonal relationship. Sifneos (1979), in fact, sets as a selection criterion that the client has experienced a meaningful relationship at some point in the past, and Strupp and Binder (1984) include basic trust as a prerequisite for time-limited dynamic psychotherapy.

Aside from selecting clients with a good capacity to rapidly form a working relationship in therapy, the brief therapist must work at establishing rapport with the client. The therapist must be more active in supporting and encouraging the alliance by statements such as "Can we look at this?" "I know this is difficult for you, but you are suffering with this problem." "You have always tried to be the good and helpful person, but it is not working for you now. Together we must see what has happened." Research informs us that indicators of the helping alliance early in therapy are very good predictors of therapy outcome (e.g., Crits-Christoph, Cooper, & Luborsky, 1988; Frieswyk et al., 1986). In one study (Hartley & Strupp 1983), it was the increase in the alliance in the first quartile of brief therapy that differentiated successful outcomes from the unsuccessful ones, in which the alliance in fact decreased. Clearly it behooves all therapists, short-term or long-term in orientation, to pay careful attention to the alliance.

In addition, it is important for therapists to make interventions along the line of a focus that resonates to client concerns. "What is crucial is a pattern of interpretation that is comprehensibly simple and that reasonably and justifiably conforms to the basic character of the patient's experiences by consistently capturing their essence" (Winokur et al., 1981, p. 140). Being understood will increase clients' motivation and engagement, thus increasing the prospects for a positive experience in brief therapy. In this connection, interventions that adhered to patients' core conflicts were predictive of good outcome (Crits-Christoph et al., 1988), and interpretations compatible with a dynamic formulation, arrived at through the Plan Formulation Method (Silberschatz, Fretter, & Curtis, 1986) predicted patient progress in brief dynamic therapy.

4. *Resistances are stubborn and tend to prolong therapy.* The traditional view of resistance is that it is understood or overcome only slowly and painstakingly through interpretation. One response to this view is that the brief therapist selects patients whose resistances can be dealt with in the time period available. For example, one of the contraindi-

cations for BPT is psychosomatic disturbance precisely because somatiz-
ers tend to be highly resistant patients since so much of their affect
is bound up in their symptoms. Brief therapists also have methods for
overcoming resistance. In Davanloo's (1980) and Sifneos's (1979)
drive/structural model, patient resistance is challenged from the start
at the same time that high levels of support and empathy are provided
to help mitigate the anxiety generated. In the relational psychodynamic model, resistance is viewed as part and parcel of the patient's interpersonal problem and is addressed as such from the outset.

5. *You cannot know the nature of the patients' real problems early on.* This
view is related to the notion of resistance as obscuring the true picture, thereby necessitating a prolonged therapy. It is true that for some
patients it takes many months before one has a reasonably good idea
of the nature of the problem. If no obvious focus is discerned after
two or three interviews, the patient is less than ideal for brief therapy,
as Malan (1976a) and others have pointed out. It is also the case that
diagnostic acumen is important in setting out to conduct BPT. Nevertheless, for many patients, one can arrive at a good understanding of the
nature of the problem quite rapidly. One of the exciting new areas of
research related to psychoanalytic therapy has been the ability to formulate patient dynamic issues on the basis of early interviews, with good
interjudge reliability. For example, Crits-Christoph and colleagues
(1988) were able to discern patients' core conflictual relationship themes
(CCRT) on the basis of relationship episodes extracted from early sessions of therapy, with high reliability. They were also able to show that
therapist accuracy in their interventions about the main wishes of patients and the responses these wishes elicited from others that were expressed in the relationship themes were positively related to outcomes
in moderate-length psychodynamic therapy.

In a similar vein, Horowitz, Rosenberg, Ureño, Kalehzan, and
O'Halloran (1989), have developed a reliable, consensual response method for arriving at interpersonal psychodynamic formulations based on
initial interviews. Furthermore, upon reading the consensual formulation, clinical raters were successful in predicting which problems would
be discussed in treatment. Silberschatz et al. (1986) reliably discerned
patients' problems and likely behavior in therapy by means of the Plan
Formulation Method, constructed on the basis of early sessions. They
reported that therapist interventions compatible with the plan were
predictive of patient progress and outcome. This line of research
demonstrates the possibility of formulating patient problems rapidly and provides evidence that doing so enhances the results of brief
to moderate-length therapy. It lends important empirical support to
a basic proposition of BPT, namely, that a focus can be arrived at ear-

ly, that it can be rated reliably, and that it is useful in the conduct of therapy.

6. *To bring about personality reorganization or structural change, therapy needs to be long.* Long-term therapy or psychoanalysis, perhaps because of the large investment each entails, aim at some rather fundamental shifts in a person's character style, be it histrionic, obsessive, dependent, or borderline. Brief dynamic therapy typically does not aspire to personality reorganization (except, perhaps, for Davanloo's (1980) intensive short-term dynamic psychotherapy). Rather than being extensive and comprehensive, it strives to be intensive and focused. One cannot range over as many domains of personality, fantasy systems, interpersonal issues, and the like, as in long-term therapy. Cure is conceived of in terms such as an increase in self-esteem, resolution of a conflict, change in an interpersonal pattern, alleviation of a symptom, an increased understanding of one's problems, or feeling and functioning better. That is, BPT is more modest in its aspirations than long-term psychoanalytic therapy.

Learning Brief Psychodynamic Therapy

The previously cited survey of psychologists in California and Massachusetts (Levenson et al., 1995) found that 37% had scant or no training in brief therapy, whether or not they were practicing it. In fact, psychologists who reported having had no training in brief treatment were conducting, on average, 10 hours of brief therapy per week. As mentioned earlier, the psychodynamic and existential–humanistic therapists stated that they had less skill in conducting it than all other therapists. Among training methods for learning brief therapy, supervision was ranked first in effectiveness, followed by self-selected reading. Since more than 80% of the participants were presently conducting some amount of brief therapy, which accounted for 40% of their clinical practice, the need for more training among students and practitioners is apparent, especially for those with a psychodynamic orientation.

There is a lively debate in the literature as to who is most amenable to learning BPT. On the one hand, the demands for a rapid evaluation of the patient's problem, the discernment of transference, and the ability to keep interventions focused requires some comfort and expertise with psychoanalytic theory and therapy (Mann & Goldman, 1982; Said, 1988). On the other hand, those who have been conducting long-term psychoanalytic therapy for some time develop habitual ways of thinking and behaving that need to be modified in switching to BPT. The novice comes to BPT with fewer preconceived ideas about what constitutes good practice and with enthusiasm and high motivation that are great assets for learning any new procedure. Flegenheimer (1982) concluded that it is best for candidates learning BPT to have some background in psychodynamic theory and therapy but not yet be habituated to the particular techniques of long-term therapy. Both he and Strupp and Binder (1984) suggest that BPT be taught at some intermediate phase of training. Our own outlook is that either group can learn BPT but the emphasis in teaching should be different for each. Didactic learning and skill acquisition are paramount for the novice, whereas overcoming resistances and intellectual preconceptions are more critical in training more experienced therapists (Winokur & Dasberg, 1983). Below we will discuss the teaching and training of both groups, taking into account their different needs.

Teaching Brief Psychodynamic Therapy to the Relatively Inexperienced Therapist

Probably the ideal time to learn BPT is at the more advanced phase of a graduate or residency program, after some helpful background courses and experience have been acquired. This would include course or practicum work in interviewing, fundamentals of psychoanalytic theory, psychopathology, and some experience conducting long-term psychoanalytically oriented psychotherapy. The fewer of these prerequisites that the student has in hand, the more time that a course in BPT should devote to this subject matter. One of us (SBM) has been teaching BPT for 15 years to clinical psychology students in the format of a full year (30-week) course, and the suggestions below are based on that experience.

There are five elements that characterize the teaching module: (1) theories of BPT; (2) videotaped illustrations of brief dynamic therapists at work; (3) supervised practice of BPT along with student in-class case presentations; (4) research pertinent to psychotherapy, especially BPT; and (5) special topics and issues that bear on BPT, such as integration/eclecticism, values and visions, curative factors, the practice of BPT in various settings, such as community mental health centers and within managed care programs, race/class/gender differences, termination, and follow up.

Theories of Brief Psychodynamic Therapy. Because we take a pluralistic view regarding the value of different approaches to theories of psychotherapy (Messer, 1992; Messer & Warren, 1990), we consider it optimal to teach several BPT approaches in one course. As is apparent from the organization of this book, we regard the major psychodynamically informed therapies as drive/structural, relational and cognitive, integrative/analytic, and eclectic. Exposure to several therapies allows students to decide which approach they find most congenial and to learn to appreciate the different facets of human functioning each illuminates. Readings include representative works of each of these approaches along with case examples. Each week the class discusses the readings with an eye to comparing and evaluating their theoretical suppositions, their strengths and weaknesses, and the clinical issues they raise. Seven weeks are allotted to this didactic emphasis, along with videotaped examples that we describe next.

Videotaped Demonstrations. Over the years we have acquired interview samples of some of the leading brief psychodynamic therapists at work that vividly illustrate their clinical approach. We also use demonstrations of our own work, which is important since we ask students to expose their interviews for public scrutiny as well. Students are enormously appreciative of the willingness of their instructors to reveal their less-than-perfect clinical style, and it gives them courage to present their own necessarily imperfect efforts. It is not necessary for these to be shining examples, since students can learn from observing and discussing errors as well as from seeing good technique modeled.

If demonstration tapes are not available, we would recommend inviting local practitioners to conduct interviews for the class. Another alternative is to analyze published case material that is readily available, and/or to role play cases in class with students alternately taking the roles of patient and therapist. The general point is for students to get an experience-near opportunity to practice BPT before taking on actual cases. At this stage of the course, the demonstrations focus on initial interviews in which a careful dynamic assessment leading to a focus is a primary goal, as well as establishing a relationship and enhancing patient motivation for therapy. With most of the videotaped cases, we have information on the course and outcome of therapy, and so we ask students to predict whether the patients, in their estimation, are suitable candidates for BPT based on the selection criteria they have read about. They can then compare their predictions to the actual results, which is often an instructive, if sobering, experience.

One of these demonstration cases is used for the purpose of a mid-semester homework assignment in which students are asked to formulate the case from three different theoretical perspectives, including the focus and the goals set for therapy.

Student Cases and Presentations. The first two components take up about 7 to 8 weeks of class time, at which point students are assigned cases through the psychological clinic attached to our program. A preliminary phone or live interview is conducted by one of the clinic coordinators to exclude grossly unsuitable cases. A patient deemed suitable by the coordinator and the course instructor is then assigned to the student, along with a supervisor who has some expertise in BPT. The latter might include staff of the college counseling center, psychologists who work at the local community mental health centers, private practitioners, or the course instructor. Whenever possible, students are assigned to supervisors with special interest or experience in a particular brand of BPT.

During the next 8 weeks of the course, each student brings to class a videotape of the initial interview just conducted, for class discussion. After receiving feedback on areas that need exploring, suggestions for alterations in technique, and so forth, students conduct a second interview, a summary of which they present in class for a determination of suitability and the formulation of a focus. In this way, students get to follow, from beginning to end, about eight to ten cases, each seen for 10 to 20 sessions. All the while, they continue to read relevant literature and to discuss it in class. By the end of the first semester, all or most of the students are engaged in conducting BPT. The major assignment in this semester is a full write-up of their own case, with formulations and foci from three different psychodynamic perspectives, as well as a statement of anticipated difficulties, and goals for the therapy.

In the second semester, students have another opportunity to present their cases, this time a middle or late session, with the focus on the particular problems that arise in the later phases of BPT. Students often comment that they rarely have the opportunity in other courses to see cases through to the end, and specifically to discuss termination issues.

Research in Psychotherapy. Throughout the course, but particularly in the second semester, articles evaluating process and outcome of BPT are assigned and discussed. We start with the research indicating that gains in global functioning come early in psychotherapy (e.g., Howard et al., 1986; Smith et al., 1980), and that comparisons of BPT with long-term psychoanalytic therapy show few differences in outcome (e.g., Piper et al., 1984). We include research on the reliability of psychodynamic formulation based on early sessions (e.g., Barber & Crits-Christoph, 1993; Crits-Christoph, Luborsky, et al., 1988; Horowitz et al., 1989; Rosenberg, Silberschatz, Curtis, Sampson, & Weiss, 1986), and the salutary effects of interventions compatible with the focus on patient progress (e.g., Messer, Tishby, & Spillman, 1992; Silberschatz et al., 1986), and outcome (Crits-Christoph, Cooper, et al., 1988). Outcome research comparing BPT with controls (e.g., Shefler, Dasberg & Ben-Shakhar, in press), or different forms of BPT (e.g., Winston, et al., 1991) are assigned. This is supplemented by research on process and outcome that helps to clarify patient or therapist factors contributing to outcome in BPT (e.g., Messer et al., 1992; Strupp, 1980a, 1980b).

Special Topics. Because this is a two-semester course, it is possible to include other topics that bear on BPT, such as the trend to integrate schools of psychotherapy; the challenge in working with the difficult patient who does not meet the selection criteria for BPT (see Chapter 6); the application of BPT to different age groups, such as children, adolescents, and the elderly (see Chapter 7); curative factors in psychotherapy (specific and nonspecific factors); the application of BPT in health maintenance organizations, employee assistance programs, and community mental health centers, with the inclusion of guest lecturers who practice BPT in those settings; brief group therapy; and special issues in working with clients of different racial, socioeconomic, or ethnic background. Of course, these topics can be altered to suit the particular interest and expertise of the instructor.

The assignment in the second semester is a substantial paper on any topic related to BPT, including the relevant literature. In one such paper, Sved (1983) evaluated the experience of 16 graduate students who had taken the course just described. Half the students had taken the course that academic year, and half were on internship, having taken the course a year earlier. All 16 viewed the course as a valuable component of their training, and stated that it helped them to become more active, focused, and flexible in conducting psychotherapy. The students agreed that some experience with long-term therapy and a good psychodynamic background were valuable prerequisites, and that the course had come at the appropriate phase of their professional development. Levenson and Bolter (1988) studied the attitudes of relatively inexperienced therapists before and after a 6-month seminar in BPT. After training, the therapists became more favorably inclined toward BPT.

Teaching Brief Psychodynamic Therapy to the Experienced Therapist

The components of training described above are also suitable for training the more experienced therapist, but the emphasis is somewhat less on skill acquisition and more on the intellectual challenges it poses to the conduct of long-term therapy. For example, Winokur and Dasberg (1983) report that, in their training group, one long-term therapist complained about the "terrible omnipotence" in conducting BPT, and another about the impossibility of getting at the "real issues," while "others contended that being an active therapist would not allow patients to reach their own insights, that the technique is disrespectful of the patient's autonomy, or that the therapist could not be responsive to new material" (p. 46). Winokur and Dasberg recommended that trainers be willing to discuss these issues, but that they should keep in mind that the process of change can arouse anxiety and that strongly held opinions often have emotional underpinnings.

We suggest that trainers should review the compendium of anxieties such as those presented above, allow them to emerge, and respond to them in an empathic, supportive, and clarifying way. They should also give intellectually honest answers to the actual questions raised as well. In a parallel process, such an approach serves as a model for the conduct of the therapy itself (Dasberg & Winokur, 1984). For training approaches focusing on Sifneos's short-term anxiety-provoking psychotherapy, see Heiberg (1981), Hougardy and Luminet (1980), and Sifneos (1978, 1992). For training in Davanloo's model of short-term dynamic psychotherapy, see Said (1988). Instruction in Strupp and Binder's time-limited dynamic psychotherapy is provided in their 1984 book and in a more recent book by Levenson (1995). For a comparison of several models of training in brief therapies of different orientations, including psychoanalytic, Jungian, behavioral, and group, see Levene et al., (1972).

Training Considerations in Clinical Settings

Although much of what is described above will apply to any setting in which BPT is taught, there are some further suggestions that are particularly relevant to practicum or internship settings, where much training in brief treatments takes place. Schneider and Pinkerton (1986) offer the following suggestions to maximize the success of brief psychotherapy training:

1. The agency, including staff and administration, should be committed to brief psychotherapy.
2. The supervisory staff should be experienced in practicing brief psychotherapy and comfortable supervising it.
3. The trainee should be motivated to learn the techniques of brief therapy, feel comfortable with a more active form of therapy and with establishing modest goals, and have sufficient background in psychodynamic theory and psychodiagnostic skills to make a rapid and early assessment.
4. Careful attention should be paid to patient selection criteria

to reduce two major errors in selection and disposition: selecting the client who should be referred for long-term psychotherapy, or, conversely, referring for time-unlimited therapy the client who is suitable for brief therapy.

Robbins and Zinni (1988) present a model to aid the assessment of factors related to the implementation of brief therapy within a university counseling center, which can apply to other settings (and a variety of theoretical models of brief therapy) as well. The first facet of their model focuses on the *motivational aspects*, such as staff knowledge of the service demands compared to the resources available and whether the administration has conveyed its support for brief therapy. The second facet consists of *technical treatment issues* that the staff needs to learn, such as client selection, focus, and the use of time, as well as the rationale presented to clients for brief therapy. The third facet comprises *evaluation and planning mechanisms* by which the effects of a switch to a brief therapy model are assessed.

The authors present an instructive case example of their role as consultants in helping a counseling center change to offering solely time-limited treatment. Their tasks included an assessment of the center's current functioning on the following three dimensions: the interventions that were made (e.g., a 2-day planning conference with the staff and a training workshop), the problems encountered, and the program evaluation that was conducted. They concluded that implementing a time-limited policy can create major organizational changes, placing stress on the system as well as providing the opportunity for agency development and individual therapist growth.

In a special section of the journal *Psychotherapy* (Binder & Strupp, 1993), researchers who had developed manuals for the conduct of psychotherapy in connection with their research projects offered recommendations for improving psychotherapy training (Binder, 1993; Dobson & Shaw, 1993; Luborsky, 1993; Moras, 1993; Weiss & Marmar, 1993). Most of their research was conducted in the context of brief psychotherapy, and thus pertains to the topic at hand. Following is our distillation of the recommendations that emerge as central to the training enterprise.

1. Select therapists who are good at relating to others, or teach them how to foster a therapeutic alliance. Those selected should have good conceptual abilities and a commitment to learn the approach at hand, and should not be too strongly wedded to an alternate therapeutic approach.

2. Teach the therapist how to diagnose and select the kind of pa-

tient considered suitable for the approach. Based on diagnosis, apply a balance of techniques that are more directly supportive and those that explore underlying issues. (For psychodynamic therapy, we may add, a psychodynamic formulation is more important than a DSM diagnosis.

3. Have the trainee read the manual and other didactic materials. The manual should include examples of common problems that crop up in therapy. Take the time in supervision to work through trainee resistance to using the manual. (We believe that there are typically hidden resentments toward "manualized" treatment which the trainee should be helped to articulate and discuss with the trainer.) Check that trainees are not slavishly following the manual in a "cookbook" kind of way.

4. Teach the trainee to formulate cases within the theoretical approach of the therapy. For brief therapies in particular, trainees need to learn how to formulate a focus, such as those described in the forthcoming chapters. They should learn how to track the focus (part of the listening process) and to offer interpretations or other interventions that relate to the focus.

5. Conduct training on case materials, using videotapes when possible, to demonstrate more and less successful examples of the application of the approach. Theory should be related to practice rather than each being taught in separate contexts.

6. Provide abundant supervision of cases, especially for novices. This should include individual and group supervision, as well as case conferences or seminars. In the supervision, emphasis should be more on therapist process than patient dynamics, and on patient-therapist interaction rather than intrapsychic dynamics. Trainees should learn proper timing of interventions, therapeutic tact, and how to change or continue a process toward some therapeutic goal. (We believe that these are the skills that manuals can only partially convey.)

7. Evaluate adherence to the manual to be sure that trainees have learned what the manual intended in areas such as patient selection, formulation of a focus, case write-ups, types of interventions, and so forth.

8. Work through the meaning of termination as a special phase of therapy. That is, the meaning of termination is best seen as it relates to the dynamic focus of the particular patient's course of BPT. This will help patients internalize their gains.

9. Evaluate the efficacy of therapy, an area that is too frequently neglected. To do this is to practice and model an important feature of the clinician as scientist-practitioner, and is not just a bow to third-party payers, such as insurance companies.

Research on Training

There is general agreement that there is a need for more research on what aspects of training are most critical in learning to conduct psychotherapy. For example, although personal therapy has often been recommended as an important part of training, there is very little research to support this contention. In this connection, a survey of practitioners revealed that 80% felt that their own therapy was a very important part of their training (Norcross & Prochaska, 1982). We will now report on the few research studies that pertain to training in BPT.

In a study by Burlingame, Fuhriman, Paul, and Ogles (1989), 12 therapists of varying theoretical orientation, including psychodynamic, were randomly assigned to treat 57 suitably selected patients in brief therapy. Therapists matched on experience level were assigned to one of three training conditions: no training; self-instruction, in which therapists were offered materials on brief therapy to read; or intensive training, in the form of a 10-hour structured training program consisting of didactic explanation, demonstration, roleplaying, and discussion of how to incorporate the model into their therapeutic style. A relationship was found between increased levels of training and decreased rates of patient attrition and recidivism, as well as with clinically significant patient improvement. The authors also found that the more experienced therapists produced better outcomes.

Hamovitch (1985) explored the effects of a 20-week training program in Davanloo's intensive short-term dynamic psychotherapy (ISTDP; see Chapter 2) for 12 relatively experienced therapists from a variety of professional backgrounds. He compared three videotapes from each: an intake session conducted prior to training, and an intake or therapy tape conducted midway through the training as well as one conducted at the end of the seminar. The competencies assessed reflected the requirements of ISTDP. Hamovitch found that, by the end of the seminar, the trainees employed more of some ISTDP competencies, such as confrontations, clarifications of defense, and transference interventions, but not others, such as interpretations connecting persons in the patient's past, current life, and in the transference. He concluded that the training program was partially successful, but that more time was needed for skill acquisition of this strongly confrontational form of brief therapy.

In a very sophisticated training study, 16 therapists were enrolled in a year-long program to learn Strupp and Binder's time-limited dynamic psychotherapy (Henry, Strupp, Butler, Schacht, & Binder, 1993; see Chapter 3). The training program successfully changed therapists' technical interventions in line with the authors' manual. At the same time, there was an unexpected deterioration in certain interpersonal aspects of the therapies the trainees conducted. The researchers observed that the therapists, in their effort to gain technical competence, became somewhat more mechanical and authoritarian in their approach, suggesting that it is easier to achieve technical adherence to a manual than to increase therapist skill in conducting brief therapy.

In further exploring the therapists' response to training (Henry, Schacht, Strupp, Butler, & Binder, 1993), the investigators found that one of the two trainers was much more successful in helping therapists to achieve adherence to the manual than the other. Based on an exploration of the observed differences in the two trainers' styles reported in this study, Binder (1993) has offered a summary of the specific supervision methods that produce increments in technical adherence to manuals of time-limited dynamic psychotherapy:

1. Scrutinize actual patient–therapist interactions as examples of broader themes in the therapy rather than conducting general discussions of these issues.
2. Structure the use of supervision by focusing on specific tasks, such as maladaptive interpersonal patterns or transference allusions. Emphasize patient interactions with the therapist rather than intrapsychic dynamics.
3. Encourage the tracking of a focal theme along with instruction in how to do this.
4. Emphasize the therapist's thought process, performance and experience more than patient dynamics: for example, "What were you thinking at that point?" or "What was your rationale for doing that?"
5. When offering supportive feedback, refer to what the therapist has done that was desirable rather than offering nonspecific praise.

It should be noted in this connection that supervision was ranked first in effectiveness among the training methods for brief therapy by a large sample of practicing psychologists (Levenson et al., 1995).

Eisdorfer (1989) developed, implemented, and evaluated a 10-week training seminar in BPT in the outpatient department of a community mental health center. She followed the principles enunciated above for the training of experienced therapists by including didactic and practice components, as well as by focusing on the resistances and reservations of the staff toward BPT. The three models included were Strupp and Binder's time-limited dynamic psychotherapy (TLDP), Davanloo's intensive short-term dynamic psychotherapy (ISTDP), and Mann's time-limited therapy (TLP; see Chapter 4). Based on pretraining and post-training questionnaires, she found that therapists' views of long-term therapy remained stable, whereas their attitudes toward BPT changed in significant ways. They became more positive toward brief therapy, believing it could bring about more change and a different kind of change than they had previously thought. The therapists also came to view curative factors in long-term therapy, such as attention to the transference, as more integral to BPT and considered BPT and long-term therapy as conceptually more similar after the seminar than at the start.

The research supports the utility of carefully designed training programs in BPT. The major caveat is that emphasis must be placed not only on adherence to the technical aspects of the particular model of BPT being taught but also on broader features of conducting therapy in a skillful and interpersonally sensitive manner (Strupp, Butler, & Rosser, 1988). It is also important to attend to the attitudinal and emotional barriers to conducting BPT.

In this chapter we have covered the main issues affecting the field of brief therapy in general and BPT in particular. The introductory section on the context of practice demonstrated that brief therapy, planned or unplanned, is what most clients receive, that it constitutes a significant part of clinicians' work, and that it is likely to increase in the current climate of managed health care. We have laid out the historical context in which BPT developed and drawn the lines of influence from the early pioneers to the present innovators. We have learned that there is substantial research supporting the efficacy of BPT, and that its effects tend to last. We have described the unique set of values embodied in BPT as understood within the romantic, ironic, tragic, and comic visions of reality. We have also spelled out the intellectual and emotional resistances and challenges involved in teaching, learning, and practicing BPT for both the student and the experienced practitioner. Finally, we have noted training considerations that must be taken into account when introducing BPT into clinical settings that have a long-term therapy orientation. We will now turn to a consideration of the BPT model that is most directly derived from traditional psychoanalytic theory.

Basic Models of Brief
Psychodynamic Therapy

CHAPTER 2

The Drive/Structural Model: Malan, Davanloo, and Sifneos

The modern era of brief psychodynamic therapy begins in the 1960s with the work of Habib Davanloo, David Malan, and Peter Sifneos. Each of these psychiatrists was working in a different country (Canada, England, and the United States, respectively), applying the principles of psychoanalysis to the treatment of patients considered suitable for BPT. They met in the early 1970s, and there followed a series of conferences organized by Davanloo at which they displayed videotapes of just what it was that they were doing in the consulting room. The proceedings of the conferences were published in two volumes edited by Davanloo (1978, 1980), which gave a close-up look at the techniques of these three innovators. Malan's (1963) volume describing the therapy that he and Balint were conducting at the Tavistock Clinic in London, and in which he reviewed earlier papers on BPT, had actually preceded these conferences by more than a decade. Sifneos's first book describing his method had appeared in 1972. These books are replete with clinical examples of Davanloo's intensive short-term dynamic psychotherapy (ISTDP), Malan's brief intensive psychotherapy (BIP), and Sifneos's short-term anxiety-provoking psychotherapy (STAPP). They include portions of transcripts (typically of initial interviews), patient selection criteria, dynamic formulations, and the techniques employed to make the therapy brief. (See also Malan & Asimo, 1992; Sifneos 1992; and Davanloo, 1988.)

At the time that Davanloo, Malan, and Sifneos were experimenting with their approaches, psychoanalysis, and its offshoot psychoanalytic psychotherapy, were at the height of their popularity, enjoying a near monopoly in psychiatry. Of course, Rogerian client-centered therapy and behavior therapy were already well known, particularly among psychologists, counselors, and social workers. These clinicians, each working in public clinics, recognized the pressing need for brief therapy and were willing to swim upstream against the prevailing view that psychoanalytically based therapy, to be effective, required several sessions a week over a long time period. It will be recalled that the last major attempt to establish a bridgehead for BPT, by Alexander and French in the 1940s, was not well received within the psychoanalytic community.

What strikes us in reading these authors' works is the rather unself-conscious way in which they employ psychoanalytic theory as a basis for understanding their patients and treating them. The model they use is Freudian in shape, without the kind of discussion of the varieties of psychoanalytic or other theories to which we are now accustomed. Neither interpersonal, object relational, cognitive-dynamic or self psychological terminology confuse or complicate their outlook. In fact, they devote rather little space to the theoretical underpinnings of their approaches, assuming their audience to be of like mind theoretically, familiar with the basics of psychoanalysis, and needing only to learn about the practical aspects of applying this agreed-upon theory to suitably selected patients. In our view, this clearly reflects the *zeitgeist* or spirit of the 1960s and 1970s and indicates how much the fields of psychoanalysis and psychotherapy have changed. It also means that, from the perspective of the 1990s, with other models available for comparison, we can more readily discern the theoretical premises upon which the early proponents of BPT were operating. In spelling out these premises, we will focus on those aspects of theory that seem most relevant to the work of these authors, and that are illustrated in their case examples. We will also see how the theoretical principles influence the technique of the therapy and its mode of bringing about change.

THE THEORY OF PERSONALITY AND PSYCHOPATHOLOGY: INTERSYSTEMIC CONFLICT

The "intersystemic conflict" model of mind begins with the concept of drive or wish. Freud's dual-instinct theory posits that the motor driving behavior consists of sexual and aggressive energies (the id) and their derivatives, such as wishes or impulses. This is first and foremost a biological theory in that the drives are inborn, bodily entities that have unrelenting consequences for the mind. It is human nature to strive for pleasure, to seek gratification of these drives in one way or another.

Because society does not condone the unrestricted expression of the drives, it is necessary that they be channeled into prosocial activities which allow for their satisfaction in derivative and partial form, known as compromise formations or sublimation.

The modulation of the drives is accomplished by "the ego," a set of *functions* that mediate between the drives and external reality. One of the key functions of the ego is to institute defenses which help to keep the drives in check. Another ego function is to produce a signal of distress or anxiety in situations of psychic danger that indicates the need to erect such a defense. Freud posited that these danger situations originated in early childhood and can be elicited by similar, perceived threats in any stage of development. The first danger is loss of the object upon whom the infant relies for its very life. The compelling cry of the infant lets the caretaker know that the distress is very real and requires immediate attention. Related to this fear is loss of the object's love, which comes a short while later developmentally (at about ages two to three), when the child is able to experience and understand such an emotion, even in primitive form. The third danger situation is some sort of physical injury, which is often referred to as "castration anxiety," a reference to a real or fantasied injury to the male genitals, or an analogous genital injury in the female (about ages two to four). The fourth is a fear of disapproval or punishment by "the superego," which produces the affect of guilt, and which appears after age five or six. These sources of danger are said to continue to threaten people unconsciously throughout their lives.

When a person is faced with a situation that recalls one of these prototypical dangers, a defense is instituted to minimize pain (in accordance with the pleasure principle) and to help maintain psychic equilibrium. If things go well, a dynamic balance is maintained among id, ego, and superego functions and a person achieves some drive satisfaction as well as a suitable adaptation to reality. In such a case, the drive energy is said to be neutralized. For example, underlying the seemingly straightforward act of reading this book may be the wish for power over others through knowledge acquisition, which would be viewed in Freudian terms as a derivative of the aggressive drive. Alternately or simultaneously, if one is a student, there may be the wish to win the approval, admiration, or even love of a professor who has assigned it, which is viewed as a derivative of the sexual drive. In addition, it may satisfy one's ego ideal of being the best-informed student or psychotherapist one can be, thereby avoiding social disapproval (superego function). Defenses such as sublimation and intellectualization (ego functions) enable one to read and learn relatively smoothly and comfortably in spite of such unconscious wishes and fears.

Things do not always go so smoothly, however. Even an innocuous act like reading can get bound up in conflict. Suppose that, along with the wish to learn something and to succeed, the student has a strong unconscious wish to defeat an authority figure, such as a professor. Because of the danger or consequences of expressing this wish directly, perhaps invoking the professor's wrath, a defense such as repression is instituted. If the defense partially fails because of the strength of the wish (a drive derivative of aggression), the ego seeks some partial gratification through the production of a symptom, which is a substitute for unachieved drive gratification. For example, one may develop a headache in reading this book or some sort of attention deficit. The drive is partially satisfied insofar as the professor's assignment is being learned only poorly, even while the wish to learn something is being partially fulfilled. It is in this sense that a symptom is a compromise formation between the reality-oriented ego and the drive content of the id. This is also an example of how symptoms and other behavior are said to carry psychological meaning.

Alternately, the failure of defense may result in vague feelings of anxiety, or in other maladaptive behavior such as procrastination. Of course, this solution does not accord well with reality insofar as the student will not get the assignment done, or will get it done in a less than satisfactory way, leading to poor grades. This may produce feelings of guilt over unachieved aspirations, which also contributes to the conflict. The superego as voice of the student's conscience may also be "demanding" punishment for the student's own aggressive impulse, which is satisfied through the untoward consequences of poor grades.

This example illustrates the dynamic that is referred to in Malan's and Davanloo's work as the triangle of conflict (see Figure 2.1, p. 82): An impulse (I) or feeling (F) leads to a defense (D), which, when unsuccessful, results in anxiety (A). Brenner (1976) expanded the motive for defense to include any kind of unpleasurable affect, but especially depressive affect. Similarly, the result of failure of defense can be any unpleasurable affect, including depression. Davanloo and Malan clearly follow Brenner's revisions in their conceptual scheme.

While this example illustrates the *structural* (id, ego, superego) and *dynamic* (conflict- and meaning-related) aspects of the drive/structural model, another component that is central to it is the *genetic or developmental* attitude. Malan (1976a) refers to the desirability in planning a brief therapy of discerning both the current conflict and the underlying "nuclear conflict" (p. 264). The latter includes the early precipitating events, such as traumatic experiences, the family constellation, and the prior instances of the problematic patterns. The important point is that the advent of the current conflict or problem is seen as a repetition of some earlier constellation of factors that occurred in the family of origin. As is well known, the terms oral, anal, phallic, latency, and genital are ways of describing the phases of life as the sexual drive changes its focus from one erogenous zone to another as its center of pleasure. Within the drive/structural model, it is not that the parents or siblings directly cause the problem so much as they constitute the supporting actors in the drama in which the vicissitudes of the person's innate drives are played out.

How do attachments to people come about? The use of the term "object" for "person" in psychoanalytic theory is not accidental. It serves to remind us that the drives seek objects for gratification. The nature of the object relationship depends upon the drive that is active and the related stage of development. Object relations are at first partial, with the infant relating to the mother, for example, as breast only. In drive/structural theory, the tie to the object is not present in the organism from the outset, as posited by the relational theorists discussed in Chapter 3 (Greenberg & Mitchell, 1983). Rather, objects emerge out of the repeated experiences of drive satisfaction and frustration with them. Social ties are secondary and are dependent on the ability of others to serve as objects for drive-related needs.

In the example above, the presumption would be that underlying the conflict over obedience to the authority of the professor is an earlier struggle with a parent. The person probably had loving feelings for the parents along with, at the same time, angry feelings, leading to an ambivalent attitude that psychoanalytic theory considers to be characteristic of human relationships. The wish to defeat the parent, if not resolved, goes underground (becomes unconscious) only to reemerge (albeit disguised and displaced) under the pressure of current circumstances—in our example, the need both to defy and submit to the authority of the professor.

The cause of this conflict would be viewed, first, as a consequence of the strength of the drives operating at the time, but also of the environmental circumstances. The notion that people adapt to their surroundings, both physical and social, is known as the *adaptive* viewpoint in psychoanalysis. Although Freud acknowledged that the reality principle serves as an aid to the pleasure principle, it was Hartmann's (1939) theory of adaptation and Erikson's (1950) model of psychosocial epigenesis, tying the psychosexual stages to the child's psychosocial development, that established the importance within psychoanalysis of human adaptation. It meant that people can only be understood in relation to their environment, on which they act and to which they adjust. It also allows for a process of differentiation from the environment. In normal functioning, there is a meshing of the child's needs and those of the caretakers at the different stages of development (Rapaport & Gill, 1959). In our example, the student, when a child, would have striven to adapt to the parents' authority, but at the same time have tried to individuate and act upon the parents in an attempt to exert his or her own drive-induced needs.

There are two other viewpoints within psychoanalysis requiring brief mention. One is the *economic* viewpoint, which posits that there is energy or excitation underlying psychological phenomena. This energy or libido has to do with people's interest in, or valuing of, objects and is especially evident when they overvalue their work or their significant others. Libido is treated as a commodity to be guarded because it is viewed as being limited in quantity and which, therefore, you don't want to "give away" to another unless you will "get it back." What is most important to understand about this energy is that it can be displaced and transformed. An erogenous zone can be suffused with energy, and objects or part objects can be cathected with energy. In the case of the symptom of stuttering, for example, the oral cavity is said to be suffused with aggressive energy, interrupting the smooth flow of speech. Normally the speech function is neutralized by the ego in the process of growth and development, but, under conflictual circumstances, can become "reinstinctualized." It should be mentioned in passing that the value and scientific status of the economic viewpoint has been a matter of considerable debate and is considered by some (e.g., Holt, 1976) to be anachronistic.

Finally, there is the *topographic* viewpoint, which refers to the layering of mental processes into conscious, preconscious, and unconscious. That which is preconscious, while not at the center of attention, can be retrieved by attending to it. What is unconscious, however, is kept that way by an active force of repression. This viewpoint is still referred to in the psychoanalytic literature but was largely replaced by the structural hypothesis (partitioning the activities of the mind into id, ego, and superego functions), which allows for a broader understanding of many mental phenomena (Arlow & Brenner, 1964).

Before we move on to the kind of brief therapy that emanates from Freudian theory there is one other key psychoanalytic concept to describe: the oedipal complex. For Davanloo, Malan, and Sifneos, the object relations of the oedipal stage are the major precursors of the kind of problems considered most suitable for BPT. In fact, Freud considered this phase to be of utmost importance in the formation of neuroses and their treatment in psychoanalysis as well. He found in the unconscious mental life of his patients a wish to possess the parent of the opposite sex and to get rid of the parent of the same sex. At the same time, there existed the inverse wish, to destroy the opposite sex parent and take his or her place with the same-sex parent. These feelings of rivalry with one parent or the other are connected with sexual sensations, the whole pattern (or complex) constituting a real, passionate love affair. Children come to fear the consequences of these wishes, which include retaliation through genital or physical injury and loss of love, which ultimately leads to renouncing oedipal wishes and seeking substitute gratifications. The wishes do not disappear entirely, but they go underground and can resurface under certain conditions. The particular form that the oedipal complex takes in any individual will depend on experiences such as the birth of siblings, the presence or absence of a parent, and the strength of the drives, which are said to vary constitutionally. (For a fuller description, see Freud, 1924b/1959, and Brenner, 1973.)

To return to our beleaguered student, whom we shall denominate as male for the purposes of this discussion, what appears on the surface as merely a struggle with authority may represent the wish to eliminate a hated rival who has the power and resources he wishes to have for himself. This may include, for example, the admiration of the female students in the class. This jealousy would be regarded as a derivative of the competition he once felt toward his father or a sibling as a rival for his mother's affections.

The instinctual renunciation required of the child in the oedipal phase is not easy to attain. Freud emphasized the importance of the child's detaching himself or herself from parents and moving from dependence to autonomy (Greenberg & Mitchell, 1983). The terms that he used to describe this developmental effort are ones that come up often in the writings of drive/structural brief therapists: the move from passivity to activity. Freud (1931/1964) wrote that "the first sexual and sexually colored experiences which a child has in relation to its mother are naturally of a passive character. . . . A part of its libido goes on clinging to those experiences and enjoys the satisfactions bound up with them; but another part strives to turn them into activity" (p. 236) in order to become self-sufficient. There often remains a conflict between active and passive sexual aims, which the relational theorists refer to in their language as the tension between individuation or autonomy, on the one hand, and merger or dependence, on the other. Remaining passive is a maladaptive way of resolving the oedipal complex, as it leaves the person fixated in the incestuous object relations of this phase. It is probably for this reason that there is such a great emphasis in Davanloo's and Sifneos's therapies on moving the person from passivity to activity (which may be aided by patients modeling the therapist's "phallic" therapeutic style).

The main point to grasp about the drive/structural model is its focus on a self-contained individual. Defense mechanisms such as repression, intellectualization, and so forth, result from internal drive forces and the dangers of their expression. The elements of conflicts are seen to reside within the person, and these get projected onto available (e.g., the therapist) or sought-after objects. It is a one-person or one-body psychology, "a biologically closed system seeking to discharge energy in order to maintain homeostasis" or equilibrium (Aron, 1990, p. 466).

THE FORMULATION OF A FOCUS

With this much theory in hand, we can now apply the model to a case summary to illustrate two important aspects of BPT, namely, the formulation of a psychoanalytically informed focus and the selection criteria for suitability. Regarding the focus, since Malan, Davanloo, and Sifneos all rely on traditional psychoanalysis and ego psychology, we may assume that they would formulate the patient's problems in a similar way. It is interesting that in spite of their emphasis on a psychodynamic formulation and focus, we could not find a fully presented dynamic formulation in their writings. They seem to take for granted that any well-trained psychoanalytic practitioner would view a patient similarly, which research has shown is not necessarily the case (e.g., Collins & Messer, 1991). The stress in their writings is more on the process of the initial interview and the therapy, and less on the explicit formulation of the dynamics. Malan (1976a), however, does spell out what he refers to as "a minimal dynamic hypothesis" to guide the therapy.

Case Illustration

Vera is a single, 22-year-old, White, Catholic, college student majoring in the humanities. She wore a serious expression in the initial interview and smiled rarely. She was not spontaneous but preferred waiting to be asked questions by the interviewer. Vera did not express emotions readily, and when she began to cry once during the two evaluation interviews, she quickly restrained herself. She comes to the clinic complaining of severe cramps that feel to her like a knife was cutting through her stomach. The attacks occurred about five times over the past several months and the pain has gotten worse. She had seen a physician, who ruled out a physical lesion as a cause of her discomfort and who prescribed a combination of a tranquilizer and an antispasmodic.

The stomach pains date back about a year, to when her fiancé, with whom she lives, was unemployed and she felt insecure financially. The cramps also occur in connection with arguments she has with him. She finds him to be slow moving, unambitious, even docile—and this bothers her. She is now considering leaving him but is having difficulty doing so. She has also been very jealous when he is engaged in photographing models in connection with his college curriculum. The stomach pains also occur when Vera is with her mother. She says that she loves her mother but feels tense when with her and finds it difficult to express feelings to her, particularly anger. She reports that her mother rarely complimented her when she was growing up.

Nevertheless, Vera recalls her early years as being happy. She was one of four children; her brothers are 29, 18, and 12-years old. She was very fond of her father and was "daddy's girl." She said he was an active, lively, outgoing man with whom she went fishing and riding in his delivery truck. She also recalls considerable bickering between her parents. Her father drank; one night he hit her mother, which shocked and disturbed Vera greatly. This occurred when she was 9 or 10 years old, at which time she took a green liquid for stomach cramps. Her father was seeing other women and even introduced her to them on occasion. Her parents divorced when she was 12, and her father has been in touch with her only rarely since then, and not in the past several years. She feels totally indifferent to him now. Several months ago she learned that he had become quite ill.

About a year after the divorce she began to feel resentful toward her mother because she had to babysit for her younger brothers while her mother went out on dates. On one such occasion, fearing that her mother might not return, she had an "hysterical fit" and was chided by her sister-in-law for being immature. In the second of the two evaluation interviews, she presented a dream in which she was in a doctor's office having an abortion. She was in great pain, and her father was nearby, asking the doctor how she was, and expressing general concern about her welfare.

Vera is currently interested in an older, married man of 36, her boss in her part-time clerical work, whom she describes as very warm, lively, and outgoing, but with whom she sees no future. She said in the interview, "I speak to him like he was my father." She has not had sex with him but does fantasize about it. She also has a good female friend who is 36 years old.

Starting with the symptom, we could postulate that Vera's stomach cramps are her way of dealing with what is quite clearly a problem she has with the expression of aggression (the drive or impulse). Rather than express her anger directly, she swallows it and turns it against herself (the defense). Thus, the symptom can be seen as a compromise between gratifying the drive and inhibiting it. Symptoms, like other features of mental life, are often overdetermined, and we may ask whether the sex drive plays a role in its formation. The dream may give us a clue, because the symptom appears in connection with an aborted pregnancy, with her father nearby offering comfort. Could this be a fantasied pregnancy by her father as a throwback to the oedipal period when, according to psychoanalytic theory, girls often experience such fantasies along with a wish to marry their father? Perhaps the abortion and pain involved are an expiation for this guilt-arousing fantasy (superego function). The occurrence of the symptom when she was a child points to the nuclear conflict underlying the current conflict, involving the threat of loss of her then-beloved father.

Like Freud before them, Davanloo, Malan, and Sifneos often focus on the oedipal features of a case, and it is certainly possible to discern Vera's entanglement in oedipal triangles. One of the main precipitating factors for her symptoms was her jealousy of her fiancé's attention to the photography models (the triangle of Vera/fiancé/female models). One wonders if her wish to leave him is a displacement of anger at father for jilting her. Another oedipal triangle includes Vera, her boss (whom she speaks to like a father, and about whom she has sexual fantasies), and her boss's wife, in which once again she is the odd woman out. This situation seems destined to be a replay of her having lost her father to another woman.

Regarding the nuclear conflict, there is the triangle of Vera (as daddy's little girl, and the only daughter among three sons), her mother, and her father—the original oedipal trio. We note that in her early years she seemed to be closer to her father than to her mother. Then there was Vera, her father, and her father's girlfriends, another potential source of jealousy and disappointment. In a later session, she referred to her high school principal as having the same last name as she, and to her being known, teasingly, as his "daughter." She reported a dream in which she was away at a resort, having an affair with him. They were dancing until her girlfriend came along and took her place. This dream provides the kind of evidence that corroborates her strong but repressed oedipal desires and her fears of coming off second best.

This brings us to another, related theme, however, that cannot be ignored even in a brief therapy, were Vera to be considered suitable for it. The theme of loss and threat of abandonment is apparent, and with good reason: Her father abandoned her when her parents divorced. Happening as it did when she was entering adolescence and puberty, the loss would have served to exacerbate earlier oedipal conflicts. She also felt abandoned by her mother, who was working and dating after the divorce. In this connection, another meaning of the symptom of stomach cramps could be her bodily way of expressing a need for nurturance, or nourishment, which was not being satisfied when her parents were constantly fighting. Currently, she feels financially insecure because of her fiancé's lack of ambition or employment, reawakening the earlier insecurities in her home. Her way of dealing with the loss has been to deny her feelings, to erase the memory of her father, never having mourned his loss openly. Her dream suggests, however, that she still longs for the love and caring of this lost relationship. Her attachment to her boss and to an older woman are also telling, in that they can be viewed as substitutes for the loss of father and the need to create an acceptable mother.

We may also wonder whether her choice of fiancé was a function of her need to attach herself to someone very unlike her father, which helps keep her longings for him repressed. But this also leaves her feeling dissatisfied with the relationship. It may be difficult for her to invest in new relationships for fear of abandonment. Some of the anger at her father's leaving may be displaced to both her mother and fiancé. As an example of one of the danger situations described above, her inability to express anger at her mother can be due to her fear of loss of whatever love she receives from that quarter.

This analysis is meant to illustrate the way that psychoanalytic theory is employed to make sense of a case, and how it sets out a course of action for the brief dynamic therapist. In fact, the ability to formulate such a focus is one of the criteria that are used to decide whether a brief therapy is possible. If there is no focus discernible in the first two or three interviews, this is a strong indication that BPT is not a treatment of choice. There are other indications and contraindications for selecting suitable patients, however, to which we now turn.

THE SELECTION CRITERIA: INDICATIONS AND CONTRAINDICATIONS

In general, brief psychodynamic therapists rule out those patients whose severity of disturbance precludes their ability to engage in an insight-oriented therapy, or who need more time to work through their problems. One way to state the contraindications is in terms of certain behaviors, which include serious suicide attempts or potential suicidality, a history of alcohol or other drug addiction, severe depression, poor impulse control, incapacitating, chronic obsessional or phobic symptoms, some psychosomatic conditions such as ulcerative colitis, and poor reality testing. With reference to DSM-IV, this would include major depressive syndrome, schizophrenia, and paranoia, as well as the more severe personality disorders such as antisocial, borderline and narcissistic. Although the latter two syndromes can be treated in brief therapy, they require modifications in focus, technique, and goals, which will be discussed in Chapter 6. In addition to the more obvious psychopathological or diagnostic exclusionary criteria, Malan (1976a, p. 69) adds the following rejection criteria:

1. Inability to make contact
2. Necessity for prolonged work in order to generate motivation for treatment
3. Necessity for prolonged work in order to penetrate rigid defenses
4. Inevitable involvement in complex or deep-seated issues that there seems no hope of working through in a short time
5. Severe dependence or other forms of unfavorable intense transference
6. Intensification of depressive or psychotic disturbance

In terms of DSM indications, those conditions included as suitable for BPT are the adjustment disorders; the milder personality disorders, such as avoidant, dependent, obsessive–compulsive, and histrionic; and the less severe anxiety and depressive disorders.

Davanloo considers his intensive short-term dynamic psychotherapy (ISTDP) suitable for patients with long-standing neurosis or maladaptive personality patterns with a focus on either oedipal or loss issues or both (Davanloo, 1980; Laikin, Winston, & McCullough, 1991). He makes specific mention of patients with obsessional and phobic neurosis as suitable.

Many of the diagnostic criteria stated above are descriptive, static, or structural, and are based largely on the patient's history, garnered from the psychiatric interview as well as the interviewer's observations. The three drive/structural therapists, however, also stress the *process* of the interview in gauging a patient's likely response to the active, frequently confrontational techniques of this model of BPT. Davanloo in particular refers to the importance of making trial interpretations in the initial interviews. He then notes whether the patient responds with deepened involvement or with some form of decompensation, such as severe anxiety, confusion, or even paranoia. If one of the latter reactions occurs, he becomes more supportive, and would consider the patient unsuitable for ISTDP. Davanloo (personal communication) regards the patient's motivation as an unimportant factor in selection because his experience is that he can break through the resistances to expose the core unconscious issues even in more fragile patients.

Sifneos (1987) lists the following presenting complaints of patients he typically sees in short-term anxiety-provoking psychotherapy (STAPP): anxiety with or without other symptoms, interpersonal problems, phobias along with obsessive thoughts, and mild depression. In terms of the process of the interview, he looks for the following (p. 27):

1. The patient's ability to have a circumscribed chief complaint
2. Evidence of a give and take, or "meaningful relationship" with another person during childhood
3. Capacity to relate flexibly to the evaluator during the interview and to experience and express feelings freely
4. Psychological sophistication—above-average intelligence and psychological-mindedness
5. Motivation for change and not (only) for symptom relief

Sifneos (1987) devotes a book chapter to spelling out and illustrating these criteria. For our purposes, a few points of clarification will suffice. Regarding the first criterion, Sifneos writes:

> The ability to circumscribe points further to the patient's capability to select a whole area of conflicting wishes rather than simply to choose a superficial symptom or interpersonal difficulty. Such a capacity, of course, demonstrates that the awareness of the underlying conflicts whose resolution will enable him to eliminate his symptoms once and for all is present and predominates at this point. (p. 28)

Regarding the nature of the focus, it is almost exclusively oedipal–genital or triangular–interpersonal in structure. Sifneos says that his form of BPT is not for patients who have suffered a loss or serious separation from a loved one and who developed grief reactions or reactive depressions.

The second criterion requires the ability to trust and to share. It represents a fairly advanced stage of object relations. The third criterion provides evidence of the second one, the ability to trust, in the interaction with the evaluator, as well as ready access to a variety of affects as demonstrated in the interview. The fourth criterion calls for the patient's ability to understand problems in psychological terms and to engage in problem solving. "For example, a patient who is convinced that a stomach pain which occurs whenever he has a fight with his supervisor at work must be due exclusively to physical factors, and who refuses to investigate the possibility that psychological issues may be associated with it, does not show evidence of psychological sophistication" (Stifneos, 1987, p. 39). The requirement for good intelligence as traditionally defined is somewhat downplayed, with the emphasis now being on the ability to problem-solve effectively (Nielsen & Barth, 1991). The final criterion includes the patient's curiosity about him- or herself, an openness to new ideas, and the willingness to make reasonable sacrifices to engage in therapy.

THE TECHNIQUES OF THE THERAPY

All of the therapies described in this volume adhere to some basic principles of psychoanalytic technique, although they are also modified in important respects. We will spell out what those fundamental techniques are, what modifications are common to the three drive/structural therapists, and what is unique to each. Some time ago, Bibring (1954) proposed a conceptual scheme consisting of basic therapeutic principles and procedures present to varying degrees in all psychotherapies, and it will serve to guide us. In fact, both Davanloo (1978, pp. 78–81) and Mann (1973, pp. 49–56) refer explicitly to the Bibring model.

Bibring (1954) refers to five groups of basic techniques: (1) suggestive, (2) abreactive, (3) manipulative, (4) clarifying, and (5) interpretive. As the latter two are the ones most characteristic of psychoanalytic approaches, we begin with them. *Clarification* involves a restatement, reflection, or reorganization of patients' statements without going much beyond the phenomenological or descriptive level. The statements are patterns or processes which patients are at least dimly aware of but which have largely escaped their attention. "They cannot recognize or differentiate adequately what troubles them, they relate matters which are unrelated, or fail to relate what belongs together, or they do not perceive or evaluate reality properly but in a distorted fashion under the influence of their emotions or neurotic patterns" (p. 755).

Clarifying interventions help patients reach a higher level of self-awareness regarding their patterns of conduct, such as how they react in typical ways to specific situations and how certain attitudes are related. Pointing out to the patient how he or she smiles when feeling anxious, comes late to a session when feeling angry, or discourses intellectually when painful matters arise are examples of clarification. Such interventions are said to help patients get a broadened sense of their feelings, impulses, traits, and typical modes of behaving in relation to themselves, others, and their environment. In this way patients have the opportunity to see their problems in a different light through their observing ego.

Interpretation goes beyond the phenomenological material and refers to what is unconscious. It includes unconscious defensive operations, warded-off instinctual tendencies, and the hidden meanings of behavior patterns. It often addresses not only what patients do, but why they do it. It is not meant to be merely an intellectual construction, but one that touches on affectively charged issues. To return to the examples above, smiling may be interpreted to the patient as a way of maintaining emotional distance from the therapist; coming late to a session, as a passive way of expressing anger to a perceived authority figure in the patient's life; and intellectualizing, as a defensive means of protecting oneself from unbearable sadness. Interpretation, according to Bibring, is more likely to encounter resistance, whereas clarification elicits surprise or intellectual satisfaction. Although it is useful for some purposes to distinguish between clarification and interpretation, in our opinion one cannot put too fine a point on the difference between them. Clarification is a continuum that shades off into reflection on the one hand and psychoanalytic interpretation on the other.

Suggestion refers to the induction of ideas, emotions, or other mental states in the patient, who is in a dependent position, by the therapist, who is in a position of authority. It is said to bypass the patient's rational, critical, or realistic thinking. To say to the patient that he or she will feel better after the session is to call on one's status as a healer and to tap into the patient's wish for a cure. The therapist may suggest to the patient, for example, that he or she will have a dream following the session, or will recall certain memories, or be able to tolerate anxiety or depression better.

A more subtle but potentially as powerful technique is indirect suggestion. The role of the therapist as healer, sanctioned by society, in itself sets up unconscious positive expectations in patients, making them feel better. Instilling hope in the patient likewise can be healing (Frank, 1974). One's demeanor or even office furnishings can be a part of "a context of healing" (Appelbaum, 1988). We know, for example, that placebos regularly lead to improvement, and we ascribe the benefit to the patient's belief in the therapist's curative power.

Abreaction refers to the patient's emotional discharge. It originally referred to the release of dammed-up tensions which were abnormally discharged through symptoms, and was considered curative in and of itself. It eventually came to mean an emotional reliving that convinced patients of the reality of their repressed feelings. As such, it was considered to be a means of acquiring insight and of having one's feelings accepted and understood by the therapist. The current emphasis on acquiring *emotional* insight in psychoanalytic therapy suggests that abreaction is once again considered a curative element when it is experienced in connection with increased cognitive clarity (but not necessarily in the dramatic way that one sometimes sees in the movies).

Manipulation draws on the therapist's understanding of a patient to get him or her to act in a way that furthers the therapeutic endeavour. To use one of Bibring's examples, if a patient comes to therapy at another's urging, and the therapist makes the patient understand that it is up to him or her whether or not to discuss his or her problems and, furthermore, that the therapist will accept this decision, the patient's freedom of choice is enhanced. This will tend to lessen the patient's resentment and fear regarding the therapy. Or, if the therapist encourages a patient to take responsibility for his or her own self, the patient may initially comply out of a desire to please the therapist, but in doing so the patient undergoes a corrective emotional and/or cognitive experience: He or she learns that self-responsibility need not have untoward consequences. "Such experience may neutralize or correct existent attitudes based on opposite (actual or imaginary) experiences in the infantile past or reinforce latent tendencies or perhaps even establish 'new' emotional systems in the patient, which would act toward adjustive change" (p. 752). This is "learning through experience" (Bibring, 1954, p. 752) or, in Alexander and French's (1946) term described in Chapter 1, a "corrective emotional experience." This principle of change is also called upon by behavior therapists when they encourage patients to try out a certain previously avoided behavior, thereby giving patients the opportunity to learn that the feared consequences do not necessarily come about.

To return to clarification and interpretation, these are the techniques that are referred to most frequently by Malan (1976a) and Davanloo (1978, 1980). They conceptualize their therapeutic work by reference to the triangles of conflict and of person (Figure 2.1). The triangle of conflict includes the impulse or feeling (I-F), the defense erected against it (D) and the anxiety (A) or symptom that results when the defense fails. The triangle of person consists of the objects toward whom the impulse is felt, namely, the therapist (T), significant people in the patient's current life (C), and significant people in the past (P), typically parents, other caretakers, or siblings.

Malan (1976a) recommends that work start with the triangle of conflict as it applies to one corner of the triangle of person, and that its

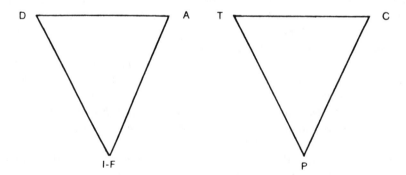

FIGURE 2.I. Triangle of conflict (left) and triangle of person (right).

elements be clarified before going on to another corner. The object is to link the pattern pertaining to one corner of the triangle of person with a similar pattern in another corner, and ultimately to link all three corners. Davanloo, however, seems to move rapidly from one corner of the triangle of person to another and back again. We will illustrate the technique and the variations of therapeutic style by examining vignettes of case transcriptions from these authors' writings.

Malan's Brief Intensive Psychotherapy (BIP)

Malan's therapy is a good place to start because, among the three drive/structural approaches, his is closest to standard psychoanalytic technique. For those with experience conducting long-term therapy, this similarity will make it the easiest to learn; a familiarity with the readings and some appropriate supervision would be all that is needed to get started. The two triangles, after all, are a way of conceptualizing any psychoanalytic therapy, including psychoanalysis. What, then are the differences between BIP and standard psychoanalytic approaches? First, the number of sessions are limited — to 20 for the healthier patient treated by an experienced brief psychotherapist, and to 30 for the less experienced therapist, or where dependency issues are strong, or when treatment is directed to more than one focus. Malan is not firmly against the patient continuing or returning if necessary (unlike Mann; see Chapter 4).

Second, the object of the therapy is to resolve as much as possible a conflict or set of conflicts which are determined after the initial interview. It is not open ended like psychoanalysis, in which the spirit of the romantic vision leads the therapist to allow for and encourage a freewheeling expansion across many domains of conflict and character. Third, and closely related to these two modifications, therapeutic interventions are focused on the previously determined conflict area. For some patients, who can remain focused on their own, the therapist hardly needs to deviate from standard technique. But for many others, the therapist will have to be more active in "*guiding* the patient during the actual sessions by means of *selective interpretation, selective attention and selective neglect*" (Malan, 1976a, p. 32; italics in original).

This is not to say that therapists need to impose wild interpretations on patients or even to insist on their own agenda. Rather, they must listen, clarify, and interpret along the lines of the focus. They select out those elements of the material presented that seem to be closely related to the focal issue. That they intervene fairly frequently is another meaning of the word "active" as applied to BPT generally. Nothing about the word "focus" should imply that the therapy is superficial. In fact, it is meant to go as deeply as possible into the patient's difficulties, with full psychodynamic understanding of the core conflicts and their origin.

In the initial interview, Malan recommends that the interviewer take a full history, formulate the psychodynamics, and test the patient's response to trial interpretations. If the response is positive, a focus or therapeutic plan is formulated and tested out. The patient's motivation is assessed and, if possible, an attempt is made to increase it. The patient should not be left with a mass of unresolved feelings at the end of the interview. Here is a vignette from an initial interview conducted by Malan (1980; the letters we have added in brackets refer to the triangles of conflict and person depicted in Figures 2.1).

The patient is a 24-year-old secretary who complained of depression and difficulties in her relationship to men. She is single but currently living with a married man, and she resents the time that he spends with his children. After checking out the severity of the depression (there had been one suicidal gesture) and the presence of any other psychopathology, and getting a picture of the situations in which the problem was manifested, Malan (1980, pp. 178–179) worked toward laying out the main elements of the conflict which would serve as a therapeutic focus:

THERAPIST: . . . You see, really your problem seems to be about sticking up for yourself [related to anger; I-F]. It seems to be about being left alone and feeling lonely [I-F], which goes way back [P]. And then what do you do about it, when you are left alone? Is it possible to do anything about it?

PATIENT: First of all in addition to my job I have joined a volunteer organization where I work once a week [D]. I am very interested in it.

THERAPIST: I am interested in that too. But it wasn't so much that I meant what you do about it in the sense of finding some substitute. . . . But what do you do about it when somebody whom you love and need neglects you?

PATIENT: What did I do? I think of what other things I can do [D]. Like . . .

THERAPIST: Yes. But that doesn't . . . that compensates your time. It doesn't deal with the basic situation. I think that your problem must be your inability to stick up for yourself and to deal with the basic situation. This is what you are asking our help for.

PATIENT: I guess so [D].

THERAPIST: Well, you say, "I guess so." You are having a problem, in a sense, sticking up for yourself with me [T], because you know, you are just agreeing with what I say [D], aren't you? What do you think?

PATIENT: But I don't see how you can fight my battle. Like, you think that I think you are going to tell me, "Do this, and do this and do this."

THERAPIST: I don't know. Do you think that?

PATIENT: I don't. Because I have heard of people going for help and you are not told what to do; you have to do it on your own. Whatever it is you might want to do.

THERAPIST: Now what is it you want to do?

PATIENT: I want to stay with him, but I don't want to keep being pushed aside.

THERAPIST: Yes, quite. And the question is, "How do you handle that," isn't it? What can you do? And I am sure that one of your fears [A] is that if you stick up for yourself, you will lose him altogether. Is that right? Or isn't it right? You see you are agreeing with me again [I-F, T].

PATIENT: That is right.

THERAPIST: Then you see, what happens is that you can't stick up for yourself [I-F] because you are afraid [A] you will lose him and then you have to hold your angry feelings inside yourself [D]. Then you get depressed [A] and then it comes out as crying.

Malan obviously is not having an easy time of it, but he persists in pursuing the focal dynamics he has discerned in this patient. She is obtuse at first, referring to activities she undertakes to make herself feel better, but eventually begins to catch on. Malan checks out whether it is just her being acquiescent, in order to assess her motivation and ability to utilize BIP.

Having clarified the pattern in relation to her boyfriend (C), and in relation to her often absent alcoholic father and hard-working mother in her childhood (P), Malan then concentrates on the corner of the triangle involving the interviewer (T). The session proceeds, and when the patient admits that she wants to cry, he explores whether there is something that she wants that she is not getting from him (p. 183).

THERAPIST: I feel that what you are doing all the time is trying to pretend you didn't want things that you haven't gotten from me [D]. . . .

You are going to go away and feel that there was something missing. . . . And don't you see that you must be showing the same pattern with me [T] that you show in your relation to Carl [C; her boyfriend]? . . .

Malan not only points out how the problem is manifested in her relationship to him, but connects it to the pattern in her relationship to her boyfriend, Carl. This is the kind of link that brief dynamic therapists consider important. The patient finally admits, in a convincing way, that she is not able to ask for what she wants from others: " . . . You just put into words what I can't do."

In commenting on his interview, Malan sees the patient's response to trial therapy as equivocal, in that she remained quite passive. He sees a necessity to break through the defensive passivity to the anger about the way that she has been neglected throughout her life, which he considers Davanloo's technique best at doing. In fact, Malan has swung over to Davanloo's approach, which he regards as superior to his own. Nevertheless, for reasons that we will discuss below, we need not agree with Malan's conclusions about the relative value of his technique, which can be described as less confrontative and more gentle than those of either Sifneos or Davanloo, to which we now turn.

Davanloo's Intensive Short-Term Dynamic Psychotherapy (ISTDP)

We start with an initial interview conducted by Davanloo (1980, pp. 47–51), as explicated by Rasmussen and Messer (1986). The patient, a 29-year-old teacher, presents problems of depression, chronic anxiety, work difficulties, and disturbances in relationships, especially with men. She has a history of disappointing heterosexual relationships, culminating most recently in a breakup with a man she had planned to marry. The session begins with the patient evading the therapist's questions, idly ruminating, and remaining preoccupied with irrelevant details. This exchange then follows. (In the following, we have labeled her passivity as a defense, but it is also a character trait, employed as a form of resistance.)

THERAPIST: How do you feel about talking to me about yourself [T]?

PATIENT: I feel uncomfortable [A]. I have never done this before, so I don't really, you know . . . I feel I don't really know how to answer some of your questions [D].

THERAPIST: Um-hum. But have you noticed that in your relationship here with me you are passive [D], and I am the one who has to question you repeatedly?

PATIENT: I know.

In the course of one interchange, Davanloo displays several crucial and pointed techniques of his repertoire. He avoids colluding with the patient's intellectualizing defenses by forcing her to examine her immediate feelings about talking with him. Only minutes into the session, he confronts her resistance and begins to work with her transference.

Davanloo also transposes the patient's view of her own behavior into ego-dystonic terms. That is, what she formulates as behavior springing from uncomfortableness and naïveté in such a new experience, Davanloo recasts into deliberate passivity, strongly implying that she is actively choosing not to involve herself. He endows the word *passive* with connotations that are less palatable than *uncomfortable*. This word choice might silently stir up retaliative anger and the wish to be more positively viewed, both of which result in what Davanloo strives for: the patient's greater involvement.

Davanloo then builds on the implications of the word *passive:* "I am the one who has to question you *repeatedly*" (p. 48, italics added). He conveys how the patient's choosing to be passive imposes demands on him. He frames her behavior in interpersonal terms intended to expose the controlling side of her passivity.

In the next exchange, Davanloo swiftly expands the focus from her passivity in the transference to her passivity in other relationships:

THERAPIST: ... Is this the way it is with other people [C], or is it only here with me [T]? ... this passivity, lack of spontaneity.

PATIENT: Yeah. To some extent. I mean, I'm ... there are a lot of things hidden, you know. Somebody once described me "like a hidden flower" or something. There are a lot of things about me that I don't think I have ever really ... uh ... explored that much.

THERAPIST: Then from what you say you are passive with others. But from what you have told me you indicated that your mother has been a passive person [P].

Davanloo's swinging from the transference [T] to past [P] and current relationships [C] begins to sketch out the "triangle of person" and, as Winokur and colleagues (1981) point out, this serves to preclude the development of excessive dependence and a transference neurosis, permitting the acceleration of treatment progress. The patient's resistance, challenged by Davanloo, has given way to a greater openness and willingness on the patient's part to consider her interpersonal reticence.

After making a fleeting connection between the patient's passivity and that of her mother, Davanloo pursues the patient's first negative self-disclosure: She does not like the passive role she assumes with men:

PATIENT: In certain situations . . . when I get involved with a man . . . I find I tend to take a passive role [D], and I don't like that.

THERAPIST: What specifically do you mean by not liking it?

PATIENT: I feel upset inside [A].

THERAPIST: What is it that you experience? You say "upset" . . .

PATIENT: Perhaps irritated [I-F] . . . something like that . . .

THERAPIST: But you say "perhaps" [D] . . . Is it that you experience irritation and anger [I-F], or isn't it?

PATIENT: Ummm. Yeah. Yeah . . . I do.

THERAPIST: You say you take a passive role in relation to men. Are you doing that here with me [T]?

PATIENT: I would say so [D].

THERAPIST: You "would" say so, but still you are not committing yourself.

Davanloo rides the patient on the question of precisely what it is that she experiences, chasing the evasiveness with forced dichotomies, and pinning her down on every noncommittal, vague response she offers. Again, he confronts the process head on:

THERAPIST: How do you feel when I indicate to you that you are passive?

PATIENT: I don't like it. (*The patient is laughing, but it is quite evident that she is irritated.*)

THERAPIST: But you are smiling [D].

PATIENT: I know. Well . . . maybe that is my way of expressing my irritation [I-F].

THERAPIST: Then you are irritated?

PATIENT: A little bit [D] . . . yeah . . .

THERAPIST: A little bit?

PATIENT: Actually, quite a bit. (*The patient is laughing.*)

THERAPIST: Let's look at what happened here. I brought to your attention your passivity, your noninvolvement [D]. You got irritated and angry with me [I-F] and the way you dealt with your irritation was by smiling [D; i.e., D/I-F/D].

PATIENT: That is right. . . .

The patient reaches a new height of emotional intensity of anger and discomfort in proportion to the degree of anxious smiling and laughter she exhibits. Davanloo's dogged pursuit of the feelings habitually avoided by the patient throws her dysfunctional defensive pattern into high relief.

After spelling out the patient's defensive pattern in her relationship to him, Davanloo moves outside the context of the transference and the immediate moment to the larger context of other relationships. He asks the patient to free associate: "What does this remind you of . . . this situation? Is there any other relationship that may have been like this?" (1980, p. 50). The patient squirms, then begins discussing her relationship with her passive, controlling mother and dominating father.

Davanloo is not simply drawing links in the triangle of person, as discussed earlier; he is also wielding a powerful device for tapping charged emotional memories, an approach related to Freud's (1914b/1958) notion that transference is a way of remembering. He brings his challenging, provocative style to the relationship, rendering the transference context affectively charged and highly stressful. There is an emotional intensity possibly unparalleled in other forms of psychoanalytic therapy.

In the last portion of the initial interview, Davanloo reiterates, clarifies, and broadens the implications of the patient's passive controlling pattern both in the transference and in relationships in general. Such careful repetition, enlarging, and educating facilitates the synthesis of so much foreign, threatening, charged material. Also, for the first time, Davanloo conveys an appreciation for the deep pain the patient has suffered in her life because of her problems, and thus provides caring support for her treatment endeavor. Such empathic support is especially needed to buoy up patients in this highly distressing treatment model (Winokur et al., 1981). By the end of the first session, Davanloo has not only determined that the patient is appropriate for his treatment model, since she proved responsive to his approach, but he has also penetrated quickly to the core problem, confronted the patient with it, undermined her resistance, interpreted the negative transference, established a working alliance, and conveyed some empathic support and understanding along the way.

In a more recent publication, Davanloo (1988) spells out the phases of the trial therapy he employs in an initial interview. Phase 1 is the initial inquiry into the patient's problems and identification of the defenses. Phase 2 involves pressure leading to resistance in the form of a number of defenses. In phase 3, defenses are clarified and confronted to get patients to turn against them. Phase 4 includes clarifying and challenging the resistance that is manifested in the transference. Phase 5 aims to bring about "an unlocking of the unconscious" (Davanloo, 1988, p. 100) and a direct view of the core neurotic structure. Phase 6 is a systematic analysis of the transference and a derepression of current or recent past conflicts. Phase 7 is the inquiry into the patient's psychopathology and history. Phase 8 relates the core neurotic structure to the patient's symptoms and character disturbances.

Sifneos's Short-Term Anxiety-Provoking Psychotherapy (STAPP)

What characterizes Sifneos's therapy is the relentless way in which he focuses on oedipal concerns in patients who are carefully selected for manifesting such issues. He claims that therapists often focus on "oral" issues because these are less of a threat to them than oedipal conflicts. Unlike Davanloo and Malan, he often confronts the impulse head on without necessarily interpreting the defense first. Here is a vignette of the fourth session of a 25-year-old male who had talked in the earlier interviews about his closeness to his mother (Sifneos, 1987, pp. 131–133; unfortunately, there is no mention of his presenting complaint). One of his fondest memories was when his mother did the washing:

THERAPIST: What was so fascinating about "washing day"? You mentioned this interest of yours before. We also know that it has something to do with your feelings for your mother.

Sifneos frequently asks pointed questions relating to oedipal issues or transference, the ones most likely to produce anxiety. As this intervention reveals, he is not content merely to ask the question, but reminds the patient that the subject has come up before. In this manner, he seems to be justifying his question, but is also educating the patient as to why he asks it. Unlike the technique of free association, he then "leads the witness," as these BPT therapists will do, by pointing him in a particular direction, namely, feelings toward his mother. The patient responds:

PATIENT: Oh, yes, indeed! It was wonderful to be with Mom. I always remember how she asked me to bring down all the dirty clothes. Then I would watch her sorting them out into those neat piles. Of course, I was most fascinated by all those feminine things that belonged to her and to my older sister . . . all the lingerie, night-gowns, stockings, panties . . . (*smiling*)

THERAPIST: Go on.

PATIENT: It was all so exciting, so much fun. It was such a "warm" feel-ing I had for my mother. (*He went on describing various details about "washing day," and then associated, smiling again, to his "sexual arousal about certain undergarments of his wife's. Soon afterward, however, he returned to the subject of his mother's washing day" and again described the "warm" feeling he had for her.*)

THERAPIST (*interrupting him*): You mean "sexual" feeling.

PATIENT (*taken aback*): No, I said "warm" feeling.

THERAPIST: Oh, yes, I heard you very well. You said "warm." It was I who used the word "sexual" because sexual was the right term, and you were using "warm" to dilute that feeling for your mother.

Note that the therapist, rather than asking further about the warm feel-ing, or even interpreting it as a defense against other unspecified feel-ings, confronts the patient head on with the sexual impulse. This is characteristic of Sifneos's technique. In spite of the patient's protesta-tions, the therapist sticks to the appropriateness of the term "sexual" and only then interprets the patient's use of the word "warm" as a defense ("to dilute that feeling for your mother").

PATIENT (*somewhat irritated*): I can use any word I wish.

THERAPIST: Of course, but if certain words tend to obscure the real meaning or the real feeling, then it's important that I bring it to your attention. You see, it was you who talked about your "sexual arousal" by certain undergarments that belonged to your wife. The word "sexual" was appropriate to your feelings for your wife, yet for the same undergarments being washed by your mother you chose to emphasize the "warm feeling." Now, I don't see why the same female undergarments should produce different kinds of feel-ings in you unless you felt that it was inappropriate to talk about sexual feelings for your mother. Is it true?

In this interchange, Sifneos brushes aside the patient's angry protesta-tion and reminds him of the importance of pursuing the truth of the

matter. He then carefully explains the basis for his confrontation, calling on logic to aid him: If A (female undergarments of his wife's)
produces B (sexual arousal), then A′ (female undergarments of his
mother's) must also produce B. (There is, of course, some slippage in
the argument, but we shall let it pass for now). The patient responds:

PATIENT: Well, sort of.

THERAPIST: No "sort of." Yes or no?

Here, we see the similarity between Sifneos and Davanloo in their
refusal to allow ambivalent responses to stand unopposed. Sifneos
makes it clear that there is to be no equivocating (which is viewed as
an intellectual defense).

PATIENT (*blushing*): Well, yes.

THERAPIST: Of course! But you see, it was quite evident that it was so,
  because when you were describing all your mother's undergarments, you said you were fascinated by them, and when you mentioned the specific items, you started to smile. Later on, while you
  were describing your "sexual arousal" at your wife's undergarments
  the same smile again appeared on your face. So I knew that "sexual" was what you were thinking about in reference to your mother
  instead of "warm," but the word "sexual" was loaded. It was much
  more anxiety-provoking so you decided to substitute another, more
  innocuous word. Your smile gave it away!

The cat has caught the mouse and there is no escape. As in this instance,
Sifneos often assumes a didactic stance in his effort to demonstrate to
the patient how he arrived at the inevitable conclusion. Sifneos in fact
emphasizes that short-term therapy is a "course tailor-made" for the patient, where the patient learns a new way of looking at him- or herself.
Interpretation provides new learning for the patient: that there are ways
of problem solving or acting in the current situation which are superi-
or to the old modes based on neurotic entanglements with nuclear
figures (e.g., mother). For a "manualized," step-by-step account of how
to evaluate patients for, and to conduct, STAPP, see Sifneos (1992).

In summary and in broad strokes, Malan's approach is based on
selective listening and interpreting along the line of the focus; Davanloo's, on the repeated confrontation of patients' defenses in order to
expose the hidden feelings and conflicts; and Sifneos's, on confronting the impulses, as well as teaching patients about their psychodynamics.

THE THEORY OF CHANGE

What is it in psychoanalytic therapy in general, and in these brief psychodynamic therapies in particular, that is said to bring about change in the patient?

General Change Factors in Psychoanalytic Psychotherapy

The Acquisition of Insight

The simplest and most frequent answer given to the question of what brings about change is the patient's acquisition of insight, aided largely by therapists' interventions, especially their interpretations and clarifications. The expansion of patients' self-understanding and awareness allows them to break out of their neurotic mode, to resolve their conflicts, and to resume growth and maturation. To state it in more technical language, Greenson (1967b) describes the goal of psychoanalysis as the attempt "to resolve the patient's neurotic conflicts by reuniting with the conscious ego those portions of the id, superego, and unconscious ego that had been excluded from the maturational processes of the healthy remainder of the total personality" (p. 773). In this quote, one can see reflected Freud's statements about the psychoanalytic aims of making the unconscious conscious (Freud, 1917/1963) and putting ego in place of id (Freud, 1933/1964).

According to this viewpoint, by becoming more fully aware of one's defenses, wishes, needs, resistances, character traits, and conflicts, one is in a much better position to exercise control over them. Otherwise they continue to exert an insidious influence beyond one's ken or control. If one has been anxious, inhibited, unproductive, or depressed, the route to overcome such dysfunctional states, according to psychoanalytic theory, is by becoming conscious of the conflicts underlying these symptoms. As expressed in terms of the economic theory of the mind, the energy bound up in defense mechanisms and in unconscious conflict becomes freed up and available for more productive, adaptive, and creative activities.

The therapist's clarifications and interpretations which aid the process of acquiring insight may refer to a defense or to the relation of a drive (or its derivatives: impulse, feeling, wish); to a defense against it (repression, reaction formation, etc.); to feelings toward the therapist, which are transferred from other important figures; to the perception of people or events in the client's current life; or to figures from the past. Interpretations may also refer to perceived parallels between the client's psychological experience of past or present figures and the way in which the therapist is viewed. These are the links in the triangle of person referred to above, the frequency of which Malan, Sifneos, and Davanloo posit is related to positive outcome in BPT. Stated different-ly, the interpretations help patients to become more aware of and to reframe certain of their own cognitive (response-produced) cues. The latter are signals that had triggered, more or less automatically, the af-fects and defenses being confronted or interpreted.

Affective Involvement

It is important to note that the process of acquiring insight is not intended to be dry and intellectual but affectively engaging, whether it involves feelings in the here and now of the transference, or a re-experiencing of infantile conflicts. As Appelbaum (1988) states it:

> the chief enemy of insight as an agent of change is intellectualizing, dealing with insight simply as information . . . insight has to be developed in tandem with the patient's readiness to accept it clearly, meaningfully, interestedly, thankfully; in short, when defenses are sufficiently worked through so as not to interfere with its acceptance and use. (p. 205)

The release of emotion was once considered to be therapeutic in and of itself and seems to be so considered once again. However, even in the context of gaining insight, it is important that there be a felt com-ponent along with the cognitive learning that takes place.

In discussing Davanloo's understanding of and approach to affect, his associate, Kalpin (1992), refers to it as

> a mixture of conflictual and painful feelings having their origins in the ear-ly part of life. Included are aggressive impulses, sexual impulses, guilt and grief. These feelings are connected to each other, and in many patients the key that first unlocks the conscious experience of this whole mixture of feel-ings is the experience of aggressive impulses toward someone about whom there are also positive feelings. (p. 245)

Davanloo (1980) refers to "releasing hidden feelings by actively work-ing on and interpreting resistance or defenses; paying strict attention to the transference relationship; and making links between the trans-ference and significant people in the patient's current life and in the past" (p. 45). It is our impression that this description applies to the change process as conceptualized by Malan and Sifneos as well. It covers the processes of interpretation, clarification, and abreaction as referred to in Bibring's (1954) scheme.

The Therapist–Patient Relationship

Insight with or without affect, however, is not enough for change to take place. From early on, Freud (1912b/1958) stressed the importance of developing rapport with the patient. He (Freud, 1917/1963) remarked:

> If the patient is to fight his way through the normal conflict with the resistances which we have uncovered for him in the analysis, he is in need of a powerful stimulus which will influence the decision in the sense which we desire, leading to recovery.... At this point what turns the scale in his struggle is not his intellectual insight ... but simply and solely his relation to the doctor. (p. 445)

We take this to mean that, aside from the technical interventions to help the patient reveal the hidden fantasies and felt conflicts, an important ingredient of change is the nature of the relationship between the therapist and the patient. In fact, the quality of this relationship may be the *sine qua non* of change in therapy. It is the soil within which insight can flourish, insofar as patients must feel that they are in the presence of a trustworthy, caring individual in relation to whom they are willing to undergo the pain and struggle that psychoanalytic therapy entails.

Greenson (1967a, 1971) proposed a tripartite definition of the therapist-patient relationship in psychoanalytic therapy. The *real relationship* is a genuine person-to-person relationship between patient and therapist, which can be characterized as appropriate, realistic, objective, and authentic. For example, a therapist may express sympathy for a loss that the patient has sustained during the course of the therapy. The *working alliance* constitutes the cooperative attitude of the patient in working with the therapist to overcome neurotic problems and to achieve the insights that analytic therapy has to offer. Even while patients are experiencing disturbing sexual and aggressive feelings or thoughts toward the therapist, this aspect of the alliance allows them to continue working with the therapist to achieve the aims of therapy. In drive/structural theory, the *transference relationship* is the inappropriate and irrational way in which the patient perceives the therapist. It is based on the patient's experience of earlier object relationships and, in this sense, is a displacement of feelings, attitudes, and impulses from the past to the therapist. (For more detail, see Messer, 1988a.) The selection criteria for BPT exclude patients who are likely to fail to distinguish between the real relationship and the transference (e.g., some borderline personality disorders), and who are therefore unable to form a dependable working alliance.

The importance of the relationship, and the ways in which it can be employed in psychoanalytic therapy, will be discussed in greater detail in the context of the relational therapies where its centrality and power are acknowledged and emphasized even more (and with a different emphasis) than in the drive/structural therapies. Suffice it to say that there is a great deal of research support for its key role in bringing about change (e.g., Horvath, Gaston, & Luborsky, 1993).

The Corrective Emotional Experience

The BPT therapists under consideration in this chapter also refer to the "corrective emotional experience" as a change factor—what Bibring (1954) calls "learning through experience." By virtue of the patients' saying what they feared to say, doing what they feared to do, and not being punished, criticized, or harmed by the therapist or others, they learn that they can think, talk, and act differently than they have before. Their ego functions are strengthened not only by the derepression of impulses and their new insight, but by the calm, accepting demeanor of the therapist in the face of "shameful" secrets. This, too, will be elaborated upon in the next chapter as a relational factor leading to change.

There remains the question of what modifications are made by Malan, Davanloo, and Sifneos that allow the psychoanalytic process to be compressed and the change factors to operate in the shorter time available.

Specific Change Factors in Brief Psychodynamic Therapy

Winokur and colleagues (1981) have proposed an explanation of how change might be brought about in the therapies of Malan, Davanloo, and Sifneos.

Focal Activity

The effort made to focus on a sector of the person's emotional life (e.g., oedipal problems) narrows the endeavor to one of manageable proportions. Long-term therapists assume that, because of the organic unity of the person, maximal benefit is achieved only if as many problem areas or fantasy systems as possible are covered. In contrast, BPT therapists propose that by sticking to and working through a focal problem, patients gain a sense of mastery over some important aspect of their life which then extends, as a ripple effect, to other domains. This change factor, however, applies less to Davanloo's ISTDP because he allows for multiple foci and claims that ISTDP's aims are as ambitious as those of psychoanalysis.

The Problem of Interpretation

Strachey (1934), in a classic paper on technique, describes the interpretive process as a gradual one: "The mutative interpretation is inevitably governed by the principle of minimal doses" (p. 144). Strachey points out that, to be effective, interpretations (1) must be emotionally immediate and experienced as something actual, (2) must be relatively specific (i.e., "accurate" or "correct"), and (3) must involve an element of abreaction (i.e., discharge of affect). Within this view, treatment based on interpretation must be long-term because if the quantity of impulse released is too large, too much anxiety is aroused, or there is real anger at the therapist, either of which may lead to a disruption of the therapeutic alliance. An examination of the case material provided by Malan, Davanloo, and Sifneos and a viewing of their videotapes suggest that these therapists have a number of ways of mitigating the impact of immediate and deep interpretation.

1. *Rapid juxtaposition of past and concurrent events with transference interpretation.* Instead of waiting for the developmental links to emerge gradually following an interpretation of a current relationship or of the transference, these therapists often encourage the patient to forge these links and actively aid the process by making a number of reconstructions of their own. This rapid juxtaposition of the developmental material with the transference interpretation insures that the feelings that emerge do not remain directed at the therapist, thereby potentially disrupting the alliance. The requisites for mutative interpretations of high immediacy and real affect can thus be realized without unduly disruptive effects. In this way, the patient's feelings toward the therapist are not allowed to develop into a crystallized attitude (transference neurosis), and the disorientation and regression that sometimes follow transference interpretations in psychoanalysis are avoided.

2. *Encouragement of neutral self-observation.* Another way the working alliance is preserved in the face of the impact of interpretation of disturbing material is through the encouragement of neutral self-observation in the patient. For instance, after a patient had been quite self-critical, Sifneos (1978) remarked, "Don't call it derogatory names, such as 'silly' and so on. Let's look at it" (p. 392). Similarly, Davanloo encourages patients to observe themselves dispassionately by the simple, repeated question "Can we look at that?" Sifneos aptly describes this approach to the working alliance as "a mutual approaching of the

problem, as something which is foreign, to be looked at and understood despite the fact that there might be pain involved" (p. 451). As Eckert (1993) has pointed out, modes of fostering the collaborative relationship through enhanced activity and dialogue have been an important contribution of brief therapy.

3. *Disconfirmation of the patient's view of the therapist.* The therapist may disconfirm the patient's transferential view of him or her by explicitly and verbally disclaiming a position, or by implicitly acting in a way contrary to the patient's expectation. For example, Sifneos (1978), in dealing with a patient's transferential view of him as an authority figure, makes it quite clear that he does not see himself that way: "If you put me, however, in the position of authority . . . by asking me questions and so forth, then you are making me something that I am not" (p. 391). This is an *explicit* disconfirmation of the therapist's role. The *implicit* disconfirmation of a transferential expectation by taking a stance contrary to what the patient might expect constitutes an important aspect of what Alexander and French (1946) called "the corrective emotional experience." Of the two modes, the latter is probably the more powerful and convincing to the patient.

4. *Active support.* In these short-term therapies, because so much intense affect may be experienced and expressed in such a short time, the therapist needs to be more actively supportive than may be necessary in long-term therapy. Therapists do not necessarily have to be seen as "nice guys" or as being in agreement with patients, but patients must come to believe that the therapist understands and accords legitimacy to their feelings, beliefs, and thoughts (an aspect of empathy; Cohen & Epstein, 1981). As we have seen, Sifneos and Davanloo in particular make very strong confrontations of resistance or impulse, which at first glance may seem to be unempathic. Both clinicians appear to mitigate the potentially negative impact of such active confrontation by providing some kind of support in the form of encouragement, praise, sympathy, challenge, or exhortation to persist. Davanloo might remind patients that they have come for their own benefit because they are suffering and that they are, therefore, defeating their own needs. Here are some comments that Sifneos (1987) makes: "You look pleased with yourself"; "I'm glad to hear about this"; "It's a good question" (p. 174).

In summary, it appears that with appropriate modifications deep and specific interpretations can be made early, can be emotionally immediate, and can elicit intense affect, thereby allowing the change factors as conceptualized within psychoanalytic theory to have effect.

REVIEW OF RESEARCH

In Chapter 1 we reviewed the general empirical literature on BPT. In this section we will describe the empirical work that pertains directly to each of the three drive/structural therapies, starting with Malan's form of BPT.

Malan's Brief Intensive Psychotherapy (BIP)

Outcome

Malan conducted research on two series of patients, which is reported in two volumes (1976a, 1976b). In general terms, he showed that a focal dynamic therapy could yield good results for selected patients. However, his design did not include control groups, and measures were based on therapist notes rather than on audiotapes or transcripts of therapy sessions. Other methodological problems limit the conclusions that can be drawn from these studies regarding the efficacy of BIP.

William Piper and his colleagues, however, have conducted two extensive, methodologically sophisticated studies of Malan's brief therapy which support its efficacy. In the first (Piper et al., 1984), which we described in some detail in Chapter 1, they showed that BIP was as effective as long-term individual and group psychoanalytic therapy and more effective than brief group therapy. Patients improved compared to their pretherapy status, and these gains were maintained on follow-up.

Piper, Azim, McCallum, and Joyce (1990) conducted a second study of 105 psychiatric outpatients whose DSM-III Axis I diagnoses comprised affective, adjustment, anxiety, and impulse control disorders. One third of the sample also received Axis II (personality disorder) diagnoses, primarily dependent and avoidant disorders. The therapists were active, interpretive, and transference-oriented. Half the sample was treated with BIP and half had their therapy delayed and served as a control group.

The treated group was significantly more improved than the controls on 10 out of 15 outcome measures, including social functioning, symptomatology, self-esteem, life satisfaction, and target problems as determined separately by both the patient and the therapist. In addition, the control group, when treated following the delay, showed considerably greater improvement after their treatment than they had following the delay, providing further evidence of significant treatment effects. Effect sizes (see Chapter 1) indicated that the average treated patients exceeded 78% of the control patients on a combined outcome measure. Five month follow-up revealed maintenance of therapeutic benefits.

These results are strongly supportive of the efficacy of Malan's BIP. We now turn to a consideration of what characteristics of patients and therapy process are predictive of a successful BIP.

Patient Predictors of Outcome

Malan correlated a variety of patient variables with outcome in his two studies of BIP. The only one that held up across both studies was *motivation for insight*. Piper and his associates have found two additional variables to be good predictors of outcome: patients' *quality of object relations* (QOR) and their *defensive style*. QOR refers to a patient's lifelong pattern of relationships, judged on the basis of behavioral manifestations, regulation of affect and self-esteem, and historical antecedents. Five levels of object relations were defined according to psychoanalytic theory, from high to low: genital, oedipal, obsessive, depressive, and narcissistic/borderline. Defense mechanisms were defined "as unconscious habitual mental processes that attempt to deal with conflict among instinctual impulses, internal prohibitions, and external reality" (Piper, de Carufel, & Szkrumelak, 1985, p. 731). The measure employed was based on Vaillant's (1971) work, in which four levels of defense are arranged in a theoretically based hierarchy of maturity (narcissistic, immature, neurotic, mature).

In one of their studies, Piper et al. (1985) correlated a long list of potential patient predictors: the two variables, QOR and defensive style, were the ones that emerged as significant predictors. The better the quality of object relations and the more a patient used higher-level defenses, the more favorable the outcome.

In a second study, Piper et al. (1990) examined the effects of QOR by means of an experimental design in which identified high- and low-QOR patients were each assigned to BIP treatment and, on a matched basis, to control (delayed treatment) groups. The effect of high versus low QOR on outcome approached but did not reach statistical significance. However, there was an additive effect of treatment plus level of QOR on outcome. In addition, when clinical (vs. statistical) significance was examined (i.e., the degree to which a pathological [patient] population, after treatment, resembles a normal [nonpatient] population), the highest percentages of patients moving into the normal range (70%–83%) were for the high-QOR/therapy group, and the lowest percentages (12%–32%) were for the low-QOR/control group. This result confirmed the additive effect on outcome of BIP treatment and QOR. In other words, patients with higher quality of object relations tend to do better in BIP.

In a third study (Piper, Azim, Joyce, McCallum, et al., 1991), QOR was found to be a significant predictor of therapeutic alliance and of outcome. It was a better predictor than measures of recent interpersonal functioning, to which it was directly compared. In addition, it was found that therapeutic alliance was a good predictor of outcome.

Høglend and his colleagues in Oslo, Norway, have also studied the relationship between patient suitability variables and outcomes in BPT (Høglend, 1993a, 1993b; Høglend, Sørlie, Heyerdahl, Sørbye, & Amlo, 1993). The therapy, administered to 43 outpatients and varying from 9 to 53 sessions (average = 27.3), was based on both Malan's and Sifneos's approaches. Outcome was assessed at 2 years and 4 years following termination of therapy.

In general, the *healthier patients,* as evaluated on the Global Assessment Scale and by DSM-III diagnosis, achieved greater change as assessed psychodynamically at follow-up. The variable *quality of interpersonal relations,* which best captured a set of five suitability criteria for dynamic psychotherapy, was an excellent predictor of dynamic change at the 4-year (but not 2-year) follow-up, paralleling Piper's findings on "quality of object relations" as a predictor of outcome.

Level of insight measured before treatment was uncorrelated with outcome at 2- and 4-year follow-up, but *gain in insight* at 2-year follow-up was strongly correlated with overall dynamic change at 4-year follow-up (Høglend, Engelstad, Sørbye, Heyerdahl, & Amlo, 1994). Also, for those patients with low levels of pretreatment insight, treatment length was correlated with symptomatic and dynamic change at both 2- and 4-year follow-up. That is, patients who start with less insight into their difficulties seem to profit from more sessions of brief to moderate length therapy.

The *presence of a personality disorder* was a negative predictor of psychodynamic change at both 2-year and 4-year follow-up. For these patients (but not for the rest of the sample), the number of treatment sessions was correlated with the acquisition of insight as measured 2 years after therapy, and with psychodynamic change at 4 year follow-up.

Relating Therapy Process to Outcome

As we discussed earlier in this chapter, the acquisition of insight through interpretation is considered to be a major way in which BPT brings about its effects. Malan (1963) studied the different kinds of interpretations involving the corners of the triangle of person (therapist, parents, and current figures) and their relation to outcome. He found a moderate but significant correlation, not for transference interpretations per se, but between transference/parent links and outcome. This result was replicated in a second study (Malan, 1976b).

Although these findings were promising in confirming a major tenet of psychoanalytic therapy, they were compromised by the data being derived from therapist notes taken from memory and by the raters' knowledge of therapy outcome. In a study that employed audio recordings, Marziali (1984) successfully replicated the finding of a moderately high correlation between transference/parent links and outcome in BIP, as well as a correlation between transference/parent/other links and outcome. In a later study, however, Piper, Debbane, Bienvenu, de Carufel, and Garant (1986) did not find such predictive relationships. None of these investigators measured the "accuracy" of the psychodynamic content of the interpretations, especially in relation to the dynamic focus of therapy. Studies performed by Silberschatz et al. (1986) and Crits-Christoph, Cooper, et al. (1988), working within other BPT models, however, did successfully predict patient progress and outcome, respectively, from therapist interpretations that adhered to the focus, as will be described in more detail in the next chapter.

In another study, Piper, Azim, Joyce, and McCallum (1991) explored the relationship between the proportion of transference interpretations and both therapeutic alliance and outcome in a brief therapy conducted in the style of Malan's BIP and Strupp and Binder's time-limited dynamic psychotherapy (TLDP; described in Chapter 3). A transference interpretation was operationally defined as one that included a reference to the therapist. The authors found an *inverse* relationship between frequency of transference interpretations and both therapeutic alliance and outcome for patients with a history of high QOR. That is, high levels of transference interpretations predicted poorer outcomes in patients with good object relations. Of course, this is the opposite of what one might expect based on the writings of the BPT therapists. A similar finding was reported in a study conducted in Norway of patients in BPT who were assessed at 2 and 4 years following treatment. For patients with a history of high quality of interpersonal relationships, high frequency of transference interpretations was associated with less symptom change at 2-year follow-up and less dynamic change 4 years after therapy (Høglend, Heyerdahl, 1993c; Høglend, Heyerdahl, et al., 1993).

Piper, Azim, Joyce, and McCallum (1991) offer two explanations for such findings: One is that high doses of transference interpretations can be toxic. The other is that therapists may have responded to their perception of a poor alliance with increased transference interpretations which did not resolve the impasse in the working relationship. Høglend (1993c) speculates that even experienced therapists may have difficulty interpreting transference with ease and mastery within a brief therapy where there is pressure for prompt intervention. As to why dosage of transference interpretations was less detrimental to low-QOR patients, he suggests that the transference pattern in these patients may be apparent earlier and in a clearer form, making it more suitable for interpretation. We note that it was also the case in these studies that the timing and accuracy of the interpretations were not assessed, nor were links studied in the same fashion as in the other articles.

In a recent study of the same patients by Piper, Joyce, McCallum, and Azim (1993), they did examine the "accuracy" of transference interpretations, which they referred to as correspondence between the content of the interpretation and the therapist's initial psychodynamic formulation. For low-QOR patients, correspondence was *inversely* related to outcome at 6-month follow-up. For high-QOR patients, there was no significant relationship between correspondence of interpretations and posttherapy outcome, but there was a significantly positive one at follow-up. Apparently the high-QOR patients were able to take from these interventions what they could later on make use of. The authors suggest, and we agree, that "low QOR patients, who report a history of relatively ungratifying relationships, may be more in need of forming a gratifying relationship with the therapist than exploring their pattern of ungratifying relationships in therapy" (p. 592). By contrast, high-QOR patients are able to to continue working through transferential projections because they can incorporate the therapist's analyzing function. Multiple regression analyses showed further that the best follow-up outcomes for the high-QOR patients were associated with a low concentration of transference interpretations which were of high correspondence with the initial formulation.

In summary, there is good evidence for the efficacy of BIP and for the importance, in selecting patients, of the presence of high quality of object or interpersonal relations and maturity of defensive style. The presence of a personality disorder may contraindicate the briefer form of this kind of psychodynamic therapy but not those extending from about 30 to 50 sessions. These data suggest to us the importance of patients' ability to form an adequate therapeutic alliance, one in which they can differentiate transference phenomena from the "real relationship." Otherwise, when the therapist does not gratify them, patients might view the therapist as really being "just like" their parents.

There is some evidence for a link between interventions involving transference/parent links and change, but there are probably moderating variables such as the timing and correspondence of interventions that need to be considered. High levels of transference interpretations, in and of themselves, are related to poorer outcomes in BIP, but those offered in low dosage and which are in correspondence with the initial formulation are associated with better results at follow-up.

Davanloo's Intensive Short-Term Dynamic Psychotherapy (ISTDP)

Although Davanloo (1978, 1980) has referred to studies that he has carried out on ISTDP, they apparently have not been published, so that we cannot evaluate them as a basis of empirical support for this mode of brief therapy. The only setting in which formal research on his method has been conducted is Beth Israel Medical Center in New York.

Outcome

There has been one controlled study of the effectiveness of ISTDP. In that study (Winston et al., 1991), 32 patients with personality disorder diagnoses were assigned either to an ISTDP treatment group or to another from of brief dynamic therapy called "Brief Adaptive Psychotherapy" (BAP). The diagnoses included compulsive, avoidant, dependent, passive–aggressive, histrionic, or mixed personality disorders. ISTDP focused more on confronting defensive behavior and eliciting affect, whereas BAP focused on the identification of maladaptive patterns as they were manifested in the triangle of person. There was also a waiting list control group. Therapy lasted 37 weeks.

Both treatment groups showed significantly greater improvement from admission to termination than the control group but did not differ from each other on the summed outcome scores. The effect size for ISTDP was .92, which is considered very substantial. When differences among the outcome subscales (both based on patient report) were analyzed, it was found that ISTDP had a more beneficial effect in relieving depression and BAP in alleviating anxiety. This study has since been extended to include 81 patients, some of whom were seen at follow-up (Winston et al., 1994). The findings at termination were the same as those with the smaller sample. The follow-up reached 38 patients at a time period of 6 months to 4½ years posttherapy (average = 1.5 years), and they were assessed on target complaints only. Both ISTDP and BAP patients maintained their posttherapy gains and did not differ from each other.

Relating Therapy Process to Outcome

McCullough et al. (1991) examined the relationship between process variables such as clarifications and interpretations as isolated variables, and the same variables considered in connection with two kinds of patient responses: affect and defensiveness. The sample included the

ISTDP and BAP groups combined. Whereas the isolated variables did not predict outcome, interventions followed by affect correlated positively with outcome, and interventions followed by defense correlated negatively with outcome. The data suggest that knowing how the patient responds to certain interventions, rather than knowledge of the interventions alone, may allow prediction of outcomes in ISTDP and BAP. In addition, as reported elsewhere (Taurke, Flegenheimer, McCullough, Winston, & Pollack, 1990), the ratio of patient affect to patient defense was found to correlate with outcome in the same sample.

Another study (Salerno, Farber, McCullough, Winston, & Trujillo, 1992) compared the effects of confrontation versus clarification of defense on patient affective and defensive responding in the minute following the intervention. The sample combined those treated in ISTDP and BAP. Contrary to what one might have expected based on Davanloo's writings, no significant differences were found between the effects of confrontation versus clarification of defense on affective responses. Furthermore, confrontation of defense resulted in more defensive responding than did clarification in the minute following the intervention. The authors pointed out that for confrontation to be effective in facilitating affective responses, it may need to be cumulative, which requires that research focus on longer time periods of therapy.

In summary, the one study conducted on outcome of ISTDP is quite promising. Unlike most studies of brief therapy in which the sample consists of DSM Axis I disorders such as depression, anxiety, adjustment, and the like, this one treated personality-disordered patients. There are several features of this study that should be noted, however. First, the kind of personality disorders treated were not the borderline, schizoid, paranoid, or antisocial types, which are known to be more difficult to treat in any therapy. Second, the average length of therapy was 37 weeks, considerably longer than in most studies but comparable to the Høglend, Sørlie, et al. (1993) study, which also found that more sessions were correlated with greater gain for the personality disorder patients. Third, outcome measures were patient self-report only, and ISTDP was not shown to be superior to another, less confrontative, form of brief therapy. Regarding the process studies, the outcome data in one were based solely on patient report, and both combined two somewhat different kinds of therapy. Clearly, the clinical development of ISTDP has far outstripped its research base, which should be expanded to establish the efficacy of ISTDP and to understand its process. (See Winston, McCullough, & Laikin, 1993, for an interesting clinical comparison of successful and unsuccessful cases of BAP and ISTDP.)

Sifneos's Short-Term Anxiety-Provoking Psychotherapy (STAPP)

Outcome

The only studies of STAPP comparing a treated and an untreated group that we could locate were conducted by Sifneos and his associates (Sifneos, 1968, 1987; Sifneos, Apfel, Bassuk, Fishman, & Gill, 1980), and the latter two studies appear to have overlapping subjects.

In the first study (Sifneos, 1968), data were available on 14 experimental patients and 18 waiting list control patients who were also treated subsequently with STAPP. Outcome measures included resolution of emotional conflicts with evidence of self-understanding, symptomatic relief, new learning, and the acquisition of problem-solving abilities. According to our calculations, 79% of the experimental group improved on an average of eight outcome measures, compared to 22% of the waiting list controls. After treatment, 86% of the controls showed improvement. On long-term follow-up of "up to four years" (Sifneos, 1987, p. 201) on 21 of these patients, 58% to 91% remained improved on the various outcome measures. (The follow-up questionnaire can be found in Sifneos, 1992).

In a second study, Sifneos et al. (1980) again compared a treated group to a waiting list control group. At the end of the STAPP treatment, 18 of the 22 treated patients were considered "recovered" or "much better" on a similar composite score, as well as on a measure of the basic predisposing factors responsible for the patients' underlying difficulties. By contrast, at the end of the delay period, among the eight patients in the waiting list control, five were "unchanged" and three were a "little better." When they were treated, six of the eight were considered "recovered" or "much improved."

In the most recent controlled study of STAPP (Sifneos, 1987), 36 patients with unresolved oedipal problems were assigned to the treatment condition and 14 to a waiting list control. Thirty of the 36 patients in the treated group were rated as "recovered" or "much better" on the composite rating of symptom and dynamic change measures. By contrast, at the end of the waiting period 11 of the 14 patients were rated "unchanged," while 3 showed some symptomatic improvement. Four then decided not to continue into treatment. All 10 remaining controls were rated as "recovered" or "much better" after treatment, for a combined figure of 86% improvement.

While these figures seem to offer substantial evidence for the efficacy of STAPP, there were several problems with these studies. The outcome measures were new and no data regarding their reliability or

validity are presented, although the positive results offer some reassurance in this regard. In the latter two studies, the measures were
based on the interviewers' subjective appraisal, with no patient or
therapist measures included. In addition, the raters were not "blind"
as to whether they were evaluating the patients pre- or posttherapy,
allowing for inadvertent biases. The numbers were rather small, and
there are no statistical comparisons of the experimental and control
groups. Follow-up was not always conducted because the patients were
students who typically left the area within the year or two following
therapy.

Relating Therapy Process to Outcome

Svartberg and his associates have conducted several studies of 13 to
15 patients treated in STAPP in Trondheim, Norway. Using Sifneos's
(1992) selection criteria evaluation form, they were selected from a larger group of 79 patients who had been referred to short-term psychodynamic therapists. Patients' mean age was 29, and their diagnoses included social phobia, panic disorder, generalized anxiety disorder and
other Axis I disorders. Relationship problems with the opposite sex
had brought most of them to treatment, which was set at 20 sessions.
Most of the therapists were midway through a 3-year STAPP training
program.

In the first of these studies, Svartberg and Stiles (1992) examined
the prediction of patient change from initial session ratings of the therapist's competence in applying the technique and the interpersonal
complementarity of patient and therapist. Complementarity referred
to how well therapist responses to patient statements were complementary on the dimensions of "control/gives autonomy" and "love/hate." Only
complementarity was a good predictor of change in symptoms and in
social adjustment at the midpoint of therapy and, to a lesser extent,
at its termination. Thus, it would seem that STAPP techniques were
of lesser importance in determining outcome in this pilot study than
the interpersonal fit between patient and therapist.

In a related study, Svartberg and Stiles (1994) found that therapeutic alliance and therapists' competence in applying STAPP each made
contributions to change in general symptomatic distress above and beyond the other. However, whereas the contribution of alliance to outcome was positive, therapist competence was *inversely* related to
improvement, which they speculate may have been due to the modest
experience level of the therapists, and/or to their applying STAPP too
rigidly. This result is reminiscent of the study by Henry, Strupp et al.
(1993), reported in Chapter 1, where it was found that in gaining tech-

nical competence, therapists became more mechanical and authoritarian in applying the therapy.

In a further analysis reported in this article, Svartberg and Stiles
found, in comparing high- to low-competence therapists, that the former
were (1) more likely to hold clients reponsible for their behavior, (2)
recapitulated the clients' material when they were resistant, and (3) were
more active and directive around the oedipal focus.

What we learn from these analyses is that applying STAPP technique competently is less important than the therapist establishing a
good therapeutic alliance and responding to the patient in a complementary fashion. However, the results on the variable of competence,
if studied in a more seasoned group of STAPP therapists, may have
been quite different.

Process of Change

In another analysis of data based on the same patients, Svartberg, Seltzer, and Stiles (1993) found significant improvement in patients' degree
of "freeing of the self" during the process of therapy. They also found
that patients continued the self-freeing process through the 24 months
in which they were followed posttherapy, which supports Sifneos's
(1979) claim that gains from STAPP are also achieved posttherapy.
Clients grew faster toward self-freeing with the more competent therapists and when there was greater initial in-treatment symptomatic improvement.

Finally, Svartberg, Seltzer, Stiles, and Khoo (1995) studied the
course of symptom improvement in STAPP. The sample as a whole improved steadily and substantially over the course of treatment, with
three out of four patients showing clinically significant improvement.
Symptom decline was much slower following termination, a not unusual finding regarding posttherapy gains in general (Lambert, Shapiro
& Bergin, 1986) and symptomatic change in particular which tends to
improve early on in treatment (Howard et al., 1993). Patients with less
ego rigidity (that is, with greater ability to invoke their repertoire of
behavioral strategies flexibly in interpersonal situations) showed more
rapid symptom improvement.

It is significant that STAPP is being studied in research centers
other than that of its developer, as there are inadvertent biases that
can operate among raters in the therapy's "home" setting. In addition
to the Svartberg and Stiles project at the University of Trondheim, in
Norway, there is another study underway at the University of Bergen,
also in Norway, comparing STAPP to other therapies, but the results
at this time are preliminary and based on very small samples only (e.g.,
Barth et al., 1988).

A CRITICAL EVALUATION
OF THE DRIVE/STRUCTURAL MODEL

Regarding the research findings, a promising start has been made but much remains to be done. Further outcome studies, especially of Davanloo's STDP, are necessary to provide a firm empirical base for practice. In addition, more studies are needed to determine the utility of the selection criteria employed and whether the techniques lead to satisfactory progress and positive outcomes.

In commenting on the approaches of Davanloo and Sifneos, and to a much lesser extent that of Malan, several authors have expressed a concern with what they view as their authoritarian cast. Moss (1985), for example, states that "the practice of brief therapy simply serves to mediate and legitimate the covert reintroduction of primitive authority into the suddenly shaken configuration of a patient's inner object world" (p. 33). In a similar vein, Westen (1986) writes, "Davanloo limits transference paradigms considerably by his relentless establishment of a dominance–submission interaction" (p. 503). Grand, Rechetnick, Podrug, and Schwager (1985) view interventions such as brief therapists' exhortations to patients to engage in self-examination as potentially leading to "a regressive passive acceptance of the therapist's authority" (p. 26). Gustafson (1986) goes further, describing Davanloo's technique as akin to religious revivalism, in which relief comes only when the patient agrees to give up his or her willful activity. It acts as a form of conversion, he says, in which passive patients, under the threat of abandonment, finally give way through emotional release and fall under the therapist's sway.

Interestingly, these critiques recall comments on brief therapy made a half-century ago by Fenichel (1944/1954):

> This is the way in which (brief) psychotherapeutic transference improvements are achieved: "If you are a good boy and don't behave neurotically, you get love, protection, participation from the omnipotent doctor; if you do not obey, you have to fear his revenge." In this respect, the (brief) therapist is in good company; he uses the same means of influence which God uses. (p. 253)

In other words, the critics regard the attitude of these therapists as "Father knows best," perhaps benign in intent, but paternal in a way that is inimical to psychoanalytic precepts. The consequences of such an authoritarian stance, if accurate, are considerable. It suggests that in this form of BPT, there is no true psychoanalytic exploration, no unfettered dialogue, no free associations, but only compliance with the therapist's view of reality. And this reality is drawn chiefly from psychoanalytic theory. It is as if the drive/structural therapists engage in the therapeutic enterprise with preset ideas, or a template which is superimposed on patients' verbalizations. In the words of one critic:

> To arrive at a prefigured point is to have been brought there, someone know-ing in advance where it was. Any such path in a therapy is vulnerable to the claim that it was charted by a covert agreement between patient and ther-apist, each of them finding pleasure in a bond marked by submission to the subtle suggestions of an authority deemed benign, an authority who shows the way. (Moss, 1985, p. 32)

Stated differently, a therapist's authoritarian posture may not suffi-ciently allow for the enhancement of the patient's initiative and self-efficacy. As Strupp and Binder (1984) have argued, "It is most impor-tant that therapists exert influence in a manner that fosters autonomy, allowing patients to discover and own their personal capacity for change" (p. 107). Thus, these authors prefer that impediments to speak-ing freely come from within the patient, not from the forcefulness of the therapist. In addition, they fear that confrontation may lead to a sacrifice of the collaborative therapeutic relationship.

A further consequence of an authoritarian posture is that the challenging style itself may be responsible for the gamut of feelings aroused in the patient, which is antithetical to the ideal of a psychoana-lytic therapist's neutral stance. In other words, it is not the patient's transference that we are witnessing but, for example, legitimate anger based on the therapist's provocation. Patients' reactions may have less to do with their early relationships and psychopathology than with the kind of therapist–patient relationship established. In this connection, Westen (1986) remarked that what does not get analyzed is why patients allow themselves to be dominated in a relationship that mirrors an earli-er one that was unsatisfactory. Similarly, there is no acknowledgment that only some elements of patients' problems and transference reac-tions can emerge because of the therapist's stance. Migone (1985) has pointed out, for example, that narcissistic and dependency transfer-ence reactions do not achieve expression.

Gustafson argues that many patients will defy the technique, thus lessening the breadth of suitability of BPT. And if the approach does not work, there is no other place for the therapist to go. He sees its forcefulness as an all-or-none commitment on the therapist's part from which there is no retreat.

Finally, there is little mention of countertransference in these authors' works. In this connection, Kupers (1986) believes that this is partly a function of brevity, since it might take 10 to 20 sessions to identify a countertransference theme. It is also due, he says, to the therapist quickly taking a stand and interpreting, leaving less time and attention for therapists to note their countertransference.

How might the drive/structural therapists respond to these criticisms? First, they would not view themselves as authoritarian so much as active, even relentless, in helping patients to face up to and wrestle with their problems. It is not the patient that they are up against, they would say, but the patient's conflicts and problems. They seek to help patients muster the courage to combat their self-deceptions, defenses, and resistances in the service of exposing and resolving what they have distorted and kept hidden from themselves and others. It is as if they are saying to the patient, "This will hurt, but it's good for you in the long run." By constantly monitoring patients' reactions to the confrontation, they mitigate its potential for damage. They would not agree with the criticism that they are *eliciting* affect rather than *observing* transferential responses and would point to the way that such responses parallel life issues that patients have struggled with, often for a very long time.

The drive/structural therapists might also say, "Watch our videotapes of live therapy sessions and see for yourselves if what we are saying is not true. The proof is in the pudding." And, in fact, the videotapes and transcripts are compelling. Patients do achieve breakthroughs and seem to be genuinely helped. Does it really matter, one may ask, whether change is forced from without, rather than gently encouraged from within?

What we seem to have here is a value dispute. The drive/structural therapists claim that challenge and confrontation in the service of the patient's becoming freer of neurotic conflict is justified. The critics contend that the putative ends do not justify the means employed because the therapists have merely imposed their view of reality on patients, thereby detracting from their autonomy. One could argue that this is a dispute subject to empirical test. The critics would have to show that the quality of the result achieved is different for patients treated by Davanloo and Sifneos's challenging techniques compared to the gentler therapies proposed by Mann, Strupp and Binder, and others.

The drive/structural therapists might also respond that suggestion is not the sole province of BPT but occurs in all forms of psychotherapy, including psychoanalysis. Grünbaum (1984) is merely the latest in a series of critics to claim that psychoanalysis is contaminated by therapists' suggestiveness, thus rendering it unsuitable as a locale for testing psychoanalytic concepts. Anything that a psychoanalyst says is a suggestion of a sort, subtly steering the patient in one direction or another. The unequal standing of psychoanalyst and patient, the status given by society to analysts as healers, and the analyst's shadowy presence all contribute to their authority and the importance attached to their words and gestures. In this light, BPT is not unique in exerting influence, but merely different in the way that such influence is applied. The BPT therapists might even argue that they are more explicit about the role of the therapist's influence, rather than claiming a neutrality, as does psychoanalysis, that is impossible to achieve.

Along these lines, they might also answer that the passive stance of classical psychoanalysis limits therapists' understanding of patients' psychodynamics and behavior. As Wachtel (1977) has argued:

> The ambiguous stance of the analyst, his efforts to minimize the kind of interaction with the patient that is characteristic of other kinds of relationships, make it extremely difficult to study, through this medium, the patient's way of responding to and affecting actual manifest behaviors of other people. (p. 50)

Although the source of the critics' claims may lie in the forceful and charismatic nature of the personalities involved, or in their confrontative techniques, a more fundamental consideration is the epistemological basis from which these three therapists operate. The air of certainty with which they formulate the patient's dynamics and interpret them suggest that they embrace the correspondence concept of truth. Within this framework, knowledge of objects and events is gained through observation of things as they are, independent of the theories of the observer. The correspondence theory is wedded to realism which assumes a world and mental events that have their own natures apart from our perceptions of them. This theory of truth was once the normative one in science, and it largely constituted Freud's view as well (Hanly, 1992). For Freud, there was one correct fit to the puzzle of the patient's symptoms, dreams, slips, and so forth.

This epistemological attitude can be illustrated by Davanloo's (1988) use of the metaphor "unlocking the unconscious":

> The process of *the unlocking of the unconscious* can be divided into a number of phases. The aim of the first of seven phases is to create an intrapsychic crisis between the patient's resistance and his therapeutic alliance, which results in the breakthrough of very complex feelings mostly in the transference. *This breakthrough represents the essential triggering mechanism for unlocking the unconscious.* Then the process enters to [sic] the interpretative phase and *the direct view of the multifoci core neurotic structure responsible for patient's* [sic] *symptoms as well as character disturbances.* (p. 99; italics added)

One gets the impression that the patients' dynamics reside in a locked box in the brain with Davanloo possessing the key (the techniques of ISTDP) to obtain access to them. They then emerge in such a form that any unbiased observer can view them directly. There is no room here for ambiguity, alternate construals, or open dialogue about its correctness.

Similarly, Sifneos regards the oedipal complex in concrete terms, not as hypothesis, metaphor, or construct, but as given—an obvious and proven fact. As is the case with unlocking the unconscious, there only remains the task of removing the veil and bringing the oedipal elements into the open. Malan's formulation of dynamics and pursuit of them in the focus also suggest that he views them as being accurate or inaccurate in some absolute sense. It is the therapist's interpretation of reality that counts, rather than a shared view of reality that emerges in the interaction of therapist and patient. For the traditional drive/structural therapist, when patients resolve the transference, they come to see the world as does the therapist, without distortion.

The underlying epistemology may also help to explain why there is so little emphasis on countertransference in these therapists' writings, and, it would seem, in their therapy. In the relational view of therapy (Chapter 3), countertransference refers to the feelings elicited in the therapist by the patient, which do not necessarily stem from issues in the therapist's past. They are used to inform the therapist about what the patient elicits in others, and are a reflection of the interpersonal climate created by the particular interaction of therapist and patient. This allows for two plausible realities, not just one. In the drive/structural therapies, the *presumption* is (and it is only a presumption) that therapists are neutral, with little necessity to ask patients how they view the therapist.

The alternative to the correspondence theory is the *coherence* theory of truth, which posits that there is more than one true description of the world. It is associated with the philosophical school of thought called idealism. The coherence theory regards the reality of objects and events as a function of how they are experienced by observers, not as they "actually are," as realism espouses. Objects only take on meaning by virtue of the theory we invent to define them; that is, they are constructed and constituted by our beliefs and ideas (Hanly, 1992). In this view, one does not "unlock the unconscious," have an unadorned view of "the multifoci core neurotic structure" or the elements of the oedipal complex, nor does one achieve an apodictically accurate dynamic focus. Rather, one constructs a narrative that pulls together the pieces of personality functioning with the knowledge that other constructions are always possible (e.g., Schafer, 1981). Narrative coherence rather than external correspondence to an actual reality becomes the criterion of truth. The way in which narrative and metaphor are manifested in the brief dynamic therapies will be discussed further in the following chapters.

CHAPTER 3

The Relational Model: Luborsky, Horowitz, Weiss and Sampson, and Strupp and Binder

In the present chapter we address a group of approaches that can be described as the second main trend in brief psychodynamic psychotherapy. Corresponding to historical developments within psychoanalytic theory, these treatments reflect a postclassical approach to clinical psychopathology, personality theory, and clinical technique (Greenberg & Mitchell, 1983). Greenberg and Mitchell have argued that there is a deeply rooted tension within psychoanalysis that divides the tradition into theory that places clinical primacy on drives and theories that view object relations as clinically central. The division places on one side Freud's drive/structural model along with its descendants within the classical American tradition of psychoanalysis, and on the other side the work of Melanie Klein, W. R. D. Fairbairn, D. W. Winnicott, and Harry Guntrip, along with their theoretical descendants. Their view is that this is a fundamental and irreconcilable theoretical schism, and that all clinical psychoanalytic theories will tend to be drawn toward one or the other of these two positions.

Mitchell (1988) characterizes what he and Greenberg have termed the "relational model" as follows:

> We are portrayed not as a conglomeration of physically based urges, but as being shaped by and inevitably embedded within a matrix of relationships with other people, struggling both to maintain our ties to others and to differentiate ourselves from them. In this vision the basic unit of study is not the individual as a separate entity whose desires clash with an exter-

nal reality, but an interactional field within which the individual arises and struggles to make contact and to articulate himself. (p. 3)

We choose to follow the position that the relational paradigm represents a fundamental alternative to Freud's drive/structural model, for reasons that are directly related to our present task. First, the distinction clearly delineates two groups of brief therapists/theorists that seem to correspond to the drive versus object relational dichotomy. In addition, the use of Greenberg and Mitchell's distinction helps to clarify what we believe are fundamental underlying root metaphors in the various models of brief psychotherapy. These include basic assumptions about the nature of psychopathology and its etiology, corresponding models of personality, and ideas about clinical technique that necessarily arise from these theoretical assumptions.

Further, the approaches we characterize as relational share certain ideas about the nature of the scientific enterprise entailed in the development of theory and practice, and are distinct from those espoused by Freud and classical Freudian theorists. In other words, the clinical assumptions made by each model reflect different worldviews regarding the nature of science and the development of theory and knowledge. Thus, Greenberg and Mitchell's use of the term "paradigm," referring to Kuhn's (1970) work on the development of scientific theories, seems appropriate in that it implies just such basic differences. These occur not only at the level of competing observations or differing explanations for the same data, but also at the deeper level of assumptions about method, the nature of data, and the nature of the relation of the psychotherapist–observer to his or her subject. Finally, it is our view that psychoanalysis at large is involved in an historical shift such that all the major trends of the psychoanalytic movement are becoming fundamentally more "relational" and less drive-oriented (Aron, 1990). By this we mean that, among other issues of importance, there is increasing interest in the relationship of transference and countertransference, the interactional components of transference, and the subjectivity of both members of the dyad.

Whereas the therapies of Malan, Sifneos, and Davanloo are clearly rooted in the classical tradition of Freud's drive theory, we will now turn to several models that are more closely aligned with the object relational tradition. While each has qualities that are distinct enough to warrant separate treatment, they also share enough characteristics to make entirely separate treatment redundant. Thus, we will attempt to address their underlying similarities and overlapping attributes, while indicating those characteristics that are distinctive to each. It should be noted that categorizing these therapies as relational and belonging together in some meaningful sense is entirely our doing, and not that of the theorists described. It is likely that not all of them would fully agree with our schema. As stated elsewhere, it is our belief that the organization of therapies which we have followed provides a unique and useful perspective on these clinical theories, and is justified even though, like all heuristic devices, it may leave certain relationships understated and others overly emphasized.

The four brief dynamic therapies that will be addressed here are (1) the supportive–expressive psychotherapy of Lester Luborsky and the Penn Psychotherapy Project; (2) the short-term dynamic therapy model of Mardi Horowitz and the Center for the Study of Neuroses; (3) the control–mastery therapy of Joseph Weiss, Harold Sampson, and the Mount Zion group; and (4) the time-limited dynamic psychotherapy of Hans Strupp, Jeffrey Binder, and the Vanderbilt group. It is interesting to note that none of these groups of theorists intentionally set out to develop or promote a model of brief therapy. Relatively less attention is paid to the issues of treatment brevity, time limits, and special patient selection which are hallmarks of the psychotherapies treated in the previous chapter. In fact, all four groups have set out to develop and research general approaches to psychoanalytic psychotherapy, rather than brief therapy in particular. However, the inclusion of these therapies in this book seems essential because of their theoretical importance and their wide applicability to brief treatment. All four groups have published research and clinical findings which have been based on brief psychotherapy. It may be that these theorists are brief therapists only incidentally, their true interest having been the facilitation of psychotherapy research and the development of general psychodynamic theory. Nonetheless, their contribution to the theory and practice of brief psychotherapy is substantial and warrants close evaluation.

It is notable that the short-term dynamic therapy of Horowitz and his associates and, to a lesser extent, the control–mastery therapy of Weiss and Sampson make use of explicitly cognitive language. Horowitz draws directly on contemporary cognitive theory and relies heavily on schematic representations that appear to have their origins in cognitive and information-processing approaches to psychology. Weiss, Sampson, and their colleagues rely centrally on concepts such as "pathogenic beliefs," which appear to be quite closely related to similar concepts arising in current cognitive therapies. In fact, we choose to include these models in this chapter because they provide a useful illustration of the intrinsic compatibility of cognitive theory and terminology and clinical object relational theories (see Singer & Singer, 1992, and Westen, 1988, for attempts to bridge the two literatures). As Westen suggests, cognitive theory provides useful models for the linguistic and conceptual representation of clinical psychodynamic ideas.

THE THEORY OF PERSONALITY AND PSYCHOPATHOLOGY

The relational conception of personality is broadly psychoanalytic, drawing on Sullivan's (1953) interpersonal psychiatry; the interpersonal tradition in psychoanalysis as developed by Erich Fromm (1944, 1947), Karen Horney (1950), Erik Erikson (1950), and others; Melanie Klein's (1950) work on the idea of internalized representations of self and object, and its further developments by Fairbairn (1952), Winnicott (1965), Guntrip (1961), Edith Jacobson (1964), Kernberg (1976), and other object relations theorists; John Bowlby's (1969) "attachment theory," and the research it has stimulated; aspects of intersubjective notions of Kohut's (1971, 1977) psychoanalytic self psychology and its recent developments (Stolorow & Atwood, 1992); and, finally, current research into the development of internalized representations of self, other, and self–other interaction by infant researchers such as Beebe (1994) and Stern (1985). Central to this approach is a shift away from drives and instinctual wishes as the primary or sole motivational construct, and a movement toward the idea of intrinsic motivations arising from the vicissitudes of human relating.

What we are calling a *relational approach* is thus actually a synthesis of several important, relatively independent traditions which have evolved out of traditional psychoanalytic views. It may be argued that the term "relational" is in fact a *point of view,* encompassing a wide range of theories and therapeutic orientations, which colors virtually all of contemporary psychoanalytic theorizing.

An Object Relational View of Mind, with Internalized Representations of Self, Other, and Interaction as Fundamental

The glue holding together this conglomeration of theories and models is the object relations emphasis on internalized representations of self and other, located at the core of personality structure. Relational views imply a concept of personality that is organized around structures of mind that are fundamentally oriented toward the object world. Relational approaches, while diverse, stand together in contrast to a more purely dynamic view of mind in which the fundamental structures of personality are drives and the defenses against their direct expression, with anxiety signaling the failure of defense structures to contain unacceptable impulses. While drive theory does offer a theory of object relations, as discussed in Chapter 2, drives remain central. For Freud, objects are the residue of attachments to lost instinct-gratifying others that have been internalized (Freud, 1905a/1958; 1917/1958). Thus, internal objects arise from the frustration of instinctual wishes.

The relational models instead rely on some notion of primary, original, and independent structures of mind that provide for the mental representation of self, others, and relating. Melanie Klein, in her paper "The Origins of Transference," states: "The analysis of very young children has taught me that there is no instinctual urge, no anxiety situation, no mental process which does not involve objects, external or internal; in other words object relations are at the *centre* of emotional life" (Klein, 1952, p. 53; italics in original). In a recent discussion, Greenberg (1991) describes such relational mental structures and their motivational value:

> People form intentions on the basis of their dominant self representations (and their attendant feeling states), which serve as indicators not only of where we are but also of where we would like to go next. Guided by these indicators, we construct wishes, which are themselves represented mentally. *The wish has three components: the self, an object, and an interactional field within which the two establish a particular sort of relationship.* The self and object components of the wish are, like all representations, complex and multiply determined. They are drawn from an experience of the need at the moment, from recollected images of self and object under similar conditions of need, and from convictions about the capacities and limits of the self as embodied in its dominant shape. (p. 171; italics added)

Each of the therapies dealt with in this chapter relies to a great extent on some similar notion of internalized representations of self, other, and relationship, in its explanation of personality structure, psychopathology, and therapeutic process.

Psychopathology as Essentially Interpersonal and Intersubjective

Mitchell (1988) explains the ubiquitous maladaptive interpersonal repetitions characterizing all forms of psychopathology in the following way: "The relational model rests on the premise that the repetitive patterns within human experience are not derived, as in the drive model, from pursuing gratification of inherent pressures and pleasures (nor, as in Freud's post-1920 understanding, from the automatic workings of the death instinct), but from a pervasive tendency to preserve the continuity, connections, familiarity of one's personal, interactional world" (p. 33).

Mitchell is delineating the fundamental shift from a drive-based conception of psychopathology (in which drives, defenses, and intrapsychic conflict are understood as central), to one rooted in interpersonal and intersubjective experience. From this latter point of view, there is always an *other* with whom we are interacting, and in relation to whom psychopathology arises and continues to manifest itself.

Each of the four therapies treated here in some way views psychopathology in terms of *recurrent patterns of interpersonal behavior which are maladaptive.* From this point of view the patient inevitably construes and contructs relationships in the context of his or her past interpersonal experience, with an emphasis on the particularly powerful shaping effects of early experience. Conflict is seen as arising in the context of interpersonal relationships as the result of conflicting wishes in relation to others. Conflict need not be related to infantile sexual impulses or primary libidinal or aggressive drives, but could instead include a wide range of affects, wishes, intentions, and subjectively experienced needs in relation to others (Sandler & Sandler, 1978). Conflict can arise in any developmental stage, and may be related to issues of separation, dependency, autonomy, and self-integration, as well as sexual or aggressive impulses (Stern, 1985). Greenberg (1991) frames conflict in terms of a need for safety and a need for effectance, or mastery. For example, later in this chapter we discuss the case of Nora, who experienced conflict between longings for her father's interest, attention, and appreciation, and the feelings of shame, humiliation, and pain around critical and rejecting aspects of her relationship with him. In this instance conflict is not thought of as arising from the expression of an unacceptable incestuous wish derived from the sexual instinct, but as a conflict between a relational need and an internally represented painful consequence.

With the deemphasis of instinctual drives as the engine of intrapsychic conflict, there tends to be an increased attention to the real failures of the environment (e.g., Kohut, 1977; Winnicott, 1965). In each of the four therapies, with the possible exception of Luborsky's group, there is much greater weight given to the role of "real experience" in the development of object relations that form the basis of pathology. There is also a much greater emphasis on the *adaptive aspects* of apparently pathological relationships, again with reference to the original developmental situation and its requirements. From this point of view defenses are understood to function not primarily as safeguards against the expression of unacceptable instinctual wishes or anxiety signaling the imminent appearance of such impulses in consciousness, but instead as adaptive mechanisms employed to minimize the experience of anticipated unpleasant affects, to control relationships so as to avoid expected traumatic or painful outcomes, and to attempt to bring about desired states of relatedness. For example, in the case of Nora, the patient relied on a superficial cheerfulness and a narrowed, rigid, and reality-directed attentional focus both to regulate her own internal states and affects (intrapsychic function) and to ward off anticipated attacks by the therapist for being self-pitying, "whining," and wrong about her private thoughts and feelings (interpersonal functions).

In addition, in these relational therapies there tends to be more emphasis on the *current maintaining factors* in psychopathological transactions, with notions like cyclical and self-perpetuating dynamics, as opposed to a strict causal emphasis on the past (e.g., Wachtel, 1987; 1993). In this sense, psychopathology is understood to be a dynamic, self-fulfilling process, in which feared and anticipated relational events tend to be elicited and enacted by the individual in his or her interactions with others, who, in turn, will tend to respond in ways complementary to the interpersonal actions of that individual.

To varying degrees, each of the following therapies being considered relies on some concept of internalized representations of self and other in their theories of personality functioning and psychopathology.

The Penn Group

Luborsky and his associates have made the core conflictual relationship theme (CCRT) method a central organizing theoretical and research construct (Luborsky & Crits-Cristoph, 1990). In clinical practice, the CCRT serves as the therapeutic focus, organizing clinical material and guiding interventions. The method involves raters evaluating "relationship episodes" from actual clinical material, and, from these, deriving the core transferential theme for that patient. The theme consists of three components: a wish, need, or intention; a response from the other; and a response of the self. A sample CCRT follows, adapted from Luborsky, Crits-Cristoph, Mintz, and Auerbach (1988).

CCRT Relationship Pattern

Wish: To not be cut off from "closeness" with others
Response from others: Excluding the client
Response from self: Anger, self-blaming

The central motivational role of the "wish" component suggests that Luborsky and his associates adopt a traditional psychodynamic notion of transference in their understanding of the CCRT (Luborsky et al., 1988). However, on closer examination, the CCRT model appears to be the expression of a relational view of psychopathology. The wish component is virtually always an implicitly interpersonal wish ("to assert myself," "to receive acceptance,"), while the other two components are explicitly relational. Drives appear to be at most secondary issues to be negotiated in the relational realm (for example, the wish to obtain sexual gratification).

Like the approach of Weiss and Sampson, described below, theirs is a conflict model, but one which emphasizes relational conflicts more than intrapsychic ones. That is, the conflicts as they are presented are between *interpersonal wishes and feared or anticipated outcomes,* rather than between parts of the psychic apparatus such as drive derivatives and the ego defenses. In this sense their approach seems quite compatible with that of the Vanderbilt group, for example, in emphasizing the anticipated response from the other and from the self in relation to some interpersonal wish or need. The Penn group is less clear about the origins of such expectations than, say, the Mount Zion group, and it appears that there is some tension in the Penn approach between a more drive-based understanding of transference, and the more relational understanding explicitly offered by the other models.

The Center for the Study of Neuroses

Mardi Horowitz relies heavily on the notion of representations of self and others, using the terminology of cognitive psychology in such concepts as "schemas," "self-schemas," "and "role-relationship models" (Horowitz, 1988). His work integrates psychodynamic theory and the tradition of cognitive psychology via Piaget's developmental cognitivism, and bears the influence of John Bowlby's work on the centrality of attachment in human development as well as the concept of "working models" (Bowlby, 1969). In a recent chapter Horowitz (1991) defined his conception of "person schemas theory": "Person schemas theory has to do with enduring but slowly changing views of self and of other, and with scripts for transactions between self and other. Each individual may have a repertoire of multiple self schemas" (p. 168).

His view is that personality represents a homeostatic mechanism by which the individual can modulate and accommodate the stresses of development as well as of external events such as losses. The individual relies upon the internalized *scripts,* or *working models,* of interpersonal situations in order to adapt to the constant flow of new situations as they arise. The quality of such working models and their flexibility are determinants of that individual's adaptability to ordinary and unusual stresses. Figure 3.1, a "configurational analysis" adapted from Horowitz, Marmar, Krupnick, Kaltreider, and Wallerstein (1984), is an example

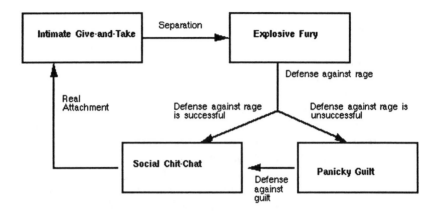

FIGURE 3.1. A simplified example of a configurational analysis of relationship structures. Adapted from Horowitz, Marmar, Krupnick, et al. (1984, p. 60). Copyright 1984 by Basic Books. Adapted by permission.

of one patient's internalized "working model" and how it represents internalized relationship structures.

The diagram depicts the patient's various modal affective states and their dynamic relation to one another, illustrating both defensive processes and underlying relational goals. This representation makes clear the cyclical aspect of such internalized working models of relationships. Other aspects of configurational analysis include identifying transference themes, common roles and their associated aims, and "story lines," which narrate the sequence of changes in role-relationship models.

Horowitz (1988) and his colleagues define psychopathology as the inappropriate application of a schema, or role-relationship model: "Persistent use of an inappropriate role-relationship model in constructing a working model will mean that the working model will deviate from the situation, or at least the other person's view of it. In spite of this fact, one may continue to use the same working model again and again. The result may be psychological pathology" (p. 76).

He notes that such inappropriate role-relationship models will be utilized "in order to undo past traumas, to make up for past deficits, or to regain some relationship they had or almost had in the developmental past" (p. 84). Problematic "script sequences" or internalized relationship scripts are characterized by rigidity as they are applied to reality, or by their inadequacy to accurately model reality.

Horowitz's theory of personality and psychopathology is a mixed model, blending some of the dynamic flavor of psychoanalytic drive theory with themes and metaphors derived from information-processing theory. However, it seems to us that his model is essentially relational in that the role-relationship schemas that he places at the center of personality are fundamental elements of personality, and not derivatives of the vicissitudes of instinctual gratification and frustration. In his model human beings seem to be relational "by design" (Mitchell, 1988); we wish to emphasize the basic relational aspect of his theory, and its connections to a larger framework of interpersonal and object relational theory.

The Mount Zion Group

Another framework, that of Weiss, Sampson, and their colleagues, uses a different language from that of object relations theories, but appears to rely upon a fundamentally relational notion of internalized representations of self and others. In their model, they refer to an individual's system of *beliefs,* partly conscious and partly unconscious, that determine his or her relation to reality:

> These beliefs . . . are central to a person's conscious and unconscious mental life. . . . They are an indispensable guide to the all-important tasks of adaptation and self-preservation. . . . They are organizers of perception. A person perceives himself and others largely as he consciously and unconsciously believes himself to be. . . . They are organizers of personality and psychopathology. It is in accordance with his beliefs about reality that a person shapes his inborn strivings and by doing so evolves his personality. (Weiss, 1990, cited in Sampson, 1992)

It would appear from this statement that the term "belief" refers to an interpersonal belief, an idea about self or other derived from experience of real interactions. An example would be a patient's belief that if he expressed angry feelings to his wife she would be hurt, arising from the patient's experience as a child with his mother, who would respond to the expression of anger by sulking. This man's pathogenic belief was extended to other significant people in his life, and was also generalized to include a variety of self-assertive behaviors. Although pathogenic beliefs are internalized based on real experience, accommodation is made in the theory for the operation of fantasy, misunderstanding, and distortion on the part of the experiencing individual. For instance, the developmentally expectable egocentricity of children reliably leads to their belief in their having personal responsibility for traumatic events actually beyond their control.

Central to the Mount Zion group's model is the idea that the individual's perception of reality is not distorted by internal, instinctual wishes, but instead by the deep motivating desire to sucessfully adapt to his or her interpersonal reality so as to minimize painful or traumatic experience (Sampson, 1992). Thus, in direct contrast to a drive/conflict model, "pathogenic beliefs" do not arise from the operation of unconscious instinctual wishes automatically seeking fulfillment, but rather reflect the internalization of actual, lived interpersonal experience and the efforts to master the traumatic aspects of that experience. For example, a young woman has the unconscious belief that competent functioning in her work and relationships will hurt her anxious and depressed mother, not because of a specific aggressive *wish* to hurt her mother, but because her actual historical experience has led her to believe that her mother cannot tolerate the patient's autonomy and will feel abandoned by her. In her effort to master this dilemma she may enact this conflict with her therapist to "test" him, to find out whether he can better tolerate her strivings toward separation and self-fulfillment.

Weiss and Sampson thus reject the drive/structural notion that instinct is the primary motivating force in personality and the development of psychopathology. Rather, "pathogenic beliefs and the fear, anxiety, shame and guilt to which they give rise provide the primary motives for the development and maintenance of repressions, inhibitions, and symptoms" (Weiss, Sampson, & the Mount Zion Psychotherapy Research Group, 1986, p. 68). Theirs is clearly a conflict model, but here conflict is not between the expression of instinctual wishes (e.g., oral or anal aggression) and their rejection as morally unacceptable, but instead between a wish to realize oneself in a particular way and the expectation of a *painful outcome based on previous interpersonal experience*. Conflict and motivation are thus understood more in terms of "goals" than drives: "A pathogenic belief is simple and compelling: It tells the person who adheres to it that if he attempts to gratify a certain impulse or to reach a certain goal he will endanger himself" (Weiss et al., 1986, p. 69). It must be emphasized that the "impulses" or "goals" referred to in this statement are not drive-based in the classical psychoanalytic sense, but rather are "ego motives" related to autonomy, mastery, and other developmentally expectable needs, more in the tradition of ego psychology.

The Vanderbilt Group

The approach of Strupp and the Vanderbilt group, in contrast to the other three, is an explicitly interpersonal model, drawing on the interpersonal psychoanalytic tradition of Sullivan (1953) and, more recently, the work of Benjamin (1982). Binder and Strupp (1991) present a view which is highly compatible with a relational perspective.

In a recent statement, Binder and Strupp (1991) define their understanding of psychopathology in terms of a recurring pattern in the patient's emotional life that is maladaptive. They have termed this the "cyclical maladaptive pattern": "The Cyclical Maladaptive Pattern (CMP) is a working model (Peterfreund, 1983) of a central or salient pattern of interpersonal roles in which patients unconsciously cast themselves; the complementary roles in which they cast others; and the maladaptive interaction sequences, self-defeating expectations, negative self-appraisals, and unpleasant affects that result" (p. 140). These organized roles are referred to as cyclical because, in Binder and Strupp's view, the patient unconsciously induces others to behave in ways that reinforce the patient's negative and painful expectations, thus leading to further establishment of those expectations and the interpersonal roles that arise from them.

They identify four categories of information, contained within their concept of the cyclical maladative pattern. We include examples of an actual clinical focus taken from a published case illustration (Binder & Strupp, 1991).

1. *Acts of self.* Included are both private and public actions. . . . Acts of self vary in the degree to which they are accessible to awareness: "The patient maintained a wary, emotionally aloof stance toward others; he felt emotionally disconnected but yearned for closeness."

2. *Expectations about others' reactions.* These are imagined reactions of others to one's own actions. Such expectations may be conscious, preconscious, or unconscious: "He expected other people to not want to be bothered with his feelings and to not like him."

3. *Acts of others toward self.* These are observed acts of others that are viewed as occurring in specific relation to the acts of self: "Other people tended to react to his emotional aloofness with reserve, which the patient interpreted as proof that they did not want to be involved with him."

4. *Acts of self toward self (introject).* This category of actions refers to how one treats oneself. . . . These actions should be articulated in specific relation to the other elements of the format: "The patient felt unappealing and uninteresting." (Adapted from Binder & Strupp, 1991, pp. 140–141)

Binder and Strupp's interpersonal tilt is conveyed in the concrete language of "acts" and "expectations" in transactions between self and other, though it is also clear that Strupp and Binder are in fact referring to *mental representations* of interpersonal acts, which locates their work in an object relations framework.

THE FORMULATION OF A FOCUS

Articulating a clinical focus or foci is a hallmark characteristic of all brief psychotherapy approaches. The approaches reviewed in this chapter each make the concept of focality a central and vital feature of their clinical theory. Two of the therapies reviewed, that of the Penn group and the Mount Zion group, take highly specialized approaches to the formulation of the therapeutic focus. In the other two therapies, there is a more general emphasis on current transactional patterns, with attention to the evolving therapeutic relationship. As a group, the four approaches apply methods to elucidate formulations which, in comparison with the previous generation of brief dynamic therapies, result in clinical foci that are more diverse, rely less on a single, a priori theoretical construct such as the Oedipus complex, and tend to be more experience near, with a here-and-now, interactional emphasis.

The Penn Group

Luborsky and the Penn group, as discussed earlier, developed the concept of the core conflictual relationship theme (CCRT) as an organizing principle of their clinical approach and research program. The CCRT can be understood as a theory-driven articulation of a central interpersonal–dynamic theme that structures patient's relationships with others across situations: "[The CCRT] captures the central pattern, script, or schema that each person follows in conducting relationships" (Luborsky & Crits-Cristoph, 1990, p. 1). This work represents the culmination of years of research into the formulation and measurement of the central psychoanalytic concept of transference (Luborsky, 1990). The process of developing a CCRT can be summarized as follows: The first step is the identification from session transcripts of "relationship episodes," which are defined as "a part of a session that occurs as a relatively discrete episode of explicit narration about relationships with others or with the self" (Luborsky, 1990, p. 16). The second step is identifying the CCRT components from the relationship episodes, and rating their qualities. These are tallied across a large number of components, and the final CCRT represents the summary of the most frequent types of components. Table 3.1 is a CCRT summary taken from Luborsky and Schaffler (1990), based on clinical material from a sample case, to exemplify the format.

TABLE 3.1. Core Conflictual Relationship Theme: Example

	CCRT component	Example
Wish	1. To be assertive by A. Exerting control over the other B. Being dominant and not dominated C. Being better than the other; not let other favor someone else	*"...I would first have to get him angry at me...."*
	2. To have more control over myself	*"...I tried to control myself...."*
	3. To be reassured; to get approval	*"...I want to be reassured you're listening...."*
	4. To be close; have physical contact	
	5. To get help from the other person	*"...I wanted his approval or direction...."*
Negative response from other	1. Dominating, controlling 2. Disapproves, doesn't reassure me	*"...he didn't [approve]..."*
Negative response from self	1. No self-control; self-blame for poor control 2. Annoyed, angry, upset	*"...so I got furious...."* *"...I was horrified that I had done this...."*
Positive response from self	1. Pleased with the other person	*"...then I would feel loving...."*

Note. From Luborsky & Schaffler (1990, p. 80). Copyright 1990 by L. Luborsky. Adapted by permission.

The table illustrates the various aspects of a final CCRT, with sample statements for each component. The patient's "wish" components represent the motivational dimension of personality as measured by the CCRT. These include the interpersonal aims or goals that the patient refers to in the scored "relationship episodes." One of the wish components is subdivided, reflecting a greater degree of specificity. The "response" components, from self and other, positive and negative, represent the patient's perceptions of or beliefs about the consequences of some wish or need. "Responses from self" typically include affect states and emotional reactions, while "responses from other" generally reflect the patient's interpretations of the other's behavior or action.

The CCRT is understood to be an empirical approach to the representation of the patient's central transference paradigm. Thus, the CCRT is the conceptual vehicle—"a guided system"—by which the Penn group arrive at their clinical understanding of the therapeutic focus for a given patient. It is worth emphasizing that all CCRT's are different, and so all CCRT-based clinical formulations will be "patient-specific." "This patient-specific appropriateness of the focus is likely to increase the patient's inclination to feel that he or she has been listened to and understood when interpretations are made" (Luborsky, 1990). The Penn group differentiates this characteristic of their supportive–expressive therapy model from other brief therapy models such as Mann's or Davanloo's, which tend to take up more general or universal issues as their foci, such as loss or oedipal conflict (Luborsky, 1990, p. 217).

Although the CCRT method is a fairly laborious system and is employed primarily in psychotherapy research, Luborsky suggests that it can be usefully applied to everyday clinical work, having advantages over unguided approaches to psychodynamic therapy (Luborsky, 1990). In particular, he notes that the methodology, because it is structured, leads to clinical formulations with greater reliability and uniformity. The method can be a guide to formulations of transference, to interpretations, and to a treatment focus, especially important for time-limited psychotherapies. Luborsky offers methods for learning to use the CCRT in practice, including use of the CCRT concept during supervision of psychotherapy, scoring practice sets of CCRT data, and a CCRT-based self-analysis exercise.

The Mount Zion Group

Weiss, Sampson, and their Mount Zion associates are the other group that has developed a formal and highly structured approach to the formulation and articulation of a clinical focus. As presented in their book (Weiss et al., 1986), and in a series of research papers (Curtis & Silberschatz, 1986; Rosenberg et al., 1986; Silberschatz & Curtis, 1986; Silberschatz, Curtis, & Nathan, 1989; Silberschatz, et al., 1986) the plan diagnostic method (or, as it is now called, the plan formulation method) is a clinical research method which is applied to actual clinical material in the form of audiotapes or transcripts to derive a patient-specific focus which can then be utilized to organize and evaluate therapist interventions.

The plan refers to the patient's intention to get better, and how he or she might accomplish this: "In its simplest form, the plan concept states that the patient enters therapy with ideas, or a plan, both conscious and unconscious, for how to overcome his or her problems with the help of the therapist" (Curtis & Silberschatz, 1986, p. 14). Four aspects of the patient's expectations or beliefs about others are generated by the method: goals, obstacles, tests and insights. The patient's *goals* refer to the conscious and unconscious goals the patient has, generally in relation to "pathogenic beliefs." The patient is motivated to be rid of such beliefs, the cause of his or her present suffering. "Goals are the attitudes, mood states, or behaviors that the patient wants to achieve or, if they are undesireable, renounce" (Curtis & Silberschatz, 1986, p. 20). *Obstacles* in this schema refer to these irrational pathogenic beliefs themselves, along with associated symptoms. They are the obstructions that prevent that individual from becoming free to attain his or her goals. *Tests* refer to the unconscious enactment within the therapeutic situation of the patient's central conflictual themes in the effort to become free of his or her pathogenic beliefs. *Insights* are the understandings that may be obtained by the patient, the result of "tests" that are "passed" by the therapist, which will help the patient to attain his or her desired goals and to modify those pathogenic beliefs that cause his or her suffering.

The following example is taken from a research paper published by the Mount Zion group:

Myra, a 30-year-old photographer, sought therapy because she was depressed about her inability to feel committed to a man with whom she had been involved for 6 years. The formulation team inferred that this was another in a series of unsatisfying, masochistic relationships and concluded that Myra's problems stemmed from her extreme worry about her boyfriend—in particular, her fear that he would be destroyed by her leaving. These concerns appeared to be related to Myra's childhood relationship with her mother, who was extremely unhappy in her marriage and constantly complained about how victimized she was by her husband. She relied on Myra as a confidante and as her primary source of emotional support. Because of these experiences, Myra had developed the unconscious belief that if she were either happy alone or fulfilled in a relationship, her mother would feel abandoned and hurt (*Pathogenic belief*). Myra therefore identified with her mother by becoming involved with men in unsatisfying relationships, and she complied with her mother's desire that she always be available to her.

The formulation team diagnosed that Myra's plan for therapy centered on her need to overcome her pathogenic identification and compliance with her mother (*Goal*). This would involve exploring the genetics of her problems and working to disavow the belief that her independence would hurt her mother (and others). She might thus *test* to see if the therapist expected her to be self-sacrificing, if the therapist was critical of her attending to her own needs, or if the therapist was hurt if she expressed disagreement. Myra would be helped by developing *insights* into her identification and compliance with her mother and, in particular, into how she had allowed herself to be victimized in order to avoid feeling blameworthy or guilty. (Silberschatz et al., 1986, p. 648)

Horowitz and the Center for the Study of Neuroses

Horowitz and his colleagues have evolved a brief psychodynamic therapy approach to the treatment of stress response syndromes. As a result, the development of a therapeutic focus takes place within a developmental, phase-oriented approach to loss and mourning. Within this context they apply what Horowitz has termed "person schemas theory," which is the expression of a relational view of personality and psychopathology arising from a conceptualization of internalized representations of self, others, and relationships, or *person schemas*. The following is a clinical vignette illustrating this cognitive-dynamic approach to the formulation of clinical material as it is crystalized around a central precipitant of loss:

> The patient was a young woman in her mid-twenties. She sought help because of feelings of confusion, intense sadness, and loss of initiative six weeks after the sudden, unexpected death of her father. Her first aim was to regain a sense of self-control. This was accomplished within a few sessions, because she had found a substitute for the idealized, positive relationship with her father in the relationship with the therapist and realistically hoped that she could understand and master her changed life circumstances.
>
> As she regained control and could feel pangs of sadness without entering flooded, overwhelmed, or dazed states, she began to wonder what she might further accomplish in the therapy and whether the therapy was worthwhile. The focus gradually shifted from recounting the story of her father's death and her responses, to understanding her past and current inner relationship with her father. The focus of therapy became her vulnerability to entering states governed by defective, weak, and evil self-concepts. These self-concepts related to feelings that her father had scorned her in recent years because she had not lived up to his ideals. He died before she could accomplish her goal of reestablishing a mutual relationship of admiration and respect through her plan to convince him that her own modified career line and life style would lead to many worthwhile accomplishments.
>
> This image of herself as bad and defective was matched by a complementary image of her father as scornful of her. She felt ashamed of herself and angry with him for not confirming her as worthwhile. . . . In this role relationship model, she held him to be strong, even omnipotent, and in a magical way she saw his death as a deliberate desertion of her. These ideas had been warded off because of the intense humiliation and rage that would occur when they were clearly represented. But contemplation of such ideas in therapy allowed her to review and reappraise them, revising her view of herself and of him. (Horowitz, 1991, p. 182)

This clinical formulation illustrates the use of person schemas theory, as we see the description of internalized mental structures interacting with the lifespan stressor of the loss of a parent. We can also see the shift from a focus on the modulation and integration of affects in the earlier phase of treatment to the reworking of internalized object relations in the latter phase.

The Vanderbilt Group

As previously described, the Vanderbilt approach relies upon the concept of cyclical maladaptive patterns to articulate the clinical focus. Strupp and Binder make use of Sullivan's (1954) idea of *participant-observation* as a means of gaining access to the structures that organize the patient's interpersonal world. For them, the patient's important relationships and the relationship with the therapist are understood to be substantially structured by internal representations of objects, self, and interactions. The formulation is thus the therapist's understanding of the central organizing interpersonal structures in the patient: the characteristic patterns of relating, involving the patient's perception of self, others, and their interaction. Strupp and Binder (1984) articulate a scheme that includes four elements:

1. *Acts of self.* These may include all domains of human action, such as affects, and motives ("I feel affectionate toward my mother" or "I wish my wife would pay more attention to me"); perceiving situations ("I sensed we were in a competition together"); cognitions ("I can't stop thinking about how ugly and inferior I am when I meet someone attractive"); or overt behaviors ("I can't refrain from avoiding eye contact with my boss when I'm angry with him").

2. *Expectations about others' reactions.* These are imagined reactions of others to one's own actions and may be conscious, preconscious, or unconscious. To achieve a transactional understanding, these should be articulated in specific relation to some acts of self. . . . Expectations about others' reactions often take a form such as: "If I speak up, I imagine that she will disapprove of me" or "If I ask her out she will just laugh at me."

3. *Acts of others toward self.* These are observed acts of others that are viewed as occurring in specific relation to the acts of self. That is, these actions of others appear (or are assumed) to be evoked by the patient's own actions. . . . Acts of others are typically expressed in a form such as this: "When I asked for the money he ignored me."

4. *Acts of self toward self (introject).* This category of actions refers to how one treats oneself (self-controlling, self-punishing, self-congratulating, self-destroying). These actions should be articulated in specific relation to the acts of self, expectations of others' reactions, and acts of others which compose the remainder of the format. An introject prototypically takes

a form such as: "When my husband praises me I feel guilty and remind myself of my shortcomings" or "When I get angry I just try to slow myself down and think things through. I give myself all the time I need." (pp. 76–77)

This emphasis on current and past interpersonal transactions assumes the centrality of internalized representations of self, other, and interaction in understanding psychopathology and the clinical process. For Strupp and Binder, the function of therapy is to identify maladaptive patterns as they appear in the patient's interactions with others and with the therapist, interpret their meaning, and enable the patient to articulate and modify these entrenched and limiting views of self, others, and their interaction. "One changes as one lives through affectively painful but engrained interpersonal scenarios, and as the therapeutic relationship gives them outcomes different from those expected, anticipated, feared, and sometimes hoped for" (Strupp & Binder, 1984, p. 35).

Therapy, in this view, is a learning process that is affectively charged and experiential, reminiscent of the notion of "corrective emotional experience" (Alexander, 1956). Like other models of brief therapy, a focus for inquiry and attention is formulated based on the clinical material obtained both from history and, particularly, from the interactional qualities of the therapeutic relationship. This "dynamic focus" helps the therapist organize and structure the complex interpersonal and historical information gathered in the early phases of treatment, enabling the therapist to guide the treatment and delimit the work as required by constraints of time. "The TLDP [time-limited dynamic psychotherapy] focus should be understood as an ad hoc individualized theory which clarifies and connects behavioral and experiential phenomena that otherwise appear unrelated and discontinuous" (Strupp & Binder, 1984, p. 67).

The following is a brief clinical example taken from Strupp and Binder (1984):

Catherine was a twenty-seven-year-old educated professional woman who entered therapy complaining of depression and of feeling that she was a freak because she devoted several hours each evening to meticulously trimming her hair. Her hair was so shortened from this activity that she felt forced to wear a wig when in public. Catherine was extremely embarrassed to even relate her presenting complaint to the therapist, and she was mystified by her compulsion to the point of seriously doubting her sanity. In seeking the transactional significance of Catherine's complaints, the therapist began by noting two features of the therapeutic relationship. First, Catherine displayed dramatic, incongruous, and repetitive changes in her emotional state and nonverbal style during the early treatment sessions. Second, she maintained an assiduoulsy professional distance from the therapist. Even when her tone of voice clearly indicated a strong emotional reaction to the therapist's comments, she steadfastly denied having any personal reaction to him. The therapist identified these features of the patient's transactional style as sources of possible hypotheses about her hair-cutting symptom.... [*Three important historical scenarios follow, including Catherine's grandmother lovingly trimming her hair, cutting her hair as a teenager to repudiate the unwelcome advances of a boyfriend, and the abrupt ending of her first deeply romantic relationship at which time her hair-trimming became compulsive.*]

Dynamic Focus

Acts of self. Catherine imagines herself to be globally flawed and defective. She spends many hours trimming her hair, and is especially prone to engage in this behavior when she is feeling distressed about herself. The activity of trimming her hair reflects multiple interpersonal actions, including: (1) symbolically making restitution for her imagined failure to prevent her lover's disappearance; (2) making herself unattractive to ward off the tempting but forbidden attentions of men and especially the possiblity of becoming intimate and having her unworthiness exposed; (3) retaining a sense of control (by perfectionistically cutting each hair to a precise length); and (4) comforting herself through the self-stroking and manipulations of her hair that accompany the trimming activity.

Expectations of others. Catherine imagines that others find her inadequate, especially with respect to her physical appearance. She believes in particular that most men will demonstrate this lack of appreciation by becoming intrusive or attempting to take sexual advantage of her.

Observed reactions of others. Catherine observes that most people have little to do with her. She interprets this as validation of her negative expectations, rather than as a reasonable consequence of her withdrawal.

Introject. Catherine punishes herself with verbal self-recriminations and by refraining from opportunities to engage in potentially pleasureable social activities in order to devote the time to trimming her hair. (pp. 84–86)

This example of a dynamic focus illustrates a number of important facets of the Vanderbilt approach. The presenting symptom is linked to important interpersonal themes, thereby connecting it both to historical relationships and to the evolving therapy relationship. The transactional significance of the symptom and other interpersonal patterns are highlighted. The cyclical aspect of the patient's interaction pattern is noted in how her behavior, based on her own beliefs and expectancies, tends to elicit the very behavior in others which is most painful to her — and confirming of her expectations in the first place. In a more recent discussion of their model, Binder and Strupp (1991) refer to the dynamic focus in terms of the cyclical maladaptive pattern which was described above. Here it can be seen that the therapeutic focus becomes the articulation of the patient's psychopathology in terms of object relational structures.

Case Illustration of a Relational Formulation

We present a vignette of a case to illustrate aspects of a relational formulation, emphasizing features that might distinguish such an approach from one based on a drive/structural formulation. The formulation is presented as the evolving focus of therapeutic activity over the course of a brief dynamic psychotherapy.

> Nora was a 30-year-old single woman who was initially referred by a nutritionist. She was significantly overweight but agreed with the nutritional counselor that she needed more attention than she could find in that setting. When she presented for treatment she described chronic dysphoria, loneliness, and conflict within her family of origin. She had never had a sexual relationship of any kind, and felt she lacked a clear direction in her career. She worked in a division of a large corporation and appeared to be competent in her work, but was prone to becoming embroiled in personality conflicts and office politics in a way that contributed to her discontent with her work situation.
>
> The focus of therapy shifted quickly to her feelings of depression. She revealed a preoccupation with suicidal thoughts dating back to the actual suicide of her college roommate. There was a striking split between her outwardly jovial, cheerful, and even Pollyanna-like demeanor, and the extent of her pain and sadness, which was only acknowledged superficially and in passing.
>
> She was well aware of difficulties in her relationship to her father, who was in some ways a loving parent but also a controlling, critical, and devaluing man prone to explosive outbursts. He seemed to value both her older and younger brothers, who were seen as smart and competent, more than her. Her older sister was developmentally delayed and had developed cervical cancer early in life, requiring the surgical removal of her reproductive organs. Nora's sister continues to live at home with her parents, able to care for herself only to a limited degree.
>
> Nora seemed unaware of the enormous impact her sister's needs had imposed on the family, and herself in particular. Although she expressed irritation at her sister's impairments, it was as if her sister was simply difficult or recalcitrant, rather than truly impaired and limited. It seemed that the family was not able to be fully aware of the extent of the sister's damage, and outwardly denied the full measure of its implications for her or for the family.
>
> Nora described her mother as a passive and even masochistic woman who put up with her father's emotional abuse by making jokes about "the W_____ temper," which allegedly "runs in the men" of the family.

In sessions, Nora uses a childlike, singsong voice, usually appearing chipper and upbeat, describing the week's events as though reciting a list. After a few moments she might stop, saying, "Well, that's it. What do I talk about next?" or "Here I go, rambling again!" Even painful experiences or feelings would be encapsulated in little "chunks" of discourse, with apparently no recognition of their having much connection to anything else in her life.

Over the course of some weeks Nora began to present dreams, recalling that some were continuous with recurrent dream images dating back to adolescence. These were terrifying dreams of being stalked by an intruder, of a man getting into her house or her room while she was sleeping, or feeling as though someone was on top of her holding her down and threatening her with rape or violence. The dreams were very disturbing, particularly because of their repetitiveness and apparent lack of connection to anything in her current life. Yet even these powerful and charged images were contained and stripped of meaning by Nora's presentation of them, minimizing them and quickly moving on to the next item. She was reluctant to discuss their possible meanings in any detailed way.

The dreams became linked with a partially acknowledged fear of her male therapist. In particular, she became afraid that if she revealed either her more disturbing thoughts and feelings, or sexual thoughts and feelings the therapist would send her away. This was initially understood in terms of a fear that her feelings were too much for her father, and that she experienced a deep fear of rejection by him which she connected to her own strong feelings of love and need. She was also frightened that she might be too disturbed for the therapist, and that he would not accept the more chaotic, disorganized and depressed parts of herself.

Now the sessions revolved around the split between her inner experience of self as depressed, rageful, and lacking in clarity and focus on the one hand, and her powerful need to present herself as cheerful, happy, and highly organized and goal-oriented on the other. She became torn between a recognition that her family environment had been profoundly unsupportive in some ways, and feelings of loyalty and protectiveness toward her parents. Nora's anxiety increased dramatically as the split began to lift, and for the first time she became capable of integrated feelings of anger, sadness, and betrayal. She began to recognize how hurt she had been by her father's critical nature and her mother's tendency to minimize the significance of Nora's emotional life, and could feel the sadness and anger connected to these realizations.

The theme of wanting the therapist to "take charge" became elaborated, with more or less direct requests either for advice about various matters or to be told what to talk about. It was as though Nora wanted to be relieved of any power or control and to submit to the therapist's will: "Ask me anything—I'll tell you!" It had to come from the therapist. These requests were made in a singsong-y, whining tone, as though both pleading, seducing, and reproaching the therapist all at once. These requests were understood in a number of ways. First, by having the therapist do the talking Nora would be led away from her own experience, and could thus isolate and contain disturbing feelings. But also she was creating a particular kind of relationship, namely, a submissive and powerless position in relation to a know-ing and powerful man. This masochistic stance was understood to be relat-ed to her deep need for contact with her father, and the feeling that a connection with him was not possible on terms in which her own power and authority would be respected. Nora wondered whether this concealed sub-missive part of herself was so disturbing to her that she had avoided all inti-mate contact with men, fearing that any such relationship would involve the same disturbing pattern as that with her father. In a way, her isolation preserved her from the pain of her relationship with her father, in which emotional abuse and love were intermingled. Perhaps love could only be had on such painful terms, terms that, thus far, Nora had rejected. She did not yet have faith that some other, more fulfilling kind of intimacy might be possible.

Much of Nora's personality then could be understood in terms of the con-flict between her longing for contact with her father and the sense of hu-miliation, self-negation, and depression that would accompany contact with him. Her problem with food seemed related both to a need for self-regulation and control, and a need to keep others at a distance, particularly in a romantic or sexual sense. The dream images depicted her experience of powerless-ness, and the violation of her sense of self and self-boundaries. That these dreams might also represent actual physical or sexual violation can only be entertained as a possibility at this point in the ongoing psychotherapy. They might represent, too, the erotization of powerlessness and fear, conveying some underlying sexual fantasy which as yet is unacceptable and only bare-ly acknowledged by the patient. More generally, her tendency toward sub-mission can be understood as the repetition of her relationship to her father, expressing both the expectation that such a relationship is the only one pos-sible with a man, and the deep longing for a more fulfilling intimacy in which love and power are not mutually exclusive choices.

This vignette is certainly not presented as a full or complete formulation—if such a thing were even possible. It is not presented as the only possible understanding of the case. But we wish to high-light some differences between a relational approach and a drive/structural one. First, the masochistic longings are not understood as derivatives of an innate aggressive instinct which has been redirect-ed toward the self (Freud, 1924/1958). In fact, here we do not find any need to rely on the notion of instinctual aggression. The masochism instead is seen as the repetition of a lived, experienced object relation-ship which has been internalized and which continues to shape the pa-tient's experience of herself, others, and their interaction. *What is internalized is a relational configuration.* We might add that the internali-zation includes images of the parental relationship, as well as her iden-tifications with both mother and father.

Second, we do not rely here on any notion of the frustration of a basic sexual drive in the context of an oedipal conflict. Although the patient struggles with oedipal and sexual issues, they take the form of seeking emotional contact with her father and the validation of her sense of herself as a person and as a female being. What is primary is her seeking recognition and connection, rather than gratification of an infantile fantasy of excluding her mother and possessing her father sexually, along with the defenses against such wishes.

Finally, the characterological aspects of Nora's difficulties can be understood as the result of her adaptive efforts to regulate herself in the context of her particular developmental environment. For example, her reliance on denial, isolation of affect, and intellectualization can be thought of as means to regulate internal states to avoid more painful or unmanageable experience. Such defense mechanisms can be thought of as the solution to a need for self-regulation that was not adequately met by her early environment; that is, self-regulation in the face of a failure of environmental regulation. Perhaps certain inner states and feelings were not "mirrored" or recognized by caretakers, and were left, thereby, unvalidated or negated. Thus, Nora came to feel she could not express negative feelings, angry feelings, or sexual feelings. In fact, this may reflect some mixture of actual and fantasied anxiety or rejection on the part of her parents in response to the expression of such feelings. A more drive-oriented model would lead to a different understanding of these defenses, emphasizing instead Nora's need to keep contained and repressed unacceptable sexual and aggressive wishes that had arisen during the course of her early development.

THE SELECTION CRITERIA: INDICATIONS AND CONTRAINDICATIONS

While the earlier drive/structural model of brief therapy places emphasis on the issues of patient selection and suitability, the relational model under consideration here on the whole does not do so. These therapies place considerably less demand on the patient, particularly in their lesser emphasis on the use of confrontation of resistances and defenses, which is characteristic of the drive/structural models. In fact, the relational approaches of brief psychotherapy tend to have more in common with the practice of dynamic psychotherapy in general, and so tend to rely on more traditional views of psychodynamic therapies regarding the issue of patient selection. Further, the relational perspective tends to place more weight on the therapist's personality characteristics, as well as the unique interpersonal and intersubjective field that emerges in the therapeutic relationship, and thus deemphasizes patient characteristics taken in isolation.

Nonetheless, Strupp and Binder (1984) list the characteristics that they associate with a successful brief treatment.

1. *Emotional discomfort.* The patient is sufficiently uncomfortable with his or her feelings and/or behavior to seek help via psychotherapy.
2. Basic trust...
3. Willingness to consider conflicts in interpersonal terms...
4. Willingness to examine feelings...
5. *Capacity for mature relationships.* The patient evinces sufficient capacity for relating to others as separate individuals so that identifiable relationship predispositions, no matter how painful and conflict ridden, can be enacted in the therapy relationship and then collaboratively examined...
6. *Motivation for the treatment offered.* ... the assessment of motivation is reflected in the judgements reflected in criteria 1 through 5. (pp. 57–58)

We can readily see from this list that more medically oriented, DSM kinds of diagnostic categories, or even more dynamically conceived categories such as "hysterical," "obsessional," "neurotic," and "character pathology," are not viewed as relevant to the expectations for the patient's success or failure in brief therapy. "The object relations capacities sought in potential TLDP [time-limited dynamic psychotherapy] patients may be detected across a broad range of formal diagnostic syndromes. Therefore, neither a presenting symptom nor the diagnosis of a specific personality disorder will itself justify exclusion from this form of treatment" (Binder & Strupp, 1991, p. 139). The criteria above are principally interpersonal and psychological, and can be assessed only from within the therapeutic situation. This is a form of interpersonal diagnosis, with the therapist's use of self as a crucial ingredient. Nonetheless, it can be noted that some of these criteria, such as "the capacity for mature relationships," must be highly correlated with the quality of object relations, and thus, with certain diagnostic dimensions such as the structural distinctions between neurotic, borderline, and psychotic personality organization (Kernberg, 1976).

Horowitz applies a rather more traditional criterion for suitability, focusing his attention on the particular group of patients to which he has tended to apply brief psychotherapy, namely, those suffering traumatic losses, with consequent stress reactions. He addresses the issue of selection in the following statement:

Time-limited psychotherapy is a useful technique if the traumatic event is relatively recent and if the person does not have an excessively conflictual or deficient personality structure. In the approach developed with my colleagues, we excluded persons with psychotic or borderline personality disorders, persons involved in litigation, and persons who had experienced a complex and long series of linked traumatic events. We focused instead on accepting for study persons who developed a neurotic level of illness. (Horowitz, 1991, p. 168)

The Penn group also tends to take a broad psychodynamic approach to the issue of patient suitability, noting that short-term supportive–expressive psychotherapy "is suitable for many kinds of patients" (Luborsky & Mark, 1991, p. 112). They, too, recommend screening out most borderline or psychotic patients, noting that patients with personality disorders may often require longer treatment. They rely on the supportive-expressive dimension to address the issue of degree of psychopathology, allowing for a greater measure of "supportive" techniques in the treatment of relatively sicker patients, and a greater measure of "expressive" techniques for healthier patients.

Published research from the Penn Psychotherapy Project suggests that treatment outcome is modestly but significantly correlelated with initial patient characteristics, most notably as rated on the Health-Sickness rating scale, a very general measure of psychological health, with healthier patients showing better psychotherapy outcomes (Luborsky et al., 1988).

The work of the Mount Zion group tends to be highly concerned with the psychotherapeutic *process,* addressing through theory and empirical research questions pertaining to the facillitation of therapeutic progress or its hindrance (Weiss et al., 1986). For this reason their work tends to have relatively little to say about patient selection or suitability, emphasizing the ongoing flow of psychotherapeutic interaction rather than initial patient characteristics. Because it is in the nature of the clinical hypotheses explored by this group, their research involves close analysis of clinical data of very small numbers of clinical cases; it does not appear possible on this basis to develop generalizations about patient suitability. It is probably safe to say that their selection criteria would overlap substantially with those of the other models presented here, tending to be broader rather than narrower.

THE THEORY OF CHANGE

In the previous chapter we discussed the principles of change as they are understood within a psychoanalytic framework in general, as well as the specific factors associated with the brief drive/structural models of psychotherapy. Here we take up those factors which are more specifically associated with the relational approaches to brief psychotherapy.

It is worth emphasizing that little is to be gained by attempting to make absolute distinctions and dichotomies. The clinical reality is that the process of change as understood psychoanalytically is sufficiently complex and multidimensional so that any theory will draw on various change processes, and great overlap exists between those therapies relying more on drive theory and those which are more relationally oriented. Rather than redundantly citing many of the same change factors, we will try to articulate the particular configuration of change factors as presented by the relational models under consideration.

From a relational viewpoint, therapeutic change is understood to rely on several related ideas in addition to traditional psychodynamic factors such as catharsis, ego support, and emotional insight. There is an emphasis on "two-person" processes in the therapeutic setting, including the use of the therapist in a therapeutic object relationship. As in drive/structural models, interpretation of transference is central; however, transference is conceptualized differently, and there is more emphasis on the "here-and-now" dimension of transference. In addition, the idea of "corrective emotional experience" is utilized, as the role of new experience in the therapeutic relationship is elevated and the role of insight diminished relative to the drive/structural model.

Shift from the Intrapsychic to Self and Other

We wish to briefly review the development of certain object relational ideas of what is curative about psychotherapy. These ideas can be counterposed to the centrality of interpretation of unconscious psychic contents, particularly genetic interpretation, which forms the core of the theory of change in more drive-based psychoanalysis and its short-term derivatives.

Melanie Klein's (1946) development of the idea of projection, and projective and introjective identification, marks the beginning of a fundamental shift in the way the therapeutic relationship can be understood. When Klein developed her concept of the infant's fantasy of expelling unwanted psychic contents into the body of the mother, she was creating the foundation for a "two-person" psychology as opposed to the "one-person" psychology that arises from more drive-oriented aspects of Freud's metapsychology (Aron, 1990). Rather than the individual struggling within him- or herself to maintain equilibrium and balance among the conflicting aspects of the personality in relation to instinctually gratifying objects, Klein's view opens up the possibility of the use of an object to serve psychic functions other than drive reduction (though the object can serve that function, too). It is these other psychic functions of the therapist that form the basis of object relations theories of therapeutic change.

Winnicott's (1965) notions of the "holding environment," the "maturational environment," and transitional phenomena are examples of the further development of "two-person" psychologies, with the basic unit of psychological experience organized around transactions of self with other. In his view what is curative is the gradual resumption of developmental processes that had been hampered or interfered with by deficient contributions of the primary maternal object. The therapist facilitates such progress to a very great extent though emotional reliability, availability, nonintrusiveness, and respect for the patient's autonomy and separateness—in short, functioning much in the fashion of a more or less optimal mother figure. In Winnicott's view, the more serious the early traumata, the less the therapist can rely on "standard" psychoanalytic techniques, and the more one relies on the relational characteristics of the therapy relationship.

Michael Balint's (1968) concept of the "basic fault" is another line in the development of object relations clinical theory. In his discussion of the "area of the basic fault," Balint delineates two levels of psychoanalytic work, the first being the "standard" level of psychoanalysis, concerning itself with oedipal difficulties and their resolution through interpretation of the transference. It is the second level, addressing more problematic areas of regression both malignant and benign, that Balint refers to as requiring the therapeutic agency of object relationship, as opposed to that of interpretation (Balint, 1968, p. 173). For the patient in a regressed state, the clinical technique is summarized as follows: "the analyst must accept the regression. This means that he must create an environment, a climate, in which he and his patient can tolerate the regression in a mutual experience" (Balint, 1968, p. 177).

Bion's (1970) notion of "the container and the contained" represents a refinement and development of the Kleinian concepts of projection and projective identification. Here again the concept arises in the context of the relationship of mother and infant. The mother serves a "containing function" for the infant by accepting the infant's projected contents, using her own psychic structure to "metabolize" them such that the transformed contents can be returned to the infant in a form which is not traumatic to the infant, and is therefore useful in the development of psychic structure. Here, the therapist can be thought of as a kind of auxilliary processor, helping to detoxify, manage, and digest the patient's experiences in a way that facilitates growth and development.

Kohut's (1977, 1984) description of "selfobject" transferences represents another kind of use of the object. In many respects similar to Winnicott's notions of the maturational environment, the selfobject concept refers to the early and ongoing experience of primary caretakers providing essential psychological functions for the individual along the lines of needed narcissistic affirmation and recognition.

For Freud, the first instinctual object is the self in the state of "primary narcissism" (Freud, 1917/1958). Thus, libido, or the sexual instinct, is first expressed as self-cathexis, or as narcissistic libido. The process of ego development proceeds along the trajectory from self to object, with the same underlying libidinal engine. Narcissistic aims are viewed as infantile and primitive in comparison to object-oriented aims in this unidirectional, temporal schema of drive theory. Kohut takes the concept of narcissism out of the context of instinct theory, and proposes instead a separate developmental line which proceeds along the dimension of the development of and vicissitudes of the self. In this view, narcissism is a lifelong aspect of human being and relating, with a progression not from narcissism to object relating, but instead from earlier, "archaic" forms of narcissism, such as unbridled fantasies of omnipotence and power, toward more mature and differentiated forms of expression, such as satisfaction in having one's work recognized and appreciated. For Freud, the object is a discovery imposed by the limitations of self-satisfaction. For Kohut, the selfobject is there from the beginning in the maturational milieu, providing regulating and organizing functions.

The selfobject relationship takes place prior to the recognition of the other as a separate object, and involves the use of needed psychological functions which the selfobject serves. This is the use the maternal figure is put to by the infant and small child, who require a particular kind of ego-centered recognition, affirmation, and "mirroring." Based on this understanding of development, the therapeutic change process involves the return to early forms of narcissistic relating as the therapist continues to provide an adequate mirroring of the patient's experience, particularly around traumas to the self and self-esteem. A consistent empathic stance enables "transmuting internalizations" to take place, with resulting development of psychic structures previously provided for by the selfobject. This permits transformation of archaic narcissistic fantasies into more adequate and mature forms of narcissism.

Each of the above are examples of therapeutic concepts that have extended psychoanalytic understanding of the therapeutic relationship and the nature of the psychotherapeutic change process. Though applicable only to varying and limited degree to each of the four short-term therapies discussed in the present chapter, they form the basis for clinical theory that places the patient–therapist relationship at the center of the therapeutic change process, and lead to clinical techiques that are complementary to interpretation as it is more traditionally understood. It might be said that object relations theories have provided us with a means for understanding how a relationship in and of itself can be therapeutic, beyond its role as a vehicle for clinical interpretation. Furthermore, these concepts lead to modifications and alterations in the clinical setup itself, the atmosphere and emotional quality of the treatment situation, and the affective coloration of the therapeutic relationship.

Although all the theorists just discussed have worked in the context of time-unlimited therapies and psychoanalysis, we shall see in the following sections how some of these ideas have been directly applied to the practice of brief psychotherapy.

Interpretation of Transference in the Here-and-Now

All four relational brief psychotherapies place emphasis on the here-and-now interaction between patient and therapist, a hallmark of the interpersonal influence to which the Vanderbilt group explicitly alludes:

> Our research has called forceful attention to the overriding importance of the dyadic *interactions* between patient and therapist over the course of therapy, with a special emphasis on the early phases. Thus, our approach forms part of a movement toward a greater integration of classical and interpersonal psychoanalytic theory and technique — in short, nothing less than a reconceptualization of transference and countertransference phenomena in interactional terms. (Binder & Strupp, 1991, p. 138)

Transference is understood not as distortion or projection by the patient onto the blank screen of the neutral analyst, but rather as the inevitable expression of the patient's construction of interpersonal reality, shaped and determined by his or her personal development and experience (Gill, 1979; 1982; Hoffman, 1983). Special attention is paid to the countertransference as a particularly valuable source of information about the patient's object relations. Countertransference is understood, in part, in terms of the therapist's feelings and reactions complementary to the patient's own. Thus, countertransference, in one of its aspects, is understood to be a kind of "interpersonal empathy," the therapist's transient participation in the enactments of the patient's inner world of representations of self and other. Drawing on Levenson (1982), it appears that Binder and Strupp (1991) view such countertransference enactments as inevitable as the patient "transforms" the therapist: "There are times when it is extraordinarily difficult for the therapist to avoid enmeshment in the patient's scenarios" (p. 146).

This view is distinct from the drive/structural model's view of transference as the transfer of drive–defense constellations from infantile situations onto the person of the therapist. Such a view implies the inaccuracy or inappropriateness of the transferred feelings and conflicts, and is consistent with the classical Freudian view of the therapist as a blank screen onto which patients project their fantasies, wishes, and conflicts. Object relational views of transference tend to emphasize the activation and repetition of internalized relationship scenarios that consist of ideas or beliefs about the self, others, and interaction between self and others. Transference in this view represents patients' return to or re-creation of previously experienced relationships, as they attempt to rectify pathogenic situations, or return to desired and longed-for states of connectedness and contact with significant others.

Corrective Experience as a Basic Curative Factor

Whereas the drive/structural model emphasizes accurate interpretation leading to insight as the chief curative factor in psychoanalytic psychotherapy, relational therapies place a higher value on corrective aspects of the therapeutic relationship and its setting. This emphasis can be traced back historically to its origin in Ferenzci's explorations of "active technique," via the reparation of developmental deficiencies and other alterations in psychoanalytic technique related to his belief in the centrality of trauma in the genesis of psychopathology (Ferenczi, 1921/1980, 1988; Ferenzci & Rank, 1925/1986). As noted previously, Balint's (1968) notion of working at the level of "the basic fault" requires at times the clinical provision of certain forms of gratification. The line of development continues in the work of Franz Alexander (Alexander, 1956; Alexander & French, 1946), who coined the expression "corrective emotional experience" and continued the earlier experiments in active techniques utilizing relational aspects of the therapeutic setting.

From this standpoint, interpretation is seen as important but other processes take on greater weight, such as the internalization of the therapist and the nonoccurrence of expected pathogenic or traumatic experiences in the therapeutic relationship. Something new occurs in the interactional sphere between patient and therapist. Mitchell (1988) describes it this way, in the context of psychoanalytic treatment: "The analyst's dogged inquiry into anxiety-ridden areas of the patient's life, and his participation in new forms of interaction, enables the patient to encounter, name, and appreciate facets of his experience unknown before. The analysand can now be a different sort of person in his experience of the analyst and others than he could allow himself to be before," (p. 289). Here it can be seen that interpretation itself is understood in a new way, not just as allowing for unconscious contents to become conscious, but as permitting new kinds of experience of one's self and others.

In Weiss and Sampson's (Weiss et al., 1986) theory, the patient "tests" the therapist in the hope of "disconfirming" pathogenic beliefs. "By such testing the patient seeks experiences with the analyst that he may use in his struggle to disconfirm his pathogenic beliefs. He seeks experiences that are new in that they are different from the traumatic experiences with his parents (or other significant individuals) from which he had inferred his pathogenic beliefs" (p. 329).

Strupp and Binder similarly refer to the importance of new experience in the therapeutic relationship, with an interpersonal focus as a reference point: "Essentially, the therapist uses the relationship with the therapist as the primary medium for bringing about change. What the patient learns in psychotherapy, what conduces to therapeutic change, is acquired primarily in and through the dynamics of the therapeutic relationship," (Binder & Strupp, 1991, p. 142).

Luborsky and his associates (Luborsky, 1984; Luborsky & Crits-Christoph, 1990; Luborsky et al., 1988) have tended to separate the supportive role of the therapeutic relationship in the form of a "helping alliance" from the insights that the patient must obtain (Luborsky, 1984). Luborsky makes direct refererence to Freud's "unobjectionable positive transference" (Freud, 1912a/1958) in his discussion of the evolution of the concept of "helping alliance" (Luborsky, 1984, p. 24), understood to be "the patient's ability to experience the relationship with the therapist as helpful" (Luborsky, 1984, p. 24). In this sense, Luborksy and his colleagues seem to propose a clinical theory more closely aligned with a traditional psychoanalytic view of an auxilliary "working alliance" which facilitates and supports the central curative power of interpretation of transference (Zetzel, 1956).

Nonetheless, the research findings of the Penn group have consistently supported the centrality of the "helping alliance" as a predictor of successful psychotherapy outcome and as the foundation of successful treatment (Luborsky et al., 1980, 1985, 1988; Woody et al., 1983). Further, Luborsky notes that "even though the two curative factors [insight and helping alliance] work in tandem, when they are isolated for the sake of comparison, the power of the relationship may prove to be the more potent of the two" (Luborsky, 1984, p. 28).

Horowitz relies on his "person schemas theory" to conceptualize the change process (Horowitz, 1988, 1991). In this view the process involves interactions with the therapist which gradually enable a shifting or evolution of structures of self and other to permit integration of new, stressful, or traumatic events. His language incorporates that of cognitive and information-processing theories, concepualizing the change process as involving modification of schemas through integration with other schemas, modification of existing schemas, or the formation of new superordinate schemas (Horowitz, 1991). "Achieving schematic change may require many repetitions in the effort to recognize new realities and practice new ways of thinking and acting. Change requires conscious and/or unconscious conceptual processing" (Horowitz, 1991, p. 168). These new cognitive structures permit more objective appraisal and interpretation of events so as to allow for more adaptive responses. The mourning process illustrates the notion of schematic change, as the survivor works and reworks his or her experience of the loss and its meaning, to gradually internalize the idea that the ongoing, living relationship with the deceased is ended. Identity must be reformed around the absence, and new patterns of relating must be devised.

Such notions of what is curative in therapy follow directly from an object relational conception of psychopathology, as opposed to one arising from a drive/structural model. If psychopathology is understood to develop as the result of unacknowledged infantile fantasies pressing on the capacities of the ego, as in drive theory, then increased awareness of such conflict will permit reorganization of these forces to the benefit of the patient's functioning. On the other hand, if psychopathology is understood to be the result of disturbed object ties and repetitive patterns of maladaptive behavior arising from particular representations of self and others, *then it follows that the treatment process must modify those representations.* The use of the therapeutic relationship thus becomes of great importance, with the *process* of that relationship being as important as the *content* of interpretations offered.

THE TECHNIQUES OF THE THERAPY

As with the theories of change, the relational approaches to brief therapy overlap greatly with the previously discussed drive/structural model in their conceptualizations of technique. Although the use of interpretation remains central, the way in which interpretation is understood to function is different in certain fundamental ways. Naturally, other psychotherapeutic techniques such as clarification, confrontation, and inquiry also have their place in relational therapies as in any psychodynamic therapy.

The present group of relational therapies place much less emphasis on specialized clinical techniques such as confrontation of resistances
or early and frequent use of transference interpretation than did the
"first generation" of brief dynamic therapies (Chapter 2). In most
respects, the four therapies discussed in this chapter represent a cross-
section of psychodynamic techniques generally practiced and, as such,
do not appear to make special or different demands on the therapist
or patient. Nonetheless, these models have elaborated technical guidelines and specific predictions about the nature of clinical interventions
and their effects on the clinical process. The following is a discussion
of general technical principles that characterize the four relational therapies as a group, as well as the formulation-specific features of each.

Attention to the Therapeutic Dyad and Interpersonal Patterns

At the level of clinical theory, each of the four relational approaches
share a number of technical principles, all more or less compatible with
the practice of psychodynamic psychotherapy in general. Based on an
interpersonal and object relational theory of psychopathology, each
therapy pays particular attention to the ongoing interactional process
in the therapeutic setting, with recognition of, and subsequent interpretation of, transactional patterns as they are manifested in the therapeutic relationship. Thus, interpretation is aimed at the clarification of and
reworking of interpersonal patterns and dynamics, linking transferential events to patterns in other current and past relationships, with a
clinical focus on recurrent and cyclical phenomena and maintaining
factors.

Shift from Therapist as Objective Observer to Participant-Observer

The epistemological status of the psychoanalyst in the psychoanalytic
situation, in Freud's view, was analogous to that of the scientist in the
laboratory. The well-analyzed therapist was expected to understand and
objectively interpret the material presented by the patient. The optimal
therapist was thought not to impinge on the therapeutic process. In
contrast, the relational therapies presented here are characterized by
a greater emphasis on the real characteristics of the therapist. Further,
the therapy situation is understood to be the product of the personality of the therapist as well as the patient, and the therapist is not accorded a radically different epistemological status from the patient. The
relationship is seen more as a dyadic interpersonal field, with the sub-

jectivity of the therapist forming an essential aspect of the treatment process. Corresponding to a greater allowance for the plausibility of the patient's perceptions of the therapist is an increased emphasis on the accuracy of the patient's experience of his early environment. This is in distinction to the drive theorist's assumption that the patient's experience of reality is primarily a function of intrapsychic processes and conflicts. Harold Sampson (1992) of the Mount Zion group describes the acquisition of pathogenic beliefs: "A child acquires (i.e., constructs) beliefs about reality by inference from experience.... The child's inferences in constructing a belief are influenced by various factors.... Beliefs about reality are, of course, subjective, but they are influenced, in most instances quite powerfully, by actual experiences" (p. 515). The characteristics of the external situation, whether the individual's early environment or aspects of the therapeutic situation, are understood to be important determinants of that experience.

This understanding, as well as the diminution of the therapist's authority as the final arbiter of reality, is expressed in the idea of participant-observation. In this view, first proposed by Sullivan (1954) and elaborated by others in the interpersonal and relational tradition (Aron, 1990; Gill 1982; Havens, 1976; Hirsch, 1985; Hoffman, 1983, 1992), the therapist is seen as inexorably involved in the interpersonal and intersubjective system of patient and therapist, and therefore is accorded no categorically distinct access to reality. The therapist is placed in the paradoxical position of observing the patient's drama, which includes the therapist, and participating in that drama in an ongoing, active way. Thus, the patient's experience always includes the characteristics of the therapist as they are construed by the patient; this is differentiated from the idea of the patient projecting onto the blank screen of the classical Freudian analyst, who can impartially observe the manifestations of the transference relationship.

Each of the four therapies, to varying degrees, implicitly or explicitly apply the notion of participant-observation. Strupp and Binder (1984) make the most direct statements in this regard, alluding to their debt to the interpersonal tradition and emphasizing, as they do, the inevitability of the therapist's participation in the patient's enactments. They also clearly articulate the idea of the therapist shifting back and forth between different modes of relating, first participating, then observing, reflecting, and interpreting that which has been enacted.

Horowitz presents an explicitly epistemological model of the mind, in which individuals come to "know" about the world of self and others not "as it is," but rather through internalized representations of self and other, within a framework he calls "person schemas theory." This constructivist theory suggests that therapists, like patients, have no choice but to construct the world in terms of particular "schemas," and by implication, the schemas of the therapist are not categorically different from those of his or her patient. Therefore the therapist does not have access to a "better" knowledge of reality than his or her patient has, although it is not likely to be limited, constrained, or structured by the same themes, beliefs, feelings, and so on.

An immediate consequence of this shift from objectivism to perspectivism is a view of therapy as intrinsically inexact, as a function of the involvement of the therapist as an imperfect agent of change. While the four therapies differ in this regard, there is a common emphasis on shifts in the quality of the patient–therapist relationship, the therapist's responses to the patient's reactions, working with mistakes and misunderstanding, and the therapist's use of self to understand what is going on in the clinical situation. The importance of making the exact, correct interpretation diminishes, as does the emphasis on nongratification of transference wishes as a means of bringing into awareness unconscious mental contents. Reenactment of troubling interpersonal scenarios within the therapeutic relationship is understood to be inevitable, and the working through of those scenarios forms a crucial part of the therapeutic endeavor. The following vignette illustrates enactment and its therapeutic use:

The patient, a bright, young, psychologically minded single professional female sought psychotherapy to deal with anxiety and grief following the breakup of a relationship. About 10 weeks into weekly psychotherapy she began to make requests of the therapist around issues like scheduling and other practical matters with very little advance notice or discussion. Each request would be conveyed with a sense of great urgency and drama. The therapist first would make unusual efforts to arrange things in accord with the request, and only later would become aware of the accompanying irritation and annoyance about the feeling that there was no choice about meeting them. Through the countertransference experience of feeling controlled, abandoned, and taken for granted, the therapist came to understand the patient's own dread and anxiety about abandonment and intrusion. Once the therapist recognized his emotional response to the patient, it was possible to raise the issue with the patient without undue anxiety or pressure. Patient and therapist began to explore the terror of intimacy, which could be broken up or disrupted by the histrionic demands made by the patient in her attempt to regain control and safety.

We emphasize that the working through of this enactment pattern could only take place *after* its relational enactment, including the complementary and convergent feelings in the therapist, with their recognition being inseparable from their enactment.

The Penn Group

The following is a list of technical principles taken from Luborsky and Mark (1991):

- Be sensitive to allowing the patient to form a helping alliance.
- Formulate and respond about the central relationship patterns.
- Attend and respond to each sphere of the relationship triad, including the one with the therapist.
- Understand and respond about where the symptom fits into the patterns.
- Responses should be timed in relation to the patient's awareness.
- Recognize the patient's need to test the relationship in transference terms.
- Frame the symptoms as problem-solving or coping attempts.
- Reflect on your usual types of countertransference responses.
- Interventions should be timed to suit the length of a session.
- Interventions should be limited in complexity and length.
- The patient's shifts in mental state can be an opportunity for responses.
- The match of patient and therapist messages is a measure of the adequacy of the therapist's responses. (pp. 120–130)

Although none of these principles are specific to the practice of short-term psychotherapy, a general adherence to these will facilitate time-limited work, since they emphasize focality and therapist activity. It should be noted that in the earlier work of Luborsky and his associates there is little reference to the time limitation of psychotherapy, and the principles of technique outlined are most properly thought of as the articulation of principles of psychodynamic psychotherapy defined more broadly. However, some principles of technique have been formulated to address the special needs of the time-limited therapy situation:

The two main distinctive qualities of SE-TL [time-limited psychotherapy] are summed up here:

1. *Time Limit.* The crucial difference between SE [supportive–expressive therapy] and SE-TL is in the time limit and its consequences. Fixing that time limit has shaping effects throughout the treatment. In SE-TL the therapist and patient agree on the time limit, sometimes with a provision for a follow-up. The limit is usually less than 25 sessions.

2. *Consistent Therapeutic Focus.* Both treatment formats, the supportive-expressive therapy (SE) and the SE-TL are "focal psychotherapies" in that a selection is made early in the treatment of a primary goal around which the therapeutic work is to be concentrated. SE-TL has more of this concentration on a particular focus. Usually, the focus is on a facet of the core conflictual relationship theme (CCRT) and the symptoms connected with it. That facet is usually related to one of the patient's goals. In its concentration on a particular goal, SE-TL more than SE is in the lineage of short-term psychotherapies which include Balint (1972), Malan (1963, 1976), Sifneos (1972), and Mann (1973). (Luborsky, 1984, p. 160)

The Penn group organizes its approach to clinical technique around the poles of "supportive" and "expressive" interventions (Luborsky, 1984; Luborsky & Mark, 1991). Although these refer to the traditional dichotomy of supportive psychotherapy versus psychoanalysis as a purely interpretive approach, Luborsky and his colleagues clearly suggest that the two are more properly thought of as elements of all therapeutic interventions. These two aspects of technique are tied directly to the Penn group's concepts of the "helping alliance" and the attainment of insight and understanding, which form the basis for their view of the curative effects of psychotherapy (Luborsky, 1984). (In a sense, the relative emphasis on the therapeutic importance of the "helping relationship" adds to our comfort in placing this therapy in the current relational context.)

Supportive techniques include the therapist conveying warmth, respect, acceptance, realistic optimism, and encouragement of self-expression, and the creation of a collaborative atmosphere (Luborsky, 1984, pp. 81–89). These items may be more properly thought of as emotional and psychological characteristics of the therapist and the therapeutic setting rather than aspects of "technique." This emphasis appears to be part of an evolution in psychoanalytic clinical theory toward the correction of earlier positions that had gone to an extreme in clinical abstinence resulting from certain narrow interpretations of Freud's own clinical recommendations (Stone, 1961). As Luborksy points out, "The concern with proper technique sometimes is unnecessarily responsible for the therapist's restraining his interest and inhibiting conformity with the usual social amenities" (Luborksy, 1984, p. 67). There has been increased interest in the "supportive" aspects of the curative effects of psychotherapy, and increased recognition of its importance in the outcome of treatment (Wallerstein, 1986). This may be part of a larger "relational shift" that has been taking place across varied psychoanalytic schools of thought.

A great deal of attention is paid to what Luborsky has termed "expressive" techniques. These have been explicated at length in Luborsky's manual of supportive–expressive treatment (Luborsky, 1984) and in a more recent discussion (Luborsky & Mark, 1991), and will be noted briefly here.

Techniques for listening mainly involve the recognition of relationship patterns and their connections to the patient's presenting problems. Naturally, the formulation of the CCRT is a central aspect of how the therapist hears what the patient is saying about his or her relationships and the symptoms which occur within that context. For instance, one technical principle is "understanding the symptoms in the context of relationships" (Luborsky, 1984). In the following example, a connection is made between past relationships and the therapeutic relationship:

THERAPIST: Each time I notice and comment that you are looking attractive or that you're doing well in your work you get tearful and cry.

PATIENT (*crying*): I feel I am not attractive. I feel I will be rejected. Father could never stand it. I won a ribbon in a race and he only could say the competition was not too great. Dad did the same restricting with Mother. She even had to limit her vocabularly for him.

THERAPIST: I see, so you feel you have some well established old reasons for feeling that way with me. (Luborsky, 1984, p. 96)

Other principles for listening and understanding clinical material address the need to attend to shifts in patient state; attending to current, past, and transference relationship spheres; understanding the patient's symptoms as attempts to solve relationship problems; and attending to the patient's perceptions of the therapist.

Principles for therapist interventions similarly are organized around the development of a CCRT. The following listing is quoted from the supportive–expressive treatment manual (Luborsky, 1984, pp. 120–141).

Principle 1. The therapist's response should deal effectively with a facet of the main relationship problem and at times relate that to one of the symptoms.

Principle 2. The therapist should recurrently recognize the core relationship theme since it facilitates the working through.

Principle 3. The therapist should recognize the patient's need to test the relationship in transference terms.

Principle 4. The therapist should recognize that both therapist and patient find it especially hard to deal with the patient's experience of the relationship with the therapist.

Principle 5. The therapist should stay with the main relationship theme because it provides a focus which furthers the alliance and sense of progress.

Principle 6. Achieving the goals of treatment requires a different degree of working through and attendant insight for each patient.

Principle 7. A matching of patient's and therapist's messages serves as a test of the therapist's response in a session.

Principle 8. Responses should be timed to take into account how near the patient is to being aware of the content of the proposed response.

Principle 9. The extensiveness and complexity of each interpretive statement should be limited.

Principle 10. The therapist needs patience and restraint about responding interpretively until the therapist's understanding is adequate.

Principle 11. Responses should be timed to take into account the length of the session.

Principle 12. Countering countertransference (alertness to the existence of countertransference).

Principle 13. "Near responding," the inclination to think of responding countertherapeutically, provides a good basis for understanding the patient (recognizing countertransference reactions before acting on them).

The Center for the Study of Neuroses

Horowitz and his associates have described psychotherapeutic techniques in the time-limited treatment of "stress response syndromes" (Horowitz, 1986, 1991; Horowitz, Marmar, Weiss, et al., 1984). These techniques are elaborations and modifications of general principles of psychodynamic psychotherapy. At their core is Horowitz's notion of "person schemas theory," discussed earlier. Therapy is aimed at the modification and realignment of internalized representations of self and others in the context of a psychodynamic information-processing view of personality.

In particular, Horowitz emphasizes the importance of phase specificity in the treatment of loss. The chief discrimination made is between the "intrusive–repetitive" phase of a stress response and the "denial–numbing" phase, each having a corresponding type of intervention. For the intrusive-repetitive phase, interventions are largely supportive and ameliorative, with the therapist taking on ego functions of regulation, control, suppression, and the reduction of internally overwhelming affect states. On the other hand, for the denial–numbing phase the emphasis is on the encouragement of the patient's emotional exploration, self-expression, catharsis, and the reduction of controls over these.

The phase-oriented approach to technique leads to a shifting of therapeutic emphasis over the course of the treatment, with a realignment of the therapeutic focus from the immediate symptoms of the stress response to the patient's schemas of self and others and of relationships. There may be an increase in confrontation of resistances and defenses and attention to the transference relationship as the scope of the treatment is expanded, though the stress event remains the core of the therapeutic focus, serving to organize these other clinical "activities" (Horowitz, 1991).

Table 3.2 identifies the therapeutic techniques associated with the various stages of therapy. The model very clearly delineates the therapist's responses to the initial stressing event as well as to underlying central conflicts that are understood in the context of the immediate life stressor. Also emphasized is attention to the transference, particularly as it arises in the context of the time limit and termination. Though it is not made explicit in the table, Horowitz's approach to formulating the patient's central conflicts, as discussed previously, is relational in nature, attending to recurring patterns of interpersonal behavior and experience and internalized representations of self, other, and interaction.

The Mount Zion Group

For the Mount Zion group, technique is related to the needs of the patient as specified by the plan (i.e., the implicit patterned program for testing the validity of the patient's pathogenic beliefs). The therapist must recognize the patient's conscious and unconscious attempts to replicate with the therapist his or her pathogenic situations with the intention of ridding him- or herself of the expectations that all interactions will be such replications. Technique is thus discussed in terms of "plan compatibility," that is, the congruence of therapist interventions with the patient's plan.

There is an emphasis on the verbal interpretation of the patient's conscious and unconscious goals and the obstacles to their attainment, with the encouragement of insight into these goals and impediments. Thus, accuracy of interpretations is a central feature of this approach, accuracy being defined in terms of the therapist's grasp of the patient's pathogenic beliefs and their origins. Another important element of the therapeutic process is the therapist's recognition of "tests," which can be thought of as interpersonal reenactments of pathogenic situations in which the therapist is "invited" to play the part either of the patient

TABLE 3.2. Sample 12-Session Dynamic Therapy for Stress Disorders

Session	Relationship issues	Patient activity	Therapist activity
1	Initial positive feeling for helper	Patient tells story of event.	Preliminary focus is discussed.
2	Lull as sense of pressure is reduced	Event is related to previous life.	Takes psychiatric history. Gives patient realistic appraisal of syndrome.
3	Patient testing therapist for various relationship possibilities	Patient adds associations to indicate expanded meaning of event.	Focus is realigned; resistances to contemplating stress-related themes are interpreted.
4	Therapeutic alliance deepened	Implications of event in the present are contemplated.	Defenses and warded-off contents are interpreted, with linking of latter to stress event and responses.
5		Themes that have been avoided are worked on.	Active confrontation with feared topics and reengagement in feared activities are encouraged.
6		The future is contemplated.	Time of termination is discussed.
7–11	Transference reactions interpreted and linked to other configurations; acknowledgment of pending separation.	The working through of central conflicts and issues of termination, as related to the life event and reactions to it, is continued.	Central conflicts, termination, unfinished issues, and recommendations all are clarified and interpreted.
12	Saying good-bye	Work to be continued on own and plans for the future are discussed.	Real gains and summary of future work for patient to do on own are acknowledged.

Note. From Horowitz (1986, p. 131). Copyright 1986 by Jason Aronson. Reprinted by permission.

or some other in an earlier traumatic situation. Here the therapeutic task of "passing" the patient's "test" can be fulfilled in a variety of clinical modalities, from verbal interpretation to nonverbal activity such as the therapist's refusal to be traumatized by the patient in the same way in which the patient had been traumatized. "The patient also works to change his beliefs by unconsciously testing them in relation to the analyst. If the patient unconsciously perceives the analyst's behavior and attitudes as disconfirming the belief he is testing, the patient will make progress. In this way, direct experiences with the analyst sometimes may lead to significant analytic progress even without interpretation" (Sampson, 1992, pp. 519–520). Thus, the nonoccurence of particular, expected painful interpersonal outcomes is in itself thought to be therapeutic, as it helps to disconfirm the patient's belief in their inevitability.

Weiss and Sampson make a major contribution to clinical technique in their development of the "higher mental functioning hypothesis," as opposed to Freud's "automatic functioning hypothesis" (Weiss et al., 1986). Their idea, derived from Freud's (1926/1958, 1933/1964) notion of unconscious control of repression, is that the patient unconsciously controls his or her thought and behavior in relation to the experience of emotional safety. This is counterposed to the "automatic functioning hypothesis," wherein thoughts and actions are determined by the outcome of instinctual urges and the drive toward their gratification as mediated by the ego and superego. In this latter scenario, the therapist's task is to avoid gratification of these urges, particularly through the management of the transference, so that the repressed thoughts or feelings can be brought into consciousness (Freud, 1914b/1958). This became an organizing structure in Freud's technical writing, out of which a variety of technical prescriptions arose, including the idea of the "blank screen," and other aspects of analytic "neutrality" (Freud, 1911–1915/1958). By contrast, the "higher mental functioning hypothesis" leads to therapeutic attention to the ways in which the patient seeks to test the therapist and the safety of the therapeutic situation, before he or she is willing to bring new memories, dreams, thoughts, and feelings into therapy.

A brief clinical vignette (Silberschatz & Curtis, 1993, pp. 407–408) helps to clarify the idea of plan compatibility and the testing of the therapist to disconfirm pathogenic beliefs. First, the patient's plan is as follows:

Broadly stated, Diane's pathogenic beliefs were that her wishes, needs, and concerns could hurt others. She unconsciously believed that if she was strong or assertive, she risked hurting others by intimidating or running over them. Thus, she felt she must tightly control and inhibit her behaviors, which she did by identifying or complying with those whom she feared she would hurt by her actions.

Next, we look at an instance of a testing sequence in which the therapist responds in accordance with the patient's plan. The patient presents herself as dependent and weak, doubtful about her ability to handle her problems when therapy ends, suggesting that she is testing the therapist to see if he requires her weakness and dependency.

PATIENT (*silence*): . . . I was just thinking about how I would cope with all my problems . . . that of course are going to come up as soon as therapy ends and . . . you know, they've all been hiding, right, for 4 months. And they'll all spring out, but I mean I'll just do it the same way I've been doing it. It's not a catastrophe; it's not the end of the world. How shall I sort this out, whatever it is? (*pause*)

THERAPIST: The problems that come up in the last couple of weeks, you seem quite comfortable in solving on your own.

The patient's response to this intervention is rated to determine the usefulness of the therapist's intervention. The therapist points to Diane's competence and strength, rather than responding to her expression of dependency. In this case, her response is clearly positive:

PATIENT: Yeah. I did. Yes, when I keep working something up to stand in front of me that will be the real test, which of course I'll fail . . . like going in, observing in court, or going to the clinic last Thursday night and I . . . it seems to me I could put up another one in front of that, you know, having a trial, but I mean they're all just steps now I think, they're not road blocks. (*pause*) So even if I hadn't gone to the clinic on Thursday night I could still go next month for example, if I hadn't . . . I mean it would not have meant the failure of my whole life, if I'd lost my nerve or thrown up or something like that, you know it wouldn't have been the end of everything. . . .

The patient projects a view of herself as weak and fragile, assuming that the therapist needs her to be this way, and the therapist responds to the test instead by affirming her competence, to which in turn she responds with self-affirmation.

The Vanderbilt Group

For the Vanderbilt group, use of the therapeutic focus is the guiding technical concept. The therapist's task is to attend to and recognize the ongoing and shifting organization of dyadic interaction between therapist and patient, and make interventions that address this interpersonal pattern so that it can be understood and worked through in the context of the therapeutic relationship. The hallmark of their work is its interpersonal emphasis, and the subsequent persistent use of the transference relationship in the here-and-now: "In each therapeutic hour the TLDP therapist attempts to identify a recurrent theme that in one way or another is related to the defined TLDP focus. In TLDP, the most important facet of a theme in any interview is its interpersonal manifestation in the therapeutic relationship" (Binder & Strupp, 1991, p. 146).

In this way, the Vanderbilt approach follows an interpersonal psychoanalytic tradition of organizing clinical activity around interpretation of transference. However, TLDP is differentiated as a brief therapy by its active use of a clinical focus, along with earlier transference interventions.

The following brief vignette taken from a case example of TLDP (Binder & Strupp, 1991, pp. 151–152) illustrates these themes. The therapist begins by addressing the patient's stated reticence to address his concerns about not being closer to the therapist, and "hanging back."

THERAPIST: Why do you think you're doing that? What do you think holds you back?

PATIENT: Some kind of risk involved, and, I'm not wanting to make (*nervous laugh*) waves and feeling like, I would rather, to an extent, adjust to what your expectations are of the situation.

THERAPIST: Why? Especially since you feel that you're dissatisfied with it.

PATIENT: (*Chuckles.*) Well, yes, I don't know. I mean all I can say is why would I be hanging back? It's because I feel like, like I said, with the thing with the names, that maybe it would develop organically. Then I wouldn't have to make a plan. And somehow that would be easier, I wouldn't have to bring up something that's uncomfortable, uh, risk your displeasure or making you uncomfortable or whatever.

THERAPIST: If we pull together some of the observations, the experiences you've described in the past few minutes, maybe it would help us understand particularly what makes you hold back. You see me as reserved and you see yourself as holding back because you're not sure what that's about and you feel at risk and anxious about it. You're also reluctant, like you said, to make waves. If you say you're dissatisfied, you don't want to make waves, you don't want to make it personal. It's hard for you to admit that you're dissatisfied with me. And once you did, of course you said, "Well, it's not really you, it's me, too."

PATIENT: (*Chuckles.*)

THERAPIST: You're not going to put all the blame on me.

PATIENT: (*Chuckles.*)

THERAPIST: I wonder if you don't read something into my reserve. And that is, that I don't like you and that I don't want to be bothered by your feelings, particularly if you've got something to complain about or fuss about . . . any feelings, whether they are feelings of wanting to be closer to me or feelings of dissatisfaction, complaints, whatever. So that you feel you need to hold back, because otherwise I'll get mad or be offended, and our relationship will be ruined.

PATIENT: Uh, I think that's true. And I think that maybe I'm waiting for you to set the appropriate level of intimacy, so to speak. If you would complain about me, then I would feel free to complain about you. If your reserve wasn't there, then I feel like maybe I would be less reserved.

This interaction, occurring in the seventh session of a psychotherapy, contains the essential elements of therapist activity, focality, and interpretation of the transference in the here and now. The therapist is persistent in his pursuit of the patient's warded-off feelings toward the therapist. The transaction is brought into the context of the patient's presenting problem, namely, insufficient emotional involvement with others. The work is an active elaboration of the patient's here and now experience of the therapist, in the effort to clarify the meaning of the current issue of wanting closeness with the therapist and fearing rejection.

REVIEW OF RESEARCH

Each of the models under discussion in the present chapter has arisen in the context of an ongoing research program of substantial depth and duration, with large bodies of published literature associated with it. This is not true for any of the other approaches to brief therapy under discussion in the present volume.

The research reviewed here can be grouped in the following ways: (1) psychotherapy outcome, (2) case formulations, (3) the therapeutic relationship, and (4) psychotherapy process, including the effects of the accuracy of the therapist's interventions and other aspects of psychotherapeutic process.

Outcome Research and Evaluation

The Penn Psychotherapy Project has generated a large and complex set of results (Luborsky, et al., 1988). In brief, they found that supportive-expressive psychotherapy resulted in substantial general improvement of the patients treated, as reported by both therapists and observers (Luborsky et al., 1980), with approximately two-thirds of the patients showing "moderate" or "much" improvement, while only 2% "got worse." When outcome was evaluated according to patient-specific complaints, 75% of patients showed "moderate" or "much" improvement. More precise measurement of outcome showed a substantial effect size for the Penn study, with patients on the average improving by a magnitude of about 1 standard deviation on a mean of pre- to posttreatment measures (Luborsky et al., 1980). These gains tended to be sustained at a 7-year follow-up, with the most improved patients maintaining their benefits, while less improved patients continued to make gains after therapy ended (Luborsky et al., 1988).

Horowitz and his colleagues have also closely studied the outcome of their psychotherapy approach using a variety of measures, including assessment of the therapeutic alliance, and various psychotherapy process scales, in the treatment of 52 cases of pathological grief reactions following the death of a family member. Significant improvement was found in all symptomatic outcome measures from pretreatment to follow-up measures (Horowitz, et al., 1981). Expressed in terms of a standardized mean difference effect size, improvement ranged from around ½ to more than 1 standard deviation across different measures of outcome.

The Mount Zion group's methodology has not relied upon large group studies. Instead, they have used single case, repeated measures designs to study the relative efficacy of various kinds of psychotherapeutic interventions. Moreover, their research has been more concerned with process than outcome, using a patient's immediate response to therapist interventions as the dependent measure in their studies. Thus, this body of work has relatively less to say about the question of psychotherapy outcome in general. On the other hand, they have documented clear evidence of clinical improvement in cases of psychoanalysis (Weiss et al., 1986) and time-limited psychotherapy (Silber-schatz & Curtis, 1993), identifying the same kind of positive patient responses to therapist interventions which adhered to the plan formulation method.

Finally, the Vanderbilt I study (Strupp & Hadley, 1979) was designed to assess the differential contribution of specific versus non-specific change factors in psychotherapy (that is, change factors such as interpretation that are specified by the clinical theory versus global change factors such as attention, emotional warmth, and supportiveness). Accordingly, there were two treatment groups, one treated by psychotherapists with clinical training, and one treated by college professors with no formal training but designated as having good interpersonal skills. Both groups were compared with a control group which received no treatment. The overall results indicated that both treatment groups showed greater improvement than the control group; however, the group treated by the untrained therapists showed as much improvement as the group treated by the trained psychotherapists. Thus, while the study provided support for the efficacy of psychotherapy, it raised significant questions about the nature of the change process. The researchers noted that the group averages obscured a wide range of individual differences in outcome, and much of the research work that followed this inital phase of the study was designed to explore these individual differences in outcome.

Global outcome can be defined as the measured change from pre- to posttreatment across a large number of patients or studies. It usually is measured with general clinical instruments that rate symptoms or tap a "health–sickness" dimension that is not theoretically specific. While the problem of psychotherapy outcome has been the central research question motivating psychotherapy research over the past 3 decades, there is currently less research into the question of global psychotherapeutic outcome. We believe this is so for two reasons. First, the results of several large psychotherapy research projects and meta-analytic studies have shown, more or less consistently, that various approaches to psychotherapy all seem to have some measurable effectiveness, though with little significant difference in outcome between treatment approaches (Kernberg et al., 1972; Luborsky et al., 1980; Sloane et al., 1975; Smith et al., 1980). Second, global outcome research tends to teach us little about theories of change or of the therapeutic process, in some ways raising more questions than it answers.

The groups under consideration have expanded research efforts from more global questions of therapeutic efficacy to the problem of relating therapeutic process to outcome. The goal is to identify factors in patient, therapist and the psychotherapeutic process that are meaningfully related to successful treatment outcome. Thus, the question changes from "does this psychotherapy work?" to "what factors make this treatment model succeed or fail?"

Research on Psychotherapeutic Formulations

Some of the relational brief therapists have systematically studied the method of clinical formulations that they employ in their treatment approach. (For a review, see Barber & Crits-Christoph, 1993.)

Penn Psychotherapy Project

The Penn Psychotherapy research group has addressed a number of interesting questions: Are there central, organizing, enduring structures of personality? Can these be reliably identified? Is the CCRT method related to the psychoanalytic concept of transference? Do such structures change during the course of psychotherapy?

Their studies show that the relationship episodes which are rated in CCRT scoring are reliably defined (Crits-Christoph, Luborsky, Popp, Mellon, & Mark, et al., 1990), and that the elements of the CCRT itself are reliably rated by trained judges (Crits-Christoph et al., 1990). (For detailed exposition of the actual CCRT scoring methodology, see Luborsky & Crits-Christoph, 1990.) The CCRT has been found to be relatively pervasive and stable, but changes in pervasiveness—that is, the frequency of conflict themes in patient narratives—were found to be correlated with measures of outcome (Crits-Christoph & Luborsky, 1990). In particular, although the "wish" component of the CCRT appears not open to change as the result of psychotherapy, the perceived expectations of others, and the emotional response from self to others are somewhat open to change, and do so in relation to other measures of therapy outcome. This study also highlighted the effect of psychotherapy on psychodynamic change versus sympomatic change, the latter being only weakly correlated with the decrease in the frequency of conflict themes.

The Penn group has also found that the CCRT for a given patient in relation to the therapist significantly parallels the CCRT for others in the patient's life (Fried, Crits-Christoph, & Luborsky, 1990), and that CCRTs derived from the therapy situation parallel CCRTs derived from the patient's dreams (Popp, Luborsky, & Crits-Cristoph, 1990), suggesting that the CCRT, like the concept of transference, is related to highly stable structures of personality.

Mount Zion Psychotherapy Project

The researchers of the Mount Zion group, including Weiss, Sampson, and their colleagues, have been studying the psychoanalytic process for over 2 decades (Weiss et al., 1986). One result of their program is the "plan diagnosis" (now plan formulation) method, a systematic approach to the development of clinical case formulations.

Substantial research suggests that the plan formulation method is highly reliable (Curtis, Silberschatz, Sampson, Weiss, & Rosenberg, 1988; Silberschatz & Curtis, 1993) as measured by the interjudge reliability for individual cases. The group has also reported significant internal consistency (Curtis, Silberschatz, Sampson, & Weiss, 1994). The method has been used reliably by other researchers (e.g., Collins & Messer, 1991), who also have supported its adaptability and stability over time. Its validity was upheld in a study which found that plan compatibility of therapist interventions was correlated with patient progress in early and middle phases of psychotherapy (Messer et al., 1992). Interestingly, the Plan Compatibility of Intervention Scale has been applied successfully to different formulations (object relations versus cognitive-dynamic) of the same case, enabling researchers to compare the utility of one formulation versus another in predicting responses to therapy interventions (Tishby & Messer, 1995).

Reseach on the Therapeutic Relationship and Therapeutic Alliance

Penn Research on the "Helping Alliance"

Luborsky and his colleagues at the Penn Psychotherapy Project have devoted much attention to the issue of the therapeutic relationship, in the form of their concept of the "helping alliance." The helping alliance is thought to include two dimensions: one, the patient's experience of the therapist as providing the help that is needed, and two, the patient's experience of the therapy relationship as collaborative. Studies have examined the relative impact of a variety of therapeutic factors, including patient factors (i.e., motivation to change), therapist factors (i.e., ability to offer a technique that is clear, reasonable, and likely to be effective), and process factors (patient's experience of a helping relationship; Luborsky et al., 1988). The measure of the "helping alliance" was found to be reliable, consistent, and, as with the Vanderbilt project, a significant predictor of outcome, even across different methods of evaluating the helping alliance. "The outstanding area of successful prediction is located within the positive relationship quallities and, inside that area, for helping alliance measures" (Luborsky et al., 1988, p. 310).

Vanderbilt Research on the Therapeutic Relationship

The work of Hans Strupp and his colleagues at Vanderbilt University over the past 2 decades can be thought of as an investigation into the contribution of the therapeutic relationship to psychotherapy outcome. Their studies have been motivated by questions raised in the late 1960s as to the relative effects of specific, technical factors, as opposed to so-called "nonspecific" factors, such as empathy, respect, genuine acceptance, interest, and other general humane aspects of human relationships, which had been identified as crucial by humanistic psychotherapists (Frank, 1974; Rogers, 1951). As described above, the first phase of Strupp's project, Vanderbilt I, was an attempt to clarify the relative importance of nonspecific factors in therapy outcome. Using nontrained but empathic listeners (selected college professors with no psychotherapy training) to treat one group of patients, as compared with patients treated by trained clinicians, it was found that patients in both treatment groups improved about the same amount (Strupp & Hadley, 1979). Both groups of patients did better than those in the control group, who received no treatment.

Attempting to clarify variability in treatment outcome within each group, Strupp used a single-case design, comparing one patient therapist dyad with another to explore hypotheses about process variables affecting outcome (Strupp, 1980a, 1980b, 1980c, 1980d). Other studies were conducted exploring the process of psychotherapy and the role of the therapeutic alliance, involving the development and application of the Vanderbilt Psychotherapy Process Scale (Gomez-Schwartz, 1978); and the Vanderbilt Therapeutic Alliance Scale (Hartley & Strupp, 1983; O'Malley, Suh, & Strupp, 1983; Windholz & Silberschatz, 1988).

A major and consistent finding was that "the quality of the therapeutic relationship, established early in the interaction, proved to be an important predictor of outcome. In particular, therapy tended to be successful if by the third session the patient felt accepted, understood, and liked by the therapist" (Binder & Strupp, 1991, p. 157). Also of importance was the observation that both trained and untrained therapists did most poorly with the more disturbed patients, those who manifested chronic interpersonal difficulties, attitudes of distrust and hostility, and lower motivation for treatment. It was hypothesized that these individuals were the most difficult to engage in a positive treatment relationship, and, specifically, that they involved therapists in counterproductive enactments involving therapist hostility, retaliation, abandonment, control, or other countertransference problems.

This latter finding led to the conclusion that a major technical goal for the psychotherapist would be to reliably identify the appearance of negative transference and interpret this actively, even early on in the treatment process (Strupp & Binder, 1984). Those psychotherapies in which negative transference (and countertransference) feelings were not clearly addressed were most likely to be unsuccessful.

Other Research on the Therapeutic Alliance

Numerous other studies by different groups of researchers have confirmed the centrality of the therapeutic alliance in psychotherapy process and outcome. Marziali has contributed to the clarification of the therapeutic alliance in a number of studies (Marziali, 1984; Marziali, Marmar, & Krupnick, 1981), concluding that both therapist and patient perceptions of their own and each other's contributions to the therapeutic relationships are strong predictors of psychotherapy outcome. Researchers associated with the Menninger Clinic have pursued the reliable assessment of the therapeutic alliance (Allen, Newsom, Gabbard, & Coyne, 1984; Frieswyk, Allen et al., 1986; Frieswyk, Colson, & Allen, 1984).

Horowitz and his colleagues have studied the changes that take place in the quality of the alliance over the course of psychotherapy. They report that therapist actions affect the quality of the therapeutic relationship, suggesting that the alliance is not fixed but is instead a function of process variables as well as pretreatment variables. They speculate that the therapeutic alliance may represent a mediating variable through which therapist interventions have their effect (Foreman & Marmar, 1985; Horowitz, Marmar, Weiss, et al., 1984).

The importance of the therapeutic relationship to psychotherapy outcome is one of the most reliable and consistent findings of empirical studies. Questions about the therapeutic alliance remain, such as the relative contributions of pretreatment patient and therapist variables, and the important technical question of how the therapist can influence the quality of the therapeutic alliance.

Psychotherapy Process: The "Accuracy" of Interpretation

The question of interpretive "accuracy" has its roots firmly in the tradition of Freud and his early followers. "The pure gold of interpretation" was the hallmark of the psychoanalytic project, distinguishing analysis from all other forms of helping and influence (Freud, 1919/

1959). The question of accurate and reliable clinical formulations, and the imparting of psychodynamic insights, obviously remains a central concern of psychodynamic psychotherapists and researchers. Malan (1976b) conducted widely-noted studies of brief dynamic psychotherapy in which the correlation of transference interpretation to therapy outcome was examined. He found that the more focused the treatment, the better the outcome, and in particular, the more vigorously the interpretive links were made between the transference relationship and the historical relationships with parents, the better the outcome. Although his work did not address the issue of interpretive *accuracy* so much as therapeutic focality, it effectively raised the issue of the effect of the content of therapeutic communication.

Among the relational approaches to brief therapy, two have placed substantial emphasis on the question of interpretive acccuracy, though from quite different points of view.

Penn Psychotherapy Project on Accuracy and the Use of the CCRT

Researchers at the Penn Psychotherapy Project have organized their investigation of the reliability and accuracy of clinical formulations around the CCRT method described earlier (Luborsky & Crits-Christoph, 1990).

The results of their studies suggest that the accuracy of interpretation, defined in terms of correspondence to that patient's CCRT, could be reliably evaluated and that such accuracy was predictive of therapeutic outcome (Crits-Christoph et al., 1988). This effect was found to be the result of accuracy independent of the therapeutic alliance. That is, therapist accuracy appears to be a specific and independent factor in the outcome of psychotherapy. A more recent study was conducted to examine the relationship between the accuracy of therapist interpretations and the state of the therapeutic alliance (Crits-Christoph, Barber, & Kurcias, 1993). The researchers found that the accuracy of early therapist interventions (as measured by congruence with the patient's CCRT) was positively correlated with the helping alliance later in treatment.

It thus appears that the accuracy of the therapist's communications to the patient, as measured by their correspondence to the patient's central interpersonal relationship themes, is predictive of the efficacy of psychotherapy, both as an independent technical variable and through its contribution to the mediating variable of the helping alliance. However, as discussed in Chapter 2, such findings may apply only to patients with a high quality of object relations.

Mount Zion Research on Therapist Adherence to the Plan

The Mount Zion Psychotherapy Research Group has also conducted studies specifically addressing the issue of therapeutic accuracy. Here, the assessment of accuracy is made in terms of the plan formulation method.

The Mount Zion researchers found, contrary to Malan's original results, that it is not the use of transference interpretations per se which predicts outcome, but rather interventions that are congruent with the patient's conscious and unconscious plan to disconfirm, in the relationship with the therapist, the pathogenic beliefs which otherwise control his or her experience of self and others and of relationships (Silberschatz, Fretter, & Curtis, 1986). Outcome in these single-case studies was defined as the immediate patient response—"mini-outcomes"—rather than the global outcome of treatment. It was found that when the therapist "passed" the patient's key interpersonal tests via plan-compatible communications, there was a significant improvement in the patient (Silberschatz & Curtis, 1993).

It is interesting to note that both the Penn and Mount Zion research groups have attempted to understand the impact of interpretive accuracy in terms of the therapeutic relationship. Crits-Christoph et al. (1993) suggest that accuracy has its effect through the mediating variable of the helping alliance, and Silberschatz and Curtis (1993) interpret their findings in terms of the importance of test passing in the therapeutic relationship.

A CRITICAL EVALUATION
OF THE RELATIONAL MODEL

We conclude this chapter with a comparative summary and evaluation of the relational approaches to brief psychodynamic therapy. We first note the commonalities of the approaches discussed here, particularly at the most fundamental level of philosophical assumptions and worldview.

We believe that the differences between the relational approaches and others described in this volume are at the level of guiding metaphors and fundamental philosophical assumptions, as much as at the level of technique or theory. We suggest that a philosophical shift which has taken place across the psychoanalytic field is manifested also in the arena of brief psychodynamic psychotherapy. We view the shift within psychoanalytically-oriented psychotherapy as part of a larger postmodernist cultural current, with its greater recognition of the context-bound nature of knowledge, the plurality of points of view, and the role of narrativity in theory and observation (see Messer, Sass, & Woolfolk, 1988; Safran & Messer, 1995). These frameworks can be counterposed to a more traditional philosophy of science, in which knowledge of the world, including the psychological world, is attained systematically and in ever greater correspondence to the way things actually are, relying on methods which assume a radical division of subject and object. The following concepts are suggested as some of the elements of this basic conceptual shift. They are not equally applicable to each of the four illustrative models addressed here, nor is the list exhaustive, but they convey the spirit of the change we wish to emphasize. Of the four, Strupp and Binder's (1984) handbook comes closest to a paradigmatic example of the relational approach from the perspective of the following principles.

• *Relational versus drive metaphor:* The guiding metaphor of psychodynamics is not based on the transformations of energy, but rather rooted in the *relationship,* or dyad. The concept of drives and instinctual strivings gives way to the motivational characteristics of affective states and of relational strivings.

• *Perspectivism versus objectivism:* The individual is seen as an active construer of his or her interpersonal world. There is less attachment to the belief in an objectively knowable reality, and neither participant is understood to have a privleged understanding of reality. Transference is viewed as comprising the plausible constructions of meaning of the psychotherapy situation by patient and therapist. The subject is considered an imperfect knower of self and others; all interpersonal knowledge is colored by one's particular experience, theory, and point of view.

• *Object relational versus structural model of conflict:* Internal object relations, including representations of self, other, and expected modes of interaction and relationship are the primary personality constructs, displacing the centrality of either the structural model of Freud's later theory or the topographic model of his earlier theorizing.

• *Use of participant observation:* The relational approach views the patient-therapist dyad as a two-person psychological field. Thus, following interpersonal psychoanalysis, the notion of participant-observation is a central metaphor for the clinical method. With the abandonment of the "blank screen" metaphor of the therapist, alternative concepts arise, tending to be more interactional and deprivileging and decentering the therapist's point of view. There is a fuller recognition that the *observer affects the observed.*

• *Process versus content:* In terms of technique, attention to interpersonal process is given greater weight. Insight and interpretation are deemphasized somewhat, while the therapeutic relationship is elevated as a curative factor. Here-and-now interpretation is emphasized more than genetic interpretation.

•*Narrative versus historical validity:* These models can be seen as more concerned with narrative truth (Spence, 1982) than the objective, veridical reconstruction of past experience.

Limitations of the Relational Model

There are a number of shortcomings that the relational approaches share as a group. All four tend to ignore the role and importance of time and time limitation as integral parts of the treatment, particularly when compared with Mann's time-limited therapy (see Chapter 4) and to some extent, others of the earlier generation of brief dynamic therapies (see Chapter 2). This is least true for Horowitz's short-term dynamic therapy of stress response syndromes, which is a specialized 12-session model (Horowitz, 1991). His therapy, more than the others, takes note of phase-specific aspects of treatment, is focused on current stressors, and is adaptation oriented.

But even Horowitz's model offers no theoretical rationale for the brevity of treatment apart from acknowledging its greater utility to the clinical researcher. In fact, in all four instances, it appears that the time limitation of therapy has been implemented largely for the purposes of research. It can be no coincidence that the four therapies discussed here represent four of the most important research programs in psychoanalytically oriented psychotherapy, and whose senior members are among those who have made historic contributions to the field of psychotherapy research. In all cases, the particular model of brief therapy is a recent outgrowth of more general, time-unlimited approaches to treatment.

None of the four adequately address the issue of curative factors specific to the context of brief therapy; that is, none suggest what might be therapeutic about the time limitation itself, as does, for example, Mann (1973). A corollary of this omission is the relative neglect of technical recommendations aimed at the problems posed by limited time, particularly in comparison with the drive/structural models. To some degree, it appears to the student of these approaches that what one does in brief therapy is more or less the same as what one does in longer-term psychotherapy as defined by these schools, but for less time. Further, it appears to us that the curative factors emphasized in these relational models, such as the therapeutic relationship, internalization of a new object, identification with therapist, and corrective emotional experience, are not necessarily well suited to brief treatment. To be fair, all strongly advocate the use of a treatment focus, which becomes the vehicle for short-term work. But questions remain as to the relationship between focality and long- versus short-term treatment. Does the use of a focus necessarily lead to shorter durations of treatment? Can one work with a focus in long-term treatment? If so, how would such work differ from the briefer applications?

Short-term models that rely more on Freud's topographic model, such as Davanloo's, or those that focus on oedipal conflict and resolution through insight, such as Sifneos's, may have a conceptual advantage in terms of therapeutic brevity. Although we are sympathetic to the richness and subtlety of the relational view of mind and of change, it appears that simplicity and certainty confer some advantage clinically, if not theoretically. Placing emphasis on retrieval of specific memories, abreaction, and resolution of psychic conflict through the making conscious of unconscious contents using special techniques to deal with resistance may all offer advantages to the short-term therapist.

Finally, we wish to note the tension between the epistemology of relational theory and the use of traditional empirical research methods. In reviewing the list of principles above, it should be clear that the paradigmatic shift which we posit as having taken place is one that poses special obstacles to the researcher. *Perspectivism* as a philosphy of science emphasizes the observer's point of view within a particular set of contexts. *Constructivism* implies that what is known about the object of study is inevitably a function of preexisting models, theories, and assumptions. The notion of "*narrativity*" suggests that acts of perception and of knowing are prestructured and actively mediated by intrinsic requirements of coherence and human sensibility. *Participant-observation* as a method likewise stresses the involvement of the subject in the object of study. All of these are problematic from the point of view of traditional empirical research methods.

Such methods, including the use of sampling and other statistical methods to establish the reliability and validity of observations and to test hypotheses, rely on more mechanistic, atomistic, and naturalistic metaphors of causality and assume a separable subject and object. Instead, from the point of view of constructivism or perspectivism, psychological concepts and constructs arise out of systems of human meaning and can be located only within particular cultural, linguistic, methodological, and theoretical frameworks. This latter view seems quite compatible with a relational view of human development, personality, and psychopathology. It seems to us that the psychotherapies described in this chapter rely on a somewhat uneasy blend of the two differing philosophies of science. We are curious to see what new kinds of research programs evolve out of the perspectival paradigm as it continues to have a growing impact on psychology in general and psychotherapy in particular.

Advantages of the Relational Model

One advantage of the relational approaches is their continuity with the broader scope of psychoanalytic theory. All make substantial contributions to the theory and practice of psychodynamic psychotherapy in general, increasing the applicablity and generalizability of their theoretical and research findings.

Relational approaches integrate and organize various currents in psychoanalytic theory: object relations theories, self psychological concepts, interpersonal psychoanalysis, developmental theories, and current models in personality theory. In the field of psychotherapy, notable for its tendency toward bifurcation and divergence of theory and practice, one must appreciate the value of systematic programs which absorb and synthesize diverse areas of work, offering convergence and common ground between research and clinical domains.

Their openness to broader currents in psychology as well as psychotherapy is commendable; it is probably a result of these models arising in academic and research contexts with a commitment to theoretical rigor and intellectual diversity. The work of all these groups is thus more accessible to a wider range of psychologists and practitioners than are some of the more specialized approaches to brief therapy, such as Sifneos's or Davanloo's (Chapter 2). Corresponding to this greater intellectual openness, these approaches tend to be less extravagant in their claims and aspirations than some brief therapy models, and certainly less dependent on the strong personality of a particular individual who originates a model.

Because the relational model tends to have greater continuity with the field of psychodynamic psychotherapy in general, the training required is more consistent with existing standards and methods for training psychotherapists. Fewer special technical demands are made on the student therapist in training, and these models do not require a kind of "conversion" to a particular approach in an all-or-none fashion.

This group of approaches is unique among the brief dynamic psychotherapies in its commitment to ongoing research programs. As the issues of outcome, accountability, and cost-effectiveness continue to permeate the social discourse on psychotherapy, the development and maintenance of a clinical research base is a significant advantage. Further, this approach to learning complements the traditional psychodynamic approach to theorizing, namely, through the description of individual cases and their interpretation. These research projects show their openness to the influence of clinical wisdom and experience, and in turn have generated findings relevant to clinical practice. This model of mutual influence between clinical and research domains is unusual and warrants the attention of both researchers and practitioners.

PART III

Integrative and Eclectic Models of Brief Psychodynamic Therapy

CHAPTER 4

An Integrative Psychoanalytic Model: Mann

In Chapters 2 and 3, we described and contrasted two major theoretical and therapeutic models within psychoanalysis—drive/structural and object relational, the latter including an introduction to the self psychological approach. Our intention was to highlight differences in the underlying theory of these models and in their application to BPT. In this chapter, we describe a version of BPT that draws on the four major constructs contained within those models: ego, drive, object, and self. It does so both in the way that it views psychopathology and in its conduct of psychotherapy. We are referring to time-limited psychotherapy (TLP), developed by James Mann (1973; Mann & Goldman, 1982). Mann's belief that these theoretical outlooks are complementary rather than mutually exclusive is echoed and developed by Pine in two volumes (Pine, 1985, 1990) and in other articles (Pine, 1988, 1989) which provide us with a useful conceptual backdrop for understanding Mann's TLP.

That a full chapter is devoted to this therapy is not meant to imply its preeminent status, but, rather, its uniquely integrative emphasis. It also affords the opportunity to present a full case with commentary.

THE THEORY OF PERSONALITY AND PSYCHOPATHOLOGY

The Four Psychologies: Drive, Ego, Object, Self

Pine refers to drive, ego, object relations, and self-experience as four "psychologies," each of which describes a significant way in which the mind functions. He views the attempt to reduce the four psychologies to a single one of them as arbitrary. Each has early origins with its own line of development; none has primacy. Each, he argues, has motivational status, that is, can arouse, sustain, and direct behavior and thus can be viewed "as an independent actor on the intrapsychic stage" (Pine, 1989, p. 32). Each may be present in relatively pure form at any one moment in infancy, but in adulthood they are interconnected and are present in all significant aspects of a person's functioning. "Gradually, as organization becomes more complex and behaviors come to have multiple functions, the phenomena addressed by the several psychologies become intertwined, and we are more likely to think of behavior now from this perspective and now from that . . . " (p. 61). For any one individual, however, they may be organized in a different hierarchy. For example, in a neurosis, drive may be the more prominent facet, whereas in a narcissistic character disorder, self issues will likely predominate.

Because the four concepts have been discussed at greater length in the previous chapters, we can summarize them briefly, drawing on Pine's writings (1989, 1990). By *drive* is meant the basic impulses of sex and aggression and their modifications through the developmental stages. Although biologically based and unfolding in a preprogrammed way, they are represented psychologically and are subject to disruptions and alterations. Drives are transformed by means of defenses such as displacement and sublimation, and take the form of wishes which are expressed in conscious or unconscious fantasies. When viewed as dangerous, these wishes create conflict, as indicated by anxiety, guilt, shame, and inhibition. Symptom formation and/or pathological character traits may result. Conscience, from the perspective of drive psychology, is aggression turned against the self. It is based on identification with parental prohibitions and aids in the control of drives through feelings of guilt.

Ego is closely linked to drive in that it refers to the function of harnessing the drives in accordance with the demands of reality. Ego psychology stresses the individual's capacity for defense, adaptation, and reality testing, which develop slowly over time. It includes the possibility of ego defect, in which such capacities as the ability to delay, affect modulation, and control of impulses are wanting in some respect.

Object relations refer to the internal representation of self and others. These are acquired in childhood, based on the affect and wishes then active in the child. These internal representations are later played out in adult relations: That is, people will often construe and experience current relationships in terms of past ones, and thus not fully experience the new ones in their current form. Individuals repeat old object relationships in an effort to remain attached to them or to master and free themselves from some of their problematic aspects.

Finally, a psychology of the *self*, in Pine's terms, refers to self-experience, especially in relation to the object. The self is a phenomenological construct emphasizing a person's perception of his or her own experience, especially in relation to the establishment of boundaries and the differentiation of self from other, or the loss of such boundaries and differentiation. It involves concerns about authenticity—the existence of a "true" or "false" self—and also includes the presence or lack of a sense of self-esteem. For Kohut, the major figure in the development of self psychology, understanding a person from this perspective leads to a therapy that is more supportive, empathic, and experiential in quality than a therapy focused more exclusively on ego/drive psychology.

Mann's Theory of Brief Psychodynamic Therapy in Light of the Four Psychologies

Mann and Goldman (1982, p. 41) state quite explicitly that their view of psychopathology draws on four perspectives: (1) the structural hypothesis, (2) the theory of narcissism and the development of self-esteem, (3) object relations theory, and (4) the developmental perspective. The structural hypothesis includes both ego and drive and the conflict that ensues among agencies of the mind. As does Pine, these authors view the vicissitudes of narcissism as complementary and not contradictory to the structural theory. Under the topic of object relations, they stress the impact of environmental failure on the etiology of psychopathology, such as the birth of a younger sibling or the death or illness of parents. Similarly, it is not just the child's drives but, for example, the seductiveness or overcompetitiveness of the parents' behavior or the latter's neglectfulness that lead to symptoms or unstable self-esteem. The developmental perspective highlights normative tasks at different stages of development and maintains that maturation can proceed once a specific conflict or developmental hurdle is overcome.

In addition to this broad, integrative perspective, Mann and Goldman highlight two issues around which TLP revolves: time and separation. In a chapter on the conscious and unconscious features of time, Mann (1973) writes lyrically about the ways in which time intrudes on the mind and affects behavior. Operating on the basis of primary process thinking, young children view time as limitless and think very little about their mortality. As an aspect of infantile omnipotence and the early fusion with mother, all things are viewed as possible; the pleasure principle predominates. As the child matures, a sense of real time develops, which Mann refers to as "calendar" or "categorical" time. It develops, along with the general maturation of the child's sense of reality, in accordance with the reality principle. Just as there is, according to drive theory, a conflict between the pleasure principle and the reality principle, there is a conflict for an individual between infinite and real time. Adults try to restore that early pleasure in the sense of timelessness in various ways. They enjoy vacations during which they are relatively free from the clock and from schedules which, in daily life, too often predominate. They may take drugs such as alcohol or marijuana to diminish the relentlessness of the passage of time. In dreams and daydreams, reality and time are overcome, even if ephemerally.

The sense of timelessness is traditionally represented in folklore by a woman, where mother and child are endlessly united (Bergler & Roheim,1946), while the ravages and ending of time are represented by the man or skeleton with the scythe who evokes the horror of time (Bonaparte, 1940), whose passage brings about the ultimate separation—death. For Mann (1973), "all short forms of psychotherapy, whether their practitioners know it or not, revive the horror of time" (p. 9). The foreshortening of therapy, then, inevitably brings into high relief the difficulty human beings experience with separation.

On the one hand, the unconscious wishes of the patient coming to therapy are to return to that period of life in which time held no sway, when omnipotence of thought was paramount, and when there were intimations of immortality. This is a drive concept because the pleasure associated with timelessness is linked to the gratification once enjoyed when the child was nestled in mother's bosom, sucking her milk. On the other hand, because therapy is specifically time limited, the reality of imminent and inevitable separation is consciously present. This points to an ego function of adapting to the external world with its time demands and the growing recognition of having to live by calendar time. "The greater the ambiguity as to the duration of treatment, the greater the influence of child time on unconscious wishes and expectations. The greater the specificity of duration of treatment, the more rapidly and appropriately is child time confronted with reality and the work to be done" (Mann, 1973, p. 11).

Time-limited psychotherapy, then, is based on "the recurring life crisis of separation–individuation" (Mann, 1973, p. 24). In life, we are constantly experiencing loss in one form or another, and thus are constantly challenged to deal with the ensuing anxiety and sadness it brings. TLP is focused on the mastery of separation anxiety, specifically failures in the effort to deal with it. It is particularly the object relations of the separation–individuation phases of childhood and their effect on ego development that Mann (1973) sees as setting the stage for the successful differentiation of self from one's love object. "The interrelationship among separation–individuation, development of reality sense, and the course of ego development will determine the adequacy of the adaptive modes that emerge as a means of managing relationships with others" (p. 25).

Mann defines four universal aspects of conflict situations which relate to the capacity to tolerate and manage object loss. These are independence versus dependence, activity versus passivity, adequate self-esteem versus diminished or loss of self-esteem, and unresolved or delayed grief. Each can be viewed as most closely associated with one or another of the four "psychologies" previously discussed.

Independence refers to the extent to which the person has achieved sufficient autonomy to weather loss without becoming overly reliant on substitute objects. *Activity* relates to the ability to pursue one's own wishes or needs with appropriate aggressiveness rather than waiting passively for others to fulfill them. Loss can foster a regressive pull or yearning toward the passive pleasures of early childhood. It can also precipitate a *drop in self-esteem* by virtue of guilt over ambivalent feelings toward the lost object. *Unresolved or delayed grief* often results from a failure to mourn a loss and the ego's effort to repress or deny the painful affect associated with it. In all these conflicts, says Mann (1973), "the loss of a sustaining object revives the anxiety which had its genesis in the separation–individuation period of development" (p. 28).

The way in which time and separation are manifested in brief therapy is best summarized in Mann's (1973) own words:

> The beginning restores to the patient the golden glow of unity with mother, preseparation in endless time. The middle brings with it the disappointment that a relationship once wholly unambivalent will once more become ambivalent. And the end introduces the unavoidable harsh reality that what was lost must be given up. In the struggle over giving up the object once more, and this time without self-defeating anger or hatred or despair or guilt, one sees in capsule form both the adaptive means used by the patient over the years to defend against the ambivalent feelings and the basic conflict situation. (p. 28)

In contrast to the drive/structural therapies, the focus of TLP is on preoedipal versus oedipal issues. Mann views the preoedipal issues of separation–individuation as incorporating and transcending the Oedipus complex. He regards conflicts around separation and loss as more accessible and resolvable through BPT but holds that only psychoanalysis can overcome the formidable resistance to accepting and understanding oedipal issues on a meaningful, affective level (Mann & Goldman, 1982, p. 29).

THE FORMULATION OF A FOCUS: THE CENTRAL ISSUE

Mann's way of thinking about and arriving at a focus for brief therapy is quite different from that presented in other models. He attempts to discern how patients have felt about themselves in relation to the painful events they describe in order to formulate a statement of their chronically endured pain. The pain is a reflection of a negative feeling about the self, which often comes with the belief of having been victimized. It is a guiding fiction in the person's life which is no longer true but is felt as if it were, a discrepancy which must be exposed in therapy. Patients feel that they have always had the pain, have it now, and will always have it. Linked to a statement of this endured pain is a recognition of patients' adaptive efforts to master it. Here are some examples of central issues presented by Mann (1991, pp. 32–33):

> You are a man of ability in your particular field and have done very well in it. Yet you feel and have always felt that there is something about you that makes you feel that you are unwanted, even irrelevant.

> You have tried hard all your life to be [acceptable] and to do the acceptable things. What hurts you now and always has is the feeling that you are stupid and a phony.

> You are a big man (physically and in his field of work) who has achieved successfully and yet when you are alone you feel helpless.

To these statements, Mann adds that how the patient came to feel that way about him- or herself will be the work of treatment. Thus, the central issue has three parts: An acknowledgment of patients' active coping efforts to gain recognition and satisfaction of their needs; the observation that this has failed and that they are left with a negative feeling about themselves; and a statement about the task of therapy.

The first part of the statement of the central issue points to the role of the *ego* in disguising and managing the chronically endured pain. It is a recognition of the ego's adaptive role in keeping the pain out of one's mind and out of the sight of others. The second part touches on painful feelings that bear on the affective coloring of the *self*, an aspect of the patient's narcissism. Note that the central issue neither touches on drive issues nor is primarily oriented to the patient's conflicts in object relations. In addition, the statement makes no specific mention of symptoms, but rather highlights the underlying affect. The focus is more global and more attuned to self-esteem than is the drive/structural therapists' conception of a focus. It is an empathic statement which is meant to bypass defenses rather than confront them in a way that might arouse anger or defensiveness. It attempts to soothe the patient's damaged self, allay anxiety, and promote a working alliance and positive transference, which is more in keeping with the relational approaches.

THE SELECTION CRITERIA: INDICATIONS AND CONTRAINDICATIONS

Mann's primary criterion for acceptance into TLP is the presence of good ego strength, especially the capacity to tolerate loss as gauged by how losses have been negotiated in the past. Because of the treatment's brevity, a patient must have the capacity for rapid affective involvement as well as for rapid disengagement. Other signs of a robust ego include success in the ability to work and to love, reminiscent of Freud's statement about the prime indicators of mental health.

In terms of diagnostic categories, individuals with adjustment disorders, such as anxiety in response to current events, and those with neurotic character structures, such as the hysterical, depressive, and obsessional, tend to be the most suitable for TLP. The problems dealt with might include "repetitive unsatisfactory love relationships, problems in work or school adaptation, or difficulty with peers" (Mann, 1991, p. 20). In terms of life developmental stages, those who are experiencing difficulty negotiating the transition from one stage to another, such as leaving home, entering college, graduating, getting married, becoming parents, having one's children leave home, and so forth are good candidates. Loss as a specific stressor is often a positive indicator for TLP because brief therapy tends to recapitulate the problem which is, therefore, available for exploration and resolution in an affectively meaningful way.

The diagnostic categories that are contraindicated include schizophrenia, bipolar affective disorder, schizoid disorders, and severe psychosomatic disorders such as rheumatoid arthritis, ulcerative colitis, regional enteritis, and severe asthma. Although the latter four conditions may be related to loss, there is often too little conscious affect with which to work in the compressed time span of TLP.

Mann also cautions about the more severe manifestations of the personality or character disorders. These include obsessional characters with almost exclusive use of the defenses of isolation and intellectualization; hysterics who cannot tolerate loss; narcissistic characters who consider "it far too little help for such important problems in such a significant person" (Mann & Goldman, 1982, p. 58); depressive characters who are full of orally based rage; and patients with borderline conditions who seek gratification of early infantile wishes and have little frustration tolerance. However, patients with milder forms of even these diagnostic categories may be able to profit from TLP, such as border-line patients who can form a rapid therapeutic alliance or patients with narcissistic disturbances who view brief therapy as a challenge.

THE TECHNIQUES OF THE THERAPY

Although Mann is an active interviewer, unlike Sifneos and Davanloo he is very gentle, especially in the initial sessions. He makes the experience as easy and comfortable for the patient as he can. The technique serves to intertwine patient and therapist in a symbiotic orbit (Rasmussen & Messer, 1986). He initiates a confirming, mirroring process, often repeating the patient's words exactly, or probing in a low-keyed way:

PATIENT: . . . the doctor . . . took tests, and when he decided that it was rheumatoid arthritis, then the nerves took over . . .

DOCTOR: And then you say that the nerves took over?

PATIENT: That's it.

DOCTOR: Do you remember in what way they took over? (Mann, 1973, p. 91)

PATIENT: During a crisis or anything I will feel worse.

DOCTOR: During a crisis you will feel worse—and which crises are you remembering?

PATIENT: Well, my father's death.

DOCTOR: That was—[*Deliberate pause in order to let the patient recall the time.*]

PATIENT: Six years ago. (p. 93)

Mann seems to be creating a kind of union, bound by the overlap of words, and his letting her complete a thought, often an emotionally significant one:

DOCTOR: They had to give you an injection because you were—

PATIENT: So upset (p. 93)

DOCTOR: I think that you are saying that you are happy *for them* but *you* are not happy—

PATIENT: For myself— (p. 98)

Unlike Davanloo and Sifneos, who would challenge the patient's somatization and preoccupation with details, Mann, with great attentiveness, conveys that he accepts her as she is. He becomes the available, confirming, attuned caretaker ready to meet needs as they arise (Rasmussen & Messer, 1986). Note how he provides nurturance and empathy:

PATIENT: That's what people can't understand. How can I get so bored or upset with having the children around.

DOCTOR: People really don't understand that six kids could tie a woman down with the same thing every day. They don't understand that. I bet you would like a vacation. (Mann, 1973, p. 100)

Throughout the initial interview with this burdened woman, Mann responds to her regressive needs for warmth and fusion, supporting her ego functioning and needs for autonomy. At the same time, he uses repetition, emphasis, and selective summary to draw connections between the patient's somatic and anxiety symptoms and critical life events such as her daughter's birth, her father's death, and her mother's illness, thus enhancing a psychological view of her problems (Rasmussen & Messer, 1986).

The 12 sessions of time-limited therapy (plus one or two in which history taking and focus setting take place) can be thought of as encompassing three phases: early, middle, and late. In the early phase (about four sessions), the therapist's emphasis is on establishing an alliance and engaging the patient in therapy through mirroring, affirmation, and respectful listening and probing. This therapeutic stance plays into the magical expectations with which patients are said to enter therapy, hoping, at some unconscious level, that "long ago disappointments will now be undone and that all will be made forever well, as they should have been so long ago. The warm sustaining golden sunshine of eternal union will be restored—and in the unconscious it is restored" (Mann, 1973, p. 33). When all is going well, the patient is forthcoming with secret feelings and fantasies and important anamnestic data. Symptoms often abate or disappear. In this stage, transference manifestations are not interpreted directly. The primary demand on therapist and patient is to keep attention focused on the central issue, which also serves the purpose of limiting the tendency to regress.

By the middle phase of therapy, some disappointment begins to set in as the patient realizes that not all problems will be solved or even discussed and that this new relationship, too, is flawed, bringing back old feelings of ambivalence, pessimism, and doubt. The honeymoon is over. There is a dawning recognition by the middle or end of this phase that therapy will soon end, with expectations unfulfilled. The therapist, at this stage, has begun to confront this patient's overcompliance and dependence on him, thus urging self-reliance. The separateness of therapist and patient becomes evident:

DOCTOR: Do you make progress to please me or to please you?

PATIENT: I have to please you . . .

DOCTOR: You feel that you have to please me.

PATIENT: Not please you but probably what would be best for myself . . .

DOCTOR: But who are you going to do it for? For you? Or in order not to hurt me?

PATIENT: No, for myself.

DOCTOR: You're sure now.

PATIENT: Mmmm. Because I feel that's what you want me to do—for myself. . . . I figure that if I am displeasing you it's still connected with me because I am not doing what I should do for myself. (Mann, 1973, p. 127)

Mann is no longer letting the patient experience him as an object with whom she can regress and merge. There is a confusion and blurring of roles and boundaries as she attempts to sort out who is doing what for whom, and with what effects on the other. Mann has become much more focused and directive than earlier. He no longer lets the patient retreat to a defensive posture, as was true in the past. He goes on to encourage her to be true only to herself and her own wishes in his attempt to enhance her sense of mastery and build up her self-esteem (Rasmussen & Messer, 1986).

In the final stage of therapy, constituting the last three or four sessions, Mann focuses on the patient's reactions to termination. In fact, if the patient has not made reference to the ending, the therapist introduces the subject. In this phase, transference plays a major role. One can expect a variety of affects to emerge, including sadness, grief, anger, and guilt, all of which must be explored in relation to people within the familiar triangle of insight, including the therapist and important figures in the present and from the past. Not to do so, says Mann, will prevent both the positive internalization of the therapist and mature separation. The disappointment and ambivalence surrounding separation from the therapist are explored in relation to previous separations and to the central issue. Resistance to separation in both the patient and the therapist are common. In spite of tugs at the therapist to prolong therapy, he or she must proceed toward the contracted ending. In this phase, Mann also attempts to inculcate a sense of mastery and competence, which buoys the patient in his or her quest for greater independence.

One can expect the patient to leave therapy with some sadness instead of depression, which allows for separation without self-injury. "Ambivalence, which previously had always led to feelings of anger or depression with concomitant self-derogation, has changed into awareness of positive feelings even in the face of separation and loss" (Mann, 1991, p. 36).

To summarize, in the early stages of therapy, the therapist fosters a kind of union or merger with the patient. Along with empathic statements are other kinds of supportive interventions which convey the message to patients that the therapist recognizes both their difficulties and their coping abilities. Questions are frequently posed to help patients explore the pertinent issues. There is little in the way of confrontation or interpretive links, but rather a gentle, lulling, holding quality to the interventions that would tend to foster regression and a sense of well-being. As the therapy progresses, there is an increase in the number of clarifications, mild confrontations, and interpretations, especially regarding the current situation in the person's life. As the termination nears, the frequency of therapeutic interventions around the concepts of time and separation increases, as does explicit reference to the central issue. There is an increase in interpretations of the transference and their link to both current and past figures. In addition, there are more directly suggestive, educative, and supportive statements meant to foster self-esteem and independence and to help the patient anticipate posttreatment reactions to the loss of the therapist.

The following section presents a full case conducted in this mode, allowing a look at the development of a time-limited therapy from beginning to end.

THE CASE OF ROSE

On a visit to the Graduate School of Applied and Professional Psychology at Rutgers University in 1980, James Mann conducted client interviews which were videotaped for training purposes. When the first appointment time arrived and passed without the client appearing, I (SBM) reached her on the telephone and she explained that she had a headache, had not gotten much sleep that night, and had overslept. Nevertheless, she agreed to come to the clinic to be interviewed by Mann, who was described to her as a visiting consultant.

In the interview it was learned that Rose is a 23-year-old, single, Asian woman engaged in graduate studies. She was casually dressed, well groomed, and can be described as attractive and petite. Rose was self-referred and had not been seen previously in a mental health setting. Mann asked her what was troubling her. When she started recounting her history, he immediately brought her back to the question of what it was that she most wanted help with, thus focusing her attention on the task at hand. She then reported that she was experiencing a great deal of distress over the breakup with her boyfriend of 7 years, which had occurred just 1 month previously. Signs of depression included crying and sadness of mood, weight loss of about 10 pounds (in a woman who probably weighed about 100 pounds), insomnia, difficulty concentrating, and somatic complaints such as headaches and vomiting. She had also been doing less well in her coursework over the past few months, as the difficulties with her boyfriend grew worse.

Rose had known her boyfriend (Lee) in Hong Kong, and when she had decided to leave home and come to the United States about 5 years ago, she knew that he was planning to emigrate to the United States. When asked about why she had left home at 18, she said that she didn't want to be treated "like a kid" and to remain dependent on her parents. In his supportive mode, Mann responded, "That was a courageous step." When learning later in the interview that she was the only one of the five siblings to leave home, he inquired, "Have you wondered what has made you different such that you left?"

Lee has been her "whole family" during the 5 years she has been here, and she relied heavily on him for support. The client started dating him exclusively when she was 16. She has been intimate only with him, and it distressed her greatly when she learned from him that he was having sex with another woman. She felt that she had been very helpful to him and his family (e.g., preparing their tax returns), who now shun her. She varies between wanting to seek revenge on Lee and wishing the relationship could be restored. She recognizes that she tends to suppress her anger and other negative feelings, and generally presents a strong, independent, smiling stance to her friends.

The client grew up in Hong Kong in a traditional Chinese family; that is, her father dominated the household, which included her mother and siblings—three brothers (ages 28, 25, and 21) and one sister (age 20). Her father, 51, is a factory worker and an alcoholic who often related to the client by screaming at her to keep out of his way. He was kinder when not drunk.

Her mother, 47, is a homemaker who has endured the emotional unavailability of her husband because of his relationship with another woman. Because of her mother's difficulties, the client felt that she could not burden her further with her own problems, although she felt that her mother was patient and kind. She and her siblings generally kept things to themselves. The parents stayed together only for the children's sake and because divorce is considered a great disgrace in Hong Kong.

Toward the end of the interview, when Mann inquired about Rose's vengeful ideas, she said it wouldn't help to dwell on them. When he responded, "So you feel you're stuck the way you are — helpful and agreeable in spite of everything," she said, "I have to stop this bullshit and be more disagreeable." Mann added, "You end up getting hurt — maybe it doesn't have to be that way." When she said that "I am emotionally stronger than most people," he countered, "How long do you want to go on being hurt?" By the end of the interview, she was crying softly, and said, "I'm crying, but I feel better. The headache is gone."

In a quiet but persistent way, Mann brought her around to seeing that she had been overly agreeable and helpful at her own expense. In a discussion with one of us (SBM) following the interview, he formulated the central issue as follows: "You have been very helpful and agreeable, but what hurts you is that your efforts are not rewarded; you end up getting hurt. The work we must do is to learn what happened that it always ends up that you get hurt." Note how this statement acknowledges her coping style — being agreeable — and the chronically endured pain — feeling unrewarded and hurt.

Could an alternative central issue be formulated? For example, her pride in her independence and tough-it-out posture are suggestive of a cover-up for, or defense against, deep-seated dependency feelings. One might then formulate a central issue as follows, "You have always prided yourself on your independence, but now you find yourself feeling hurt and needy of help and this bothers you a lot." Although such a dynamic issue seems to be present, Mann might argue that it is not conscious and would arouse resistance rather than be readily accepted by the patient. The question of whether only one "story line" or central issue can be formulated will be taken up later in this chapter. Bearing on this matter is whether different clinicians observing an initial interview would arrive at the same central issue. This question is currently being explored by Gaby Shefler and Orya Tishby at the Student Counseling Center of the Hebrew University of Jerusalem.

Suitability

In considering whether Rose is a good candidate for TLP, we would first ask whether any obvious contraindications are present. A perusal of the list above suggests that there are not any. However, one might question the motivation of someone who does not appear for her first session and who complains of psychosomatic symptoms such as headaches and nausea. In such instances one would want to note carefully whether there is enough available affect to accomplish the work of therapy in 12 sessions. Mann was able to reach her on an affective level in the interview, which was reassuring in this regard.

On the positive side, she is a woman of some accomplishment, who was able to strike out on her own. However, her leaving Hong Kong seemed to be contingent on Lee's presence in the United States, suggesting that she substituted one kind of dependency for another. Her depression is related to loss, considered a good indicator for TLP. She does not report any previous loss that would have allowed us to gauge how she has responded to such trauma in the past. It was possible to formulate a central issue and to the extent that Mann touched on it in the interview, she responded positively. It was Mann's view that she was a suitable candidate and therapy was begun with one of us (SBM) as the therapist.

Session 1

When Rose has not arrived 10 minutes after her scheduled appointment time, I begin to wonder whether she will show up at all. However, she does come — explaining that she had been grading exams — and says that she is doing better, keeping her mind off Lee and concentrating on her studies. She feels that Mann was on the right track and says she felt much better after the interview. In the session she struggles to hide her hurt and the anger that she feels toward Lee, and acknowledges that expressing feelings is hard for her. She likes to see and present herself as a strong, smiling person, not weak, angry, or vulnerable, so that her friends don't know her true feelings. With some encouragement on my part, she admits to vengeful feelings and talks about her fantasy of calling Lee's new girlfriend and revealing that Lee has been seeing both of them at the same time. She says that she had depended a great deal on Lee and that now she will have to take care of herself. She is glad that I was persistent in calling her to set up the initial interview because she finds it helpful to be listened to and to express herself here. I present the central issue and the 12-week contract, to which she readily agrees.

Commentary

In spite of my initial concern about her lateness being due to resistance, she seems to have become engaged in the process. I wonder if her ready agreement to the time-limited contract is her way of being agreeable with me, or whether she feels reassured that her independence will be preserved.

Session 2

Rose says she feels good about coming to therapy as it allows her "to shelve" her feelings during the week and concentrate on her work. I ask about her reticence to express her feelings. In her family, she explains, feelings were not expressed. She didn't want to trouble her family and took care of everything herself. She talks about her father's drinking, his having a lover, and his screaming at her. In the session, she adopts a very forgiving attitude toward him but is clearly upset. When she says, "I figured he didn't mean it," or "He treated me best of all," I point out that she is crying as she said it, so that it couldn't have been too good. She responds that it's hard for her to cry here, that it makes her feel stupid, but that she has kept her feelings inside too long, and is learning to let them out. Even with Lee she tried to make herself believe that she was a happy person but then would cry when she was by herself.

Commentary

Rose is responding well to therapy, exploring both her current and past difficulties in an affectively meaningful way. I ask myself why she had put up with a man who has another lover. Was she identifying with her beleaguered mother? Did she feel that she doesn't deserve better? Was an implicit bargain struck with Lee in which he satisfied her unfulfilled dependency needs while she put up with his two-timing?

Session 3

She is trying to be more open with her friends but is afraid that she will be a burden to them. She likes to be rational and logical with others. She presents a dream in which Lee comes for his belongings and cries when they meet, and she comforts him. A friend who is with her (in the dream) is so upset with her that the friend leaves. Because of the obvious connection of the dream to the central issue, I focus the session on her associations to and feelings and thoughts about the dream. It's important to know that Lee still cares for her, she says. Further, she is afraid of her violent feelings. Part of her loves Lee and part hates him, and these feelings are in conflict. "Sometimes I can't stand myself for being so understanding and forgiving, but anger is a very disturbing emotion for me."

In her childhood, she saw her parents fight a lot and even throw things at each other. In the session, each time that she changes the subject or softens her reaction, I interpret it as a defense against deeper feelings. She says, "I'm afraid my anger would get uncontrollable and I would do something with Lee like what my parents did." What do you imagine doing, I ask. "I couldn't kill him — the most I could do is throw things. My parents loved each other even while fighting. It's disturbing to think that people who love each other can be so violent with each other."

Commentary

Note how her characteristic inclination to be agreeable is becoming somewhat more ego dystonic, as suggested by her comment that she can't stand herself at times for being so understanding. With regard to anger, Rose seems to have no expectation for using it constructively. In her mind and experience, anger leads either to violence or to no change. She seems hardly to know how to be disagreeable.

Incidentally, when patients have not brought in a dream spontaneously by the third or fourth session, I will ask them if they have had a dream. Note, too, that the emphasis in this first stage of therapy is on the current conflict and the past, with no attempt to focus on any transference manifestations. My object is to help her express herself as freely as possible and to establish a therapeutic alliance.

Session 4

She looks forward to coming here and is feeling good, she tells me. She went to the beach with a girlfriend and a fellow by the name of Stanley. She is avoiding having a romantic relationship with him because he is leaving the area at the end of the summer and she doesn't want to get hurt. I reflect that she is very worried about getting hurt, and she responds that she wants to prove to herself that she can be fully independent and that she doesn't need a man in her life.

She talks about how she can only curse in English, not Chinese, and that she never confronted her parents or disobeyed them because of her conception of what it was to be a daughter in a Chinese family. She feels there are two sides to her: the Chinese side, which is passive, obedient, holds back feelings, and the like, and the "social" side, which can get angry at men because she trusts them more than women. She treats her male friends like brothers and they treat her like their little sister. She is trying to be independent, but there are times when she feels vulnerable and needs someone to help her. Her friend Stanley listens to her. But, I commented, you're not sure how far to let it go. "I have this fear of being left behind," she responded.

Commentary

Here we see transference elements at work in which she is developing an attachment to me and is fearful of the inevitable consequences, namely, being abandoned. She is enjoying being listened to and getting things off her chest. Her mood has lightened. All of this fits quite nicely with Mann's description of the first phase of therapy as re-creating the golden glow of childhood. She is probably experiencing a sense of oneness with me, which I have fostered by being generally supportive, nonconfrontative, empathic, and exploratory. In line with the central issue, she is able to look at the way in which she has always been so agreeable, and has begun recognizing its origins in her relationship to her parents.

Session 5

She has been feeling good, is no longer depressed, and has gained back the 10 pounds she lost. She wants to forgive Lee but also to hate him. She feels that breaking up with him was a very good thing because she is learning to be self-sufficient emotionally. She sees the need not to be so forgiving, but does not want to make a 180-degree switch. She now wants to treat the men in her life as equals, a thought which scares her. The following dialogue ensued:

PATIENT: When I was with Lee, I was like a little sheep or goat and he was the shepherd. But when I was with others I tried hard to prove to them I was not subservient. I was only 16 when I met him and I let him guide me. All along I have wanted someone to love me and care for me and to guide me. My family didn't give it but he did (*all said in a shaky voice*).

THERAPIST: You wanted to be loved as a little girl by Daddy, as a little sister by your brothers and you weren't getting it, so you turned to Lee.

PATIENT: That's why I wanted to leave home so strongly at the time. (*Upset*) I didn't think I needed anything from my family. I tried to prove that I could do without them. I wanted them to feel unhappy. I wanted them to feel they needed me. Now that I'm gone, even if they wanted to give me the love and attention, they couldn't.

THERAPIST: It was a way of getting revenge wasn't it?

PATIENT: I did it in an indirect way.

THERAPIST: You've managed very well, but that doesn't mean there wasn't all along a feeling of dependence which Lee satisfied, so losing him is a very big loss for you, and you reacted strongly.

She acknowledges this. Toward the end of the session I ask her if she knows how many sessions we have left. She responds, "six or seven," then says that she is losing track and wonders if she will run out of things to say here.

Commentary

Running out of things to say may be of concern to her because it would mean not being able to please me. Her sense of child time, tied to dependency wishes, is illustrated in her getting lost in the flow of time. But her adult time sense knows of the planned ending, and she may be preempting the separation by hinting that she has said all there is to say, that she feels well enough to be on her own. She may be testing out her ways of being with me — dependent and independent. Even if I am like a "father" who guides her and allows her to be dependent, can and will I also tolerate her autonomy?

Session 6

This session starts with the reporting of a dream:

PATIENT: I had a dream in which Lee called me up and told me his girlfriend committed suicide. I told him it was none of my business and why had he called? Because he had no one to talk to, he said. I was very angry and hung up, but later regretted it because I had no way of contacting him. I ran out of the apartment to find him. . . . I guess I want to be part of his life even though consciously I try not to be. I want to forgive him but resent myself for being so forgiving.

THERAPIST: You fear that if you cut him off because of your anger you won't be able to reach him.

PATIENT: The last time I had a dream was also the night before coming here. There must be something disturbing about coming here. In the past 2 weeks I try to make up an excuse not to come — it's emotionally disturbing to sit down and talk to you this way. Yet I feel a lot better. On Friday, I try not to think about coming here in the afternoon. I tell you things I have never told anyone. I don't even know you; the one-way communication disturbs me. I feel a pressure to talk or this will be useless. Maybe I'm distrustful.

THERAPIST: What are your thoughts?

PATIENT: When I was in grade 8, I had a friend I was very close to. She convinced my other friends that I am a terrible person. Even though I don't look forward to coming, I know it helps me. It's not pleasant for me to cry in front of you. I must say you have some significance in my life, but I have two feelings about coming here— one positive, one—not negative, but not positive—the anxious part. Maybe I have to define a new role towards this person who is my therapist, who listens to me, and I don't know how to define it.

Commentary

Expressing anger in the dream leads to the loss of the object, which upsets her. The fact that I am different from her usual social contacts seems to worry her. Perhaps the problem for her is that she can't control me by taking care of me as she had done with others, and that she knows that she is going to lose me. There are some negative feelings about therapy beginning to surface. In the meantime, she is working on the central issue in noticing herself being so forgiving and berating herself for it.

Session 7

She has had Lee on her mind all week and is disturbed and disgusted by it, and wonders if therapy is not helping her now. When I ask her if she is disappointed with therapy or with me, she responds that she can't blame it on me, but blames it on herself— her lack of sufficient effort. I point out how her tendency is to blame herself, and that she is reluctant to express negative feelings to me just as she was reluctant to do so with her parents and friends.

Since last week she has had the thought that the source of her anxiety in coming to therapy is her increasing reliance on me. She likes to see herself as an independent person who should be responsible for herself. Admitting that she is, in fact, quite dependent— if not on Lee, then on me— worries her. I point out that this is the seventh session, so we're closer to the end than to the beginning of therapy. This might be why her thoughts are drifting back to Lee, her former source of support. She feels she shouldn't be comparing her relationship with Lee to that with me, but she is.

PATIENT: I have a spontaneous idea. I know it's going to come to an end and I know how I felt when my relationship with Lee ended. The same could happen here. . . . I may get depressed. . . . I'll have nowhere to unload my thoughts so I'll have to make it on my own. That's what I was practicing during the week. I'm even more open with you than I was with him.

THERAPIST: You felt good at first coming here and now you feel depressed and ambivalent about coming because it's too strong a dependency. Do you see a pattern here?

PATIENT: If that is the case, it means that I have been quite dependent all my life. I am exasperated. I don't want to think about it. . . . All my life I have convinced myself I am more independent than others. Now I see it's not true. I don't even want to know about this side of me.

THERAPIST: What is so disturbing about relying on someone?

PATIENT: Whoever you rely on can come and go . . . not be there when you need them.

Commentary

The disappointment so aptly described by Mann as inevitable in TLP is now apparent as time marches on and the pain of separation looms. There is a different tone in the last two sessions compared to the optimism of the first phase. The transference is becoming clearer. She has come to rely on me as she did on Lee, and she fears the dependence because it will lead to disappointment.

The countertransference that I experience here is that the therapy is going downhill; it may be a failure. The early gains are merely a transference cure, based on her having a substitute object from whom to draw some strength on a very temporary basis. But it can't last. I have drawn her in and will indeed abandon her, an unpleasant and guilt-arousing prospect. Should I be helping her to cover up the dependency or encourage her to struggle with it? I will be letting her down just like Lee and her parents did before me. The challenge for the therapist is to stick with the negative feelings and to trust the process, to recognize that there is an opportunity for a new learning experience here in which the patient can be helped to deal with separation on better terms than in the past.

Rose cuts out and withdraws as a way of dealing with her anger and feared loss. She did this in leaving Hong Kong and in her dream, when she hung up the phone on Lee. She is now trying to do the same with me, that is, to stop therapy prematurely. She can't get angry at me for the disappointment she is experiencing in therapy until she can stop blaming herself for it. She constantly protects the object by blaming herself. She sees her dependency as bad and I have to try to convey that it is not.

Session 8

Rose reports that she had lots of dreams this week. One involved a male friend of hers, a young professor whom she had gone to see to say good-bye before he left. He is someone who refers to her as his adopted sister. In the dream, he is going away and they share a long kiss. In reality, when he had left this past week, he had kissed her on the cheek in a friendly way and she had kissed him back on the cheek. She is very confused about the dream. She wonders if she feels the need for a romantic relationship, but doesn't feel ready. I asked her what might happen in a romantic relationship, and her first thought is that she will get hurt. Then she tells me that she will be going to Tokyo for a year at the end of the summer. She had applied for a job there some time ago, 2 weeks after breaking up with Lee. At that time, she had been inclined to leave immediately, but decided to finish her thesis first. Besides, she doesn't want to return to Hong Kong and be a burden on her family. I point to her fear of dependency and relate it to her anxiety about relying on me too. She then refers back to her friend Stanley, the young professor in the dream, and wonders if she has hesitated to get involved with him because he is leaving as well. I suggest that she is afraid to become dependent on him when he is about to leave, just as she is afraid to rely on me and then get cut off. She replies that she has come to realize that she can have lots of nice relationships and that most of them end. That's life; You have to cope with it, she says.

Commentary

Does she feel that it is only by being a little sister that she can get her dependency needs met with men? There was a pulling back from me in this session because of her fear of being hurt. She has to learn that she can get involved in relationships and handle the separation, which this therapy is ideally suited to deal with. She also has to learn that dependence and independence can coexist; her fear seems to be of going to one extreme or the other—needing to be supremely independent or to be a needy child subject to being left and hurt. One can expect these themes to be paramount as we enter the third and final stage of therapy.

Session 9

She tells me that she is relaxed here, that I am her instructor and she is my student, and that she is learning how to open up. She doesn't want to get too attached because it will end soon. I say to her that she is backing off from therapy. She says she has to prepare herself for the end, otherwise she'll get depressed, and that she has always done it this way. She would like the therapy to taper off to once every 2 weeks and then once a month. She reviews her gains in therapy, such as being able to accept the darker side of herself. I point out how she seems to be wrapping it up although this is only the ninth session. She says she is building a wall around herself and wants to pack up everything in a box. Including your emotions, I add. She admits in a tearful way that she is escaping and that, by leaving, she wants to make Lee feel bad. She intended to do the same to her parents when she left for the United States. She also admits to being scared about leaving and going to Tokyo. I say that her first attitude today was to tough it out, to have a stiff upper lip, and now she is being more honest with herself and with me. Is it so awful to feel this way? She says it is, for her. By going to Tokyo, she wants to show that she can do without anyone, but it's a crazy way to do it, she adds. I comment, "You go from one extreme to the other; is this the only way possible?"

Commentary

She is trying to cast our relationship in the familiar pattern—I, as guide; she, as student. In this way I become a big brother for her, as have other men, and she is subservient. Her defenses are not working quite so well now. She recognizes her escapism and the price in loneliness and fear that it brings. She is trying to leave therapy in the same way that she left Hong Kong. She is running from her anger and dependency. Going to Tokyo allows her to cut off her feelings about leaving me and her friends. Is she able to gain further recognition of what she is running from, namely, her fear of getting close and getting hurt? Can she verbalize the feelings instead of running from them?

Session 10

PATIENT: I have the feeling of wanting to get this over with. I have benefited a lot and I want to see how I will be at the end. I'm feeling fine.

THERAPIST: A part of you wants to put your emotions in a box and be strong and independent, but you're afraid that if you allow yourself to experience the other part, it will dominate you.

PATIENT: You know that part of me. I don't see the point in going further with it. I should not let myself depend on you permanently. Maybe 9 weeks of therapy is enough for me.

THERAPIST: You want to pull away from me just as you've done with others in the past.

PATIENT: I know I can handle my emotions much better now. I know I'm withholding somewhat but I need to stand on my own feet. I need a few weeks to adjust. It works for me.

THERAPIST: But you pay a price for it—headaches, stomachaches, and depression.

PATIENT: I know now that I want an equal relationship with a man, not to be a little sister or sheep. I don't have to provide all the emotional support. I picture you as helpful and that helps me. I have given out a lot of my emotions. I want to store what I've learned like a book on a shelf.

Commentary

Rose seems to be in full retreat, back to her independent, tough-it-out stance. She seems to be trying to mollify me with praise, and to keep things cool and intellectual. What she is not doing is talking about how she will miss me when she does not have me available, and the concomitant sadness. Perhaps she wants to make me feel badly by leaving prematurely, as she had wanted to do with her parents and with Lee. The therapist's temptation here is to go along with her request and let the therapy peter out by diminishing the frequency of visits or even stopping it at this time.

Session 11

Rose reports a dream in which Lee is being nice to her. She says her defenses are down, that she has been thinking about Lee and has not gotten enough sleep. I ask about her feelings in the dream:

PATIENT: I felt very protected, safe, and good. . . . I feel better having unpleasant dreams.

THERAPIST: This kind dream disturbs you because it interferes with your image of yourself of not wanting or needing protection.

PATIENT: I have been thinking of the good times with Lee, reading my diary, and crying. I have to free my emotions.

THERAPIST: You have a longing for the good times, the feeling of protection and security that Lee provided, but you struggle against those feelings.

PATIENT: Yes, I try to let the rational side of me predominate.

THERAPIST: It seems hard for you to accept yourself as having both kinds of feelings—that you are equal to others, able to cope, strong, but also needing friends to rely on, to be protected and secure in a relationship with a man. This is the side we see in the dream.

PATIENT: (*She laughs*) You know both sides of me. It's hard for me to admit that side outside this room. The two sides are so different. I want to be as hard as a rock so I can't be hurt any more. I feel relieved to admit it.

THERAPIST: You protect yourself against that side. You felt yourself withdrawing from me in the past few sessions. How did it feel to come in today?

PATIENT: In the last few sessions I was looking forward to therapy ending, but this week I find I can't pack up my emotions—there are things I have to reconcile with. I realize I don't always have to put up a pleasant front for my friends. I feel safe with you, but I don't want to be too dependent on you—the same old thing. But in thinking about it this week, I feel that it's okay to feel that way, to have someone provide the comfort I need, but also to feel I'm strong enough to do without you around, without these sessions.

THERAPIST: What is it like to recognize that we have just one more session?

PATIENT: I feel a little bit depressed about it but I feel I'll be okay, that I've done a good thing for myself in coming here. . . . (*a little later*) Today I am very depressed about the fact that we have just one session. Maybe I'm growing up slowly. I now believe there will always be an end to something. Before I used to believe that things never had to end. Now I have to come to terms with it.

Commentary

The theme of this session was loss and depression. In the previous session, she wanted to end therapy in a "feel good" state, and my effort to undermine this strategy seems to have paid off. She is getting in touch with her truer and deeper feelings about her need to be taken care of, and is coming to recognize that she can live with it. She is acknowledging what needs to be acknowledged in TLP, namely, the inevitability and pain of separation, which she verbalizes so well and feels very deeply. It is also instructive to see what the time limit brings to the surface—her childlike notion of time going on forever with no endings necessary. She is indeed maturing in recognizing that everything comes to an end, but that she can handle it.

Session 12

PATIENT: I feel I have gained something by coming here. I look upon you as a father figure—someone I can rely on and trust with my innermost feelings. This week I was able to cry in talking with a friend about Lee. She was surprised. I hope I'll be able to continue expressing my feelings so openly.

THERAPIST: That was a big thing for you.

PATIENT: Yes, and it felt okay. Before I came here I kept everything to myself. I shouldn't try to be a superwoman.

THERAPIST: You had to be agreeable and helpful to everyone, but you were getting nothing for yourself.

PATIENT: I now feel real friendship is a give-and-take affair, though I still like to be agreeable and helpful. I'd like to be friends with you even after today. In a way, you're my best friend at this point

THERAPIST: So it would be nice to have it continue, but here we are at the 12th session and it will stop. What is it like to lose your father figure, your best friend?

PATIENT: You can be away from your friends and still cherish the relationship. I don't have a sad feeling about the end.

THERAPIST: Your face looked sad.

PATIENT: I feel a little bit depressed.

THERAPIST: You can take away the positive memories, but this doesn't mean you don't have negative feelings which you are quick to dismiss.

PATIENT: It's embarrassing to admit I have these feelings. I feel I have been the taker, not the giver. It's a new kind of relationship for me. Most of the time I don't need anyone to give me anything.

THERAPIST: That started way back with your parents—you felt you couldn't call on them, so you became very independent, left home, and managed on your own. You've come to realize that there is another side of you, the side that would like to have gotten more from your parents, the side that felt awful when you lost Lee's support and security and the side that is depressed about losing that kind of support from me.

PATIENT: I accept that side of me. It makes me, me. But I want to be able to rely on myself.

She then tells a story about getting lost when driving home from a party this past week, not asking for directions, and then realizing how stupid it was, and telling a friend about it. She laughs and says:

PATIENT: I have too much pride in myself. The strong part of me still predominates but now I can see that it's okay to be weak, not so brave. It's a relief to admit those feelings. It's a new kind of strength I've gotten here, to admit weakness.

I ask her about the symptoms she had when she started therapy, and she responds that she feels fine, there is no nausea, and she has gained back the weight she had lost. Now and then she has trouble falling asleep, however.

PATIENT: I feel fantastic. I cried last night about leaving my friends and you. I thank you for all the help you have given me although you always said that I've been helping myself.

At the end of the session I wish her well and tell her that it has been a pleasure working with her.

Commentary

Aside from the symptom remission, that she is now able to show her vulnerable side to others is a good sign that she has changed in some important respect. In other words, she doesn't have to be only agreeable with and helpful to others, but can also look to them for support. She seems to be quite convinced that she need not be subservient in a relationship, although I note that she sees me as a "father figure" and regards me as her best friend. This, of course, tugs at me not to abandon her but to continue to provide the benefits of the relationship. However, she seems to be saying that she can now be both dependent and independent in a relationship. Perhaps this has come about because she has seen how she was able to express both needs in her relationship with me, without untoward consequences, and that this has been a corrective emotional experience for her. In retrospect, I wonder if more emphasis might have been placed on her expression of anger. Note that I worked with her on her issues and conflicts until the very end. One feels the press in TLP to make each session count. The question naturally arises as to whether the gains were lasting.

Follow-Up

Mann will often conduct a follow-up either by interview or letter to assess the patient's status 6 months to 1 year or more following the con-

clusion of therapy. He does not forewarn the patient at the time of termination so as not to dilute the effect of the work of separation. Here
is the letter I wrote to Rose at her home in Hong Kong 1 year later:

Dear Rose,

It is now almost a year since I saw you in therapy, and I thought this
would be a good time to follow up on the work we did together at that
time. How are things going for you, and what have they been like this
past year? I would also be interested to know what the impact of your
therapy was and how you view it and our relationship in retrospect.

What kinds of experiences have you had this past year, e.g., in dating men, making friends, etc., and was therapy at all helpful in these
respects? Were there ways in which therapy was detrimental?

What are your plans at this time? If you are coming back to the Rutgers area, I would like to arrange an interview with you to discuss these
matters. If you will not be back, then would you please write me as long
a letter as you like in response to the above questions. I would be pleased
to hear from you.

Three weeks later I received the following letter:

Dear Dr. Messer,

I was ecstatic — perhaps a bit surprised — to receive your letter. Since
it is quite impossible for me to go back to the United States in the near
future, I shall attempt to write you a long letter.

Basically, my life in the past year has been fairly good, though hec-
tic. My job and my traveling took most of my time. I recently settled
in a new job which took less traveling. Hopefully, I will have more time
to develop my interests outside the job. Of course, there were times
in the past year that I wished I still had therapy sessions so that I could
talk freely of my emotional disturbances. I managed to get through those
moments by concentrating on work, reading books, or going out with
friends. Sometimes, I like to walk on the beach and think quietly, trying to untie some of the knots from my past. I realize that the memories
of my relationship with Lee and his family are slowly fading away. I
ran into Lee's brother in Hong Kong back in March and chatted with
him for a while. The brief encounter did not stir anything in me. I must
admit that I was a little bit astonished by that. Our conversation on
how Lee and I broke up did not upset me at all. I think the therapy
sessions we had last summer definitely help me to get over the bitterness I had of the entire matter. Time and distance certainly help in
this case, too.

I did and still do value very highly our therapy sessions and our doctor–patient relationship. During that time I had told you that I had been slightly bothered by the one-sided communication. But now when I look back on those days, I know I could not have handled it if other people unloaded their problems on me. Maybe I felt guilty of being entirely dependent on your counseling and guidance. I am not sure whether I am now totally free of the guilt. At least I know for sure that I did the right thing in seeking help. I also thank you for your persistent calling on the morning that our initial interview was scheduled. Had it not been for those calls, I might not have been in sessions with you and it might have taken me a longer time to bounce back from my lowest ebb.

For me, our relationship was the first all-take-and-no-give relationship. I felt that I was the only one who benefited from our Friday afternoon sessions. In fact, I still believe such is the case. I have gradually learned to accept that I cannot be helpful sometimes and I am not as independent as I would like myself to be. This is a big discovery for me. I don't feel ashamed of asking for help now. Perhaps I expected too much of myself. Ever since last summer I realized that I need others' help every now and then. In a way this realization has released a lot of the pressure I exert on myself.

On making friends, I never feel that I have any troubles. But I do have difficulty in trusting them. Especially the friends I make on the job, I take every precaution [not] to reveal my true self to them. Even if I had not had the bad experience with Lee's family, I would have done the same thing with the people I met in the commercial field. I am well aware of the wall that I build to protect myself and the distance that I keep. Frustrated? Disheartened? Not really! I have at least one friend I can rely on. Though she is Japanese and we only see each other occasionally, she is my confidante and my best friend. I don't feel guilty of troubling her with my problems because we have a mutual understanding that we can help each other emotionally. I stayed with her family in Tokyo last month. That was probably the happiest month in my life. We both feel revitalized and have regained our enthusiasm toward life. We have known each other for a few years. It is not until recently that we discovered that we have overcome the language barrier, our cultural differences and the background ethnic rivalry between Chinese and Japanese to be friends with each other. This is something that we both feel [to be] comforting. Life itself is full of obstacles. I am ready to overcome them with the same kind of spirits. For sure I will encounter failures. But I am determined to make myself happy no matter what happens. It seems a bit egocentric. But I have no apology to make. Happiness is self-made. Do you agree?

As much as I value our therapy sessions, never have I mentioned the word "therapy" in front of anyone after coming back to the Far East. I do feel badly about it. As I had told you a year ago, Asians are still not used to the idea of "psychiatry," "therapy," or "psychological counseling." This is the only contradiction I have inside me. My overall assessment of therapy was absolutely positive—helpful and constructive. I learned an immense lot about myself. Yet, I cannot bring myself to tell anyone of my educational experience.

When it comes to dating men, I must say I have [had] a wide range of experience in the past year. Whether I am in Hong Kong or Tokyo, I have a very active social life. This is certainly one of the many reasons that the memories of Lee do not bother me often. Before, my male friends [were] confined to the nice and single-minded students of my peer group. Now, they are from all walks of life. I am not eager to settle down in a relationship. Though I had a brief romance which ended in pain not long ago, I recovered quickly. Sometimes I enjoy the freedom I have right now. I can pack up my bags and go off to Tokyo tomorrow without any worries. This is something that was quite foreign to me, say, a year and a half ago.

I believe that everything has its cause and effects. As one Japanese philosopher puts it, a man who cannot turn pain into gain is forever a slave to himself. Now it is only the beginning of my life. I do not intend to be a lifelong slave. This sums up my feelings.

Finally, as a matter of curiosity, I want to know whether the videotape of my initial interview has been useful as an instructing medium. I would also like to keep up the correspondence with you if at all possible.

Thank you and with best regards,

Rose

Commentary

Assessing the outcome of psychotherapy is not a simple or straightforward task, especially when we do not rely solely on objective measures. By her own account, Rose has profited from therapy, at least in getting over the loss of Lee and all that he meant to her. She does not mention any of the symptoms that disturbed her when she started therapy, and we can presume that she is free of them. Regarding her agreeableness and her dependency needs, she seems to be able to engage in a give-and-take relationship with her Japanese friend without feeling guilty, which is a new experience for her. She has been able to date, to have had a romantic relationship, and to have bounced back from its breakup. She can now acknowledge the difficulties life presents and be willing to face them with a certain spirit of optimism and strength.

On the other hand, she still feels guilty over being the taker and not the giver in our relationship. In this connection, she needs to know if she has been helpful to me in providing a videotape for instructional purposes. This suggests that she still needs to feel that she is helpful to others, perhaps more than is good for her. There is a hint of an unresolved positive transference or a transference cure in her very rapid response to my letter, its length, her being "ecstatic" in hearing from me, and in her wanting to keep up the correspondence. There is something positive she has internalized from our sessions and our relationship, yet we can ask whether she is still overly dependent in some fashion on me or her memory of me. Has this prevented her from becoming attached to another man? Would a longer therapy, were it possible, have been more helpful in fully resolving these issues? All we can do is raise these questions to illustrate the difficulty of assessing, in an all-or-none fashion, the effects of a brief, intense therapy, or any therapy for that matter.

What happens in this kind of therapy that allows change to come about? We turn now to a brief consideration of the theory of change according to Mann's integrative/analytic time-limited therapy.

THE THEORY OF CHANGE

For Mann (1991), it is the combination of the therapist's statement of the central issue and the setting of the termination date at the start of treatment that provide the therapeutic structure that leads to change. The way in which the central issue is stated by the therapist fosters the development of a therapeutic alliance and a positive transference which allows patients to experience and explore the negative feelings about the self that have dogged them throughout their lives. According to Mann, these feelings typically stem from their inability to separate from others without suffering undue damage to their evaluation of self. Patients are helped to work toward facing up to the past in order to gain some mastery over the present and, in this way, to be freer to shape their future.

The patient enters treatment with the magical expectation that time will be turned back and everything made right. Child time, hearkening back to a state of fusion with mother and to the expectation of unending time and pleasure, must give way, under the imposition of a time limit, to calendar, or adult, time. Separation and loss will occur whether the adult likes it or not, and there is work to be done in coming to terms with the reality of finite time. By constricting the parameter of time through the use of a fixed termination, Mann determinedly guides his patients through the experience of separation and loss. He maintains that the fixed time limit forces both patient and therapist to confront this issue with minimal evasion or denial. There is no therapeutic retreat back to the sense of "oneness." Patients are thus prodded once more into facing reality on their own.

During the termination phase, the patient will react with the same affect that characterized earlier separations and losses, including anger, disappointment, sadness, and guilt. Interpretations link the loss of the therapist with past losses, when misconceptions about the self and maladaptive behavior ensued. Change occurs by helping the patient achieve separation with a degree of resolution that allows for a new kind of internalization, freer of the negative emotions that previously prevailed. According to Mann (1973), it is this process that results in a stronger ego, a more benign sense of self, and a modified superego that allows patients to regard themselves more charitably. "This time the internalization will be more positive (never totally so), less anger-laden, and less guilty, thereby making separation a genuine maturational event" (p. 36).

The theory of change in time-limited psychotherapy, then, includes an integration of several elements, including *induced hope and optimism* stemming from the time limit and the therapist's show of confidence in the patient's ability to master conflict; *insight* derived from clarifications and interpretations around the central issue and its relation to separation anxiety, as well as insight about defenses against feelings; *incorporation of a more benign introject,* brought about by the kind of relationship established by the therapist; and patients' *use of the therapist as a selfobject,* thereby enhancing their self-regard.

REVIEW OF RESEARCH

Outcome

There has been only one controlled study of the effects of Mann's TLP, which was carried out by Shefler, Dasberg, and Ben-Shakhar (in press) in a Jerusalem mental health center. Thirty-three patients were selected on the basis of a variety of criteria, such as level of ego functioning, expression of a circumscribed problem, ability to express affect, and the like. Most had DSM diagnoses of anxiety, depressive, or adjustment disorder, with nine not carrying any psychiatric diagnosis. Excluded were patients with schizophrenia, schizoid character disorder, borderline and psychosomatic disorders, and other severe conditions. Because the study employed a wait-list control design, the patient's ability to delay therapy for 3 months was also considered.

Patients were randomly assigned either to an experimental or control condition. Patients in the experimental condition (12-week TLP) were assessed on a battery of general and individualized tests, both pre- and posttherapy and at 6- and 12-month follow-up. Controls were assessed at the start of the waiting period, after 3 months, at posttherapy, and at follow-up. In other words, the controls were given the same therapy as the experimental group after waiting 3 months.

Significant improvement in target complaints, symptoms, social functioning, and self-esteem was achieved in the treated group, whereas there was no change in the wait-list control group. Similarly, the wait-list control group improved on these dimensions after therapy, even more than had the experimental group. The average effect size, measured by the difference between the gain scores of the experimental versus control subjects, was a substantial 0.99. Clinically significant change was achieved by about two-thirds of treated patients. Furthermore, patients in both treated groups maintained their gains on 6-month and 12-month follow-up. The authors concluded that the outcomes were consistent with TLP's rationale, namely, improvement in self-esteem, social functioning, and target symptoms. While these results are impressive, it should be noted that the patients were highly selected, constituting about 11% of the patients screened for TLP.

In a study largely concerned with the process of TLP (Joyce & Piper, 1990), 14 patients complaining of issues related to separation-individuation were treated in TLP. Although there was no control group comparison, the authors were able to compare patients' pre- and posttherapy scores on a symptom check list (SCL-90) and on level of adaptive functioning across seven dimensions, such as self-esteem and dependence-independence (the Progress Evaluation Scales [PES]). Significant pre- to posttherapy improvement was shown on almost all SCL-90 scales, and on five of the seven PES variables. Results held at 6-month follow-up. In addition, whereas at pretreatment patients differed from nonpatient norms on 12 of the 13 SCL-90 dimensions and on all seven PES scales, at posttreatment they differed on only three of the former and none of the latter. These results provide good support for the efficacy and durability of TLP in this small but well-selected sample.

In another study relevant to the outcome of therapies that are time-limited, Sledge, Moras, Hartley, and Levine (1990) examined the dropout rate for 149 new clinic patients at a large community mental health center. Patients had been assigned by the evaluating clinician either to long-term psychodynamically oriented therapy, Mann's TLP, or a nonspecific, brief, psychodynamically oriented psychotherapy that lasted about 3 to 4 months but had no specific termination date. In TLP, unlike the case for the other brief therapy, the therapist set a specific number of sessions and a termination date at the start of therapy and, in some cases but not always, a central issue or focus.

The dropout rate for TLP was 32%, which was about one-half the rate both for the brief dynamic therapy that had not set a specific termination date (67%) and for long-term therapy (61%). The difference in dropout rates could not be explained by the patients' severity of impairment, therapists' status as trainees or staff, or differential lengths of treatment. Regarding the latter, patient dropout in the long-term therapy tended to occur before most of the brief therapies had ended. Although it is difficult to draw conclusions about Mann's TLP specifically from this study, the results do suggest that setting a time limit influences the patient to stay with therapy for the contracted time period, which has important implications for practice in similar clinical settings.

Relating Therapy Process to Outcome

A study conducted at a university mental health service investigated the relationship between patients' session-by-session evaluations of Mann's TLP and outcome (Bernard, Schwartz, Oclatis, & Stiner, 1980). Patients' in-session evaluations made in the early and in the final phases of treatment correlated with raters' judgments of patients' goal achievements and with patients' positive evaluation of the treatment experience. The authors postulated that patients are most aware of their goals in treatment in the initial and final phases of TLP and hence judge the value of sessions falling in these phases on the basis of how much they contribute to these goals.

Wiseman, Shefler, Caneti, and Ronen (1993) compared patient and therapist ratings of therapy process surrounding discussion of the central issue in each of the three phases of Mann's TLP. From the larger outcome study discussed above, they selected the cases of two 30-year old female patients, one with dependent and histrionic traits whose treatment was unsuccessful, and another with passive and depressive features, whose treatment was successful. Both were treated by the same female therapist. Qualitative and quantitative examination (by means of the Vanderbilt Psychotherapy Process Scale) of the processes surrounding the discussion of the central issue revealed the following differences between the successful and unsuccessful case:

1. In the successful case, the instances of the emergence of the central issue were spread evenly across the three phases, whereas in the unsuccessful case, they occurred largely in the initial phase of therapy.
2. While both patients were able to explore the feelings raised by the central conflict, only the successful patient was able to stay with the feelings and explore various sides of the conflict, including possible alternatives and solutions.
3. The successful patient's participation increased with time and her exploration remained steady, whereas the unsuccessful patient's participation and exploration declined with time.
4. In the successful case, the therapist's exploration reached a peak in the middle phase, whereas for the unsuccessful case it was lowest in this phase.

It would seem that in the unsuccessful case, once ambivalence set in, the central issue lost its potency as a focus, suggesting the need, as the authors point out, for increased therapist effort at this time. It is also, possible, however, that the differences in the nature of the patient problems led to their quite different reactions to the therapist or to TLP.

Process Studies: The Dynamic Sequence

Two studies have explored hypotheses regarding the dynamic sequence that is said to take place across the three phases of TLP. Schwartz and Bernard (1981) posited that patients would evaluate the early and termination phases of TLP in a consistent manner (i. e., similar from session to session), whereas the ambivalence of the middle phase would lead to a lack of consistency in their evaluation of the sessions comprising this phase. Therapist session evaluations were expected to remain consistent throughout the therapy because therapists are presumed to have an image of what the entire course of therapy will entail. In addition, therapist and patient views of the middle sessions were expected to be less congruent with each other than in the early and final phases because of the ambivalence and disappointment which is said to set in at the middle stage.

Contrary to prediction, it was found that patients showed decreasing consistency over the three phases, and therapists showed only modest and largely nonsignificant consistency. Congruence did fall off in the middle phase, but, again contrary to prediction, remained low to moderate in the final phase.

Joyce and Piper (1990) repeated this study with the small sample of 14 patients referred to in the section on therapy outcome above, but with better validated measures of session evaluations. Measures of both patient and therapist consistency and congruence failed to support Bernard and Schwartz's hypotheses. Rather, both patients and therapists evidenced an increase in their ratings from phase to phase on such variables as session accomplishment, positive feeling, and patient clarity of expression. Patients who were viewed as attaining good treatment outcomes were significantly more likely to evidence the trend toward progressively more positive session evaluations.

In summary, there is good initial support for the efficacy of TLP and for the durability of its effects. Setting a time limit appears to be very helpful in retaining clinic patients in treatment. Patient awareness of goal achievement in the early and later stages of TLP is predictive of patients' positive evaluation of outcome, suggesting that it is useful for therapists to remain attentive to patient goals. There are some very preliminary leads as to the nature of central issue events in successful and unsuccessful cases, and there is no corroboration for the middle stage of TLP differing substantially from the other stages. Nevertheless, it should be noted that the latter results may be a function of the inability of the instruments employed to pick up the ambivalence depicted by Mann; the absence of observer ratings of the actual interaction of patient and therapist; and the small samples employed.

A CRITICAL EVALUATION OF AN INTEGRATIVE PSYCHOANALYTIC MODEL

Mann's TLP, as noted above, is based primarily on an object relations theory which emphasizes anxiety and sadness over loss stemming from life events requiring separation and individuation. Neurotic conflict, in this view, results from the wish to unite with the object, thereby recreating the original mother-infant bond, alongside the contrary wish to become a separate, independent being. Psychological development is viewed as proceeding from a state of merger with the other to a state of separateness.

Can all psychopathology be encompassed within this single theme? As Westen (1986) has pointed out, "Mann has isolated one type of pathological and therapeutic process and generalized it to all neurosis" (p. 502). Similarly, Grand et al. (1985) argue: "To the extent that Mann's approach holds specific assumptions about universal prototypic relationship conflicts, his active, manipulative stance runs the risk of imposing such conflicts on the patient whether or not they are salient for the patient at a particular time" (p. 27). In other words, one critique of Mann's approach holds that it is a Procrustean bed, with one size fitting all. All of the four aspects of basic conflicts outlined by Mann and described above reduce to the patient's capacity to tolerate and manage object loss. Westen (1986) has summarized the difficulty as follows: "Single-cause theories of neurosis are intellectually appealing, but they are very likely inaccurate. . . . To the extent that separation-individuation and loss are not a patient's central dynamics, Mann's theory sheds little light on therapeutic change" (p. 502).

Implied in these criticisms is the underlying belief that there is one correct formulation and understanding of a patient's problems, and, therefore, that the theme of separation-individuation may or may not be accurate for any particular individual. In Chapter 2 we began exploring the implications of two quite different ways of understanding clinical material. We referred to one as based on the correspondence theory of truth, in which there is posited to be an objectively correct, underlying structure of psychopathology, which it is the clinician's job to discern and bring to light. The other was the coherence theory which assumes that there is more than one way to understand and interpret a patient's verbal productions. Truth is not discovered, as within an objectivist framework, but is constructed along certain lines. It is narrative truth, not historical truth, that emerges in the therapist–patient dialogue (Spence, 1982). "Narrative truth is what we have in mind when we say that such and such is a good story, that a given explanation carries conviction . . . " (p. 31).

Along these lines, Sarbin (1986) has suggested that a person's life can be viewed as a story or narrative that gives shape to, and organizes, human action. Similarly, McAdams (1993) posits that each of us is engaged in a lifelong task of creating our unique personal myth. "Stories slice the world up (or urge us to view the world) from a variety of different perspectives, points of view, and value positions, and thus construct noncomparable frames of reference through which reality might be grasped" (Howard, 1991, p. 191). Howard sees the work of therapy as life-story elaboration or repair. A life becomes meaningful when a person sees him- or herself as an actor within the context of a story. Although patients come into therapy with their own story, it gets elaborated and focused by therapist and patient in such a way that it comes to sustain "a better self-image and a more hopeful future" (Frank, 1987). In the case of Rose, for example, we saw how the story line of her agreeableness and strongly independent stance in life, and the price she was paying for it, formed the basis of a significant life story and its repair.

Omer (1993) refers to the story in the various forms of brief therapy as a life sketch. It involves renarrating the client's life story into a highly condensed psychobiography. For example, the narrative line of

Strupp and Binder's TLDP includes acts of self, expectations about other's reactions, acts of others toward self, and acts of self toward self. Omer's "integrative focus" combines and coordinates a symptomatic perspective (the immediate complaint), and a person-centered developmental task which is presented to the patient in a brief life sketch. In a postmodern spirit, he asserts that the value of a particular focus should be assessed, not in terms of its truth value, but its appeal, and capacity to involve, charm, or provoke.

Short-term therapy may be compared to a short story—a piece of written or therapeutic work that typically focuses on a single theme, a few characters, and one slice of life. Long-term therapy is more akin to a fully developed novel, incorporating plots and subplots, a panoply of characters, and a great variety of situations in which human drama unfolds. Both can be valued for what they uniquely offer.

Viewed from within a narrative understanding of psychotherapy, Mann's TLP can be characterized as a way of constructing a patient's problems along the lines of an object relations theme or story line. The story line is union and separation, and their vicissitudes in a particular person's life. Mann might argue that, since separation is a central and universal facet of human life, this particular story line is bound to be relevant in some important way, as it was for Rose. But, as we have seen, it is not the only story that can be told.

Nor is separation–individuation the only possible story line that one may discern in TLP. Gustafson (1986), for example, discerns an evangelical theme. There is the recognition of patients' chronically endured pain, in which they see themselves as stupid, unattractive, or incapable. They try hard to overcome this feeling but keep slipping back into it. The TLP therapist comes along, arousing hope and inspiring the willingness to try once more to overcome. Then follows the disappointment and deterioration of progress as termination looms. Says Gustafson (1986), "The evangelical churches are familiar with this rise and fall: first the revival; then, hard work from the convert, while he or she is full of the love of God; but finally a backsliding" (p. 155). Not everyone will accept this message, says Gustafson. Furthermore, if the pull from the family is very strong, he regards the method as too weak to be effective without addressing current systemic issues within the individual therapy (see Chapter 5).

As we have learned, Mann views the termination phase as a crisis for clients due to their loss of an important object, namely, the therapist. Clients are expected to respond with a variety of unpleasant emotions, prompting therapist countertransference reactions. In this connection, we witnessed Rose's distress at the prospect of losing her therapist, and the emotions this aroused in him as well. Quintana (1993) has challenged the notion of termination-as-crisis, pointing to empiri-cal literature (e.g., Marx & Gelso, 1987) which suggests that most clients and therapists are satisfied with therapy termination, with little evidence of a crisis over loss. When there was a crisis, it was due more to the disappointing level of therapy outcome than to loss per se.

It appears that most therapists defuse termination by inviting clients to return on an as-need basis. Quintana justifies this practice, citing investigations (Geller, 1987) which suggest that it is not neces-sary to relinquish relationships in order for them to be internalized. He recommends the metaphor of termination-as-transformation, view-ing termination as a transition phase that can promote changes in how clients view themselves and their therapists. Drawing on the develop-mental literature that conceptualizes the child's maturation as occur-ring through parental encouragement and support, he suggests that therapists need to acknowledge, review, and support clients' sense of accomplishment in therapy and the steps they have taken toward health, independence, and maturity. It is this stance that will lead to internali-zation, he asserts, rather than the prospect of definitive separation and loss, as argued by Mann. Perhaps both points of view have some validi-ty, such that the sense of accomplishment along with the struggle over separation can contribute to internalization.

There are other criticisms of TLP that we will mention briefly. Be-cause of its brevity and rigid time limit, TLP may be suitable only for a limited range of patients in comparison to other BPT approaches. In this connection, it will be recalled that the successful trial of TLP conducted by Shefler et al. (in press) focused on a highly selected sample.

Mann claims that the therapeutic benefit of TLP derives in part from the internalization of the therapist as a benign object. Westen (1986) questions whether internalization of the therapist as a replace-ment for previous less- than-benign objects is possible in a 12-session therapy. Similarly, it can be asked whether individuation can take place in such a relatively short time. On the other hand, Mann's goals for this therapy are more modest than are the claims of the drive/structur-al therapists. Mann does not suggest that it strives for, or achieves, the same goals as psychoanalysis. The question of what, if anything, gets internalized in a brief therapy appears to be an area ripe for empiri-cal investigation. (See Quintana & Meara, 1990, for some promising results regarding internalization of the counseling relationship in clients who experienced about eight sessions of various kinds of brief thera-py, including psychodynamic therapy of an unspecified kind. The authors found that clients' intrapsychic dispositions became more simi-lar to their counselors' interpersonal dispositions by the end of brief therapy.)

There is a paucity of research on TLP. As reviewed above, there are only two studies assessing the outcome of this therapy, and very few examining its process. More research needs to be carried out to put this therapy on a firmer empirical footing.

On the positive side is the relative ease with which those trained in long-term psychoanalytic therapy can learn and practice this mode of brief therapy. Its techniques are not radically different from those of long-term psychodynamic therapy. What differs is its time structure and focus. Empathy, warmth, and joining — characteristic of TLP — are more consonant with most therapists' inclinations than are challenge and confrontation which typify Davanloo's and Sifneos's brief therapies.

Also appealing is TLP's integrative psychoanalytic stance, which allows for a broader based therapy than any one variant of psychoanalysis, as Pine's work attests. It is in the spirit of the times to look not only within variants of one school of therapy but across therapies in general for commonalities and points of integration, which is the topic of the next chapter.

CHAPTER 5

Eclectic Approaches: Garfield, Bellak, and Gustafson

In recent years efforts have been made to incorporate techniques or concepts from different therapeutic traditions within psychoanalytic therapy. In adding elements of other therapies, the object has been to improve its efficacy and range of applicability. Such integrative or eclectic efforts in respect to psychoanalytic therapy are part of a larger trend in the field to look across therapies and to attempt different types and degrees of synthesis. A survey of mental health practitioners from a variety of disciplinary backgrounds found that 68% consider themselves to be eclectic (Jensen, Bergin, & Greaves, 1990). Just as current varieties of psychoanalytic theory have led to the existing models of BPT, so has the eclectic trend influenced some forms that brief therapy has taken.

Such an integrative or eclectic thrust has not emerged in a vacuum but is a response to several developments in the broader mental health field. One factor has been the increasing interaction in medical schools, graduate schools, and clinics of mental health professionals, of different orientations—such as behavior therapy, family therapy, psychopharmacological therapy, or psychoanalytic therapy. Psychoanalysts, for example, moved from their institutes, which tend to be narrowly focused in outlook, into university settings which thrive on an exchange of competing ideas. In the case of behavior therapists, as they took on more complex and problematic cases, they cast about for concepts that they could add to their repertoire to improve their results (Gold, 1993). Such exposure to the ideas and approaches of others inevitably leads to a questioning of one's own cherished beliefs and, frequently, a willingness to consider the validity of other frameworks.

A second factor promoting rapprochement has been the climate of mental health practice, which has been increasingly concerned with cost and, therefore, with the most effective and efficient therapies available to address specific problems. As insurance companies, government, consumer groups, and others have become involved in paying for mental health service delivery or influencing its policy, they have been insistent on demonstrations of efficacy, which has led mental health professionals to a greater level of cooperation to meet the needs of clients and the demands of third-party payers (Brown, 1983).

A third element contributing to the eclectic/integrative thrust has come from the research community which, in the face of Eysenck's (1952) claim of little unique benefit ensuing from psychotherapy, mounted many studies that compared therapies with each other and against no-treatment or wait-list controls. Although the upshot of this research on differential efficacy among the therapies is still controversial (e.g., Elliott, Stiles, & Shapiro, 1993), the consensus at present is that the different therapies are more or less equally effective in improving clients' lives (Lambert & Bergin, 1994; Lambert et al., 1986). This finding has come most persuasively from meta-analyses that statistically combine the effects of many studies and which have led to the conclusion (with some exceptions; e.g., Giles, 1993) of little outcome difference among therapies (Shapiro & Shapiro, 1982; Smith et al., 1980).

If this finding is accurate, it forces us to consider seriously—despite our allegiances to one or another model of therapy—the proposition that the efficacy of the various psychotherapies lies more in their *common features and concepts* than in the mechanisms of change unique to each (Beitman, Goldfried, & Norcross, 1989). This hypothesis has led to a search for factors that cut across the many varieties of psychotherapy (400 by one author's count; Karasu, 1986), such as the nature of the relationship established between therapist and client and the ways in which it helps clients heal and change. The finding of equal outcomes has also led to the attempt to combine techniques from different sources known as *technical eclecticism* (e.g., Lazarus, 1992), and to *integrate different theories* in order to capitalize on their separate virtues (e.g., Safran & Segal, 1990; Wachtel, 1977). By wedding one therapy to the other, the hope is to achieve a more perfect union, to the betterment of the client's condition.

There is also a growing consensus that there is no single approach that is adequate for all clients, and that there should be consideration given to *matching the therapy to the client*. That is, even if the overall outcomes of the different psychotherapies are similar, an enhanced result may be obtained by tailoring the therapy to the client rather that fitting him or her into the mold of one mode of therapy (e.g., see Beutler & Consoli, 1992; Jones, Cumming, & Horowitz, 1988). This issue is particularly pertinent to BPT because of the fairly stringent standards for suitability set by some of the models. In order to be more inclusive, some degree of eclecticism may be desirable in allowing for a range of practice within psychoanalytically based brief therapy. Of course, this may involve trade-offs which must be considered as well.

To summarize, there are three major ways in which the terms integration and eclecticism have been used to describe rapprochement among the therapies: (1) common factors, (2) technical eclecticism, including prescriptive matching, and (3) theoretical integration. These terms will help to serve as an organizing framework to guide our presentation of examples of brief psychodynamic therapies that have integrative elements. Although these different approaches to integration may be considered separately for didactic purposes, it is clear that there is overlap among them.

COMMON FACTORS

The common factors approach seeks out those processes or elements that are shared by different therapies. Proponents of this approach believe that what moves therapy forward are not the factors unique to each therapy but those that cut across the separate domains. What has often been referred to as "noise" when it comes to conducting research on the different models of psychotherapy in fact may be the "signal" that common-factor therapists attempt to amplify. For example, Alexander and French's (1946) term "the corrective emotional experience" was an early and influential concept highlighting a common factor:

> In all forms of etiological psychotherapy, the basic therapeutic principle is the same: To re-expose the patient, under more favorable circumstances, to emotional situations which he could not handle in the past. The patient, in order to be helped, must undergo a corrective emotional experience suitable to repair the traumatic influence of previous experience. (p. 66)

In an important effort to specify common factors, Goldfried (1980) argued that to reach consensus at either the level of theory or clinical technique would be less acceptable to proponents of the separate schools than would intermediate clinical strategies or principles. The two strategies that he proposed were (1) having patients/clients engage in new, corrective experiences in order to recognize that their fears were groundless, and (2) offering feedback to patients/clients to help them become more aware of their actions, thoughts, or feelings.

Perhaps the best known attempt to present the common factors of psychotherapy, and one that is a predominant influence in Garfield's brief therapy, described below, is that of Frank (1982; see also Frank & Frank, 1991). According to Frank, the patient enters therapy in a state of demoralization — that is, disheartened and dispirited. All therapeutic systems, he postulates, combat demoralization through the provision of four effective features:

(1) *An emotionally charged, confiding relationship with a helping person,* that inspires confidence and increases expectancies of success, thereby improving morale;

(2) *A healing setting,* which provides safety, and other special attributes which distinguish it from the rest of the person's surroundings (e.g., a hospital, clinic, or consulting room, which carry the aura of science);

(3) *A rationale or conceptual scheme* that provides a plausible explanation for the patient's symptoms which can include, for example, psychodynamic explanations;

(4) *A ritual or procedure that requires the active participation of both patient and therapist* and that is believed by both to be the means of restoring the patient's health. In psychoanalytic therapy, this may be free association and the therapist's clarifying or interpreting the patient's verbal productions. (Frank & Frank, 1991, pp. 42–44)

As we turn to Garfield's brief psychotherapy, the influence of Frank's common factors outlook will be apparent.

Garfield's Brief Psychotherapy

Garfield (1989) believes that brief therapy is the treatment of choice for most clients who can profit from psychotherapy at all. He sees its general goal as helping clients to overcome the problems or discomforts that lead them to seek help. The brief therapist does not strive for personality transformation (which in any case, he claims, is rare), but for repair of psychological damage. An additional goal is the development of coping skills and the possible prevention of future upset. Emphasis is on the here and now of the problems versus their there-and-then origin. What makes brief therapy different from long-term therapy is the specificity of goals, the active role of the therapist in helping patients achieve their goals, and the expectation that the therapy will be short. The therapist is more directive in Garfield's brief therapy than is true in psychoanalytic or existential-humanistic client-centered therapy.

As for suitability, anyone who is in touch with reality, is experiencing some discomfort, and has made the effort to seek help is eligible. Garfield sees the client's problems as interrelated and, in this sense, the therapist is dealing with one problem only—namely, manifestations of less than adequate adjustment. The therapy is clearly not meant to be an intensive reconstructive therapy with the goal of significant insight or personality change but, rather, it is an attempt to help the person solve a specific, manifest problem.

Mechanisms of Change: Garfield's List of Common Factors

The therapeutic relationship. A good relationship is the *sine qua non* for successful brief therapy, according to Garfield. It should be characterized by trust and confidentiality, which allows the client to reveal previously undisclosed thoughts and feelings. It also allows the therapist to act as an agent of persuasion or reinforcement for the client. "Suggestions, interpretations, homework assignments, and other activities of the therapist are more likely to be accepted and complied with than if such a relationship did not exist" (1989, p. 27). A good relationship increases the chances of clients modeling themselves after the therapist and taking on the therapist's values.

Interpretation, insight, and understanding. For Garfield, as for Frank (1982), the value of interpretation lies not in its accuracy or scientific validity but in its plausibility and its acceptance by the client. The nature of the explanation of the problem, therefore, is secondary to the therapist's presenting it in a confident and knowledgeable manner and the client finding it meaningful. In terms of our earlier discussion of the truth value of psychoanalytic explanations, it is narrative truth, not historical truth, that matters.

Emotional release. The client has the opportunity to express feelings such as guilt or sadness in a nonjudgmental, accepting atmosphere.

Reinforcement. Whether deliberately or unconsciously, psychotherapists reinforce desired behaviors in a positive manner and use negative reinforcement or extinction procedures for undesirable behaviors, according to Garfield. Even if only by a head nod or smile, such behavior can serve as a differential reinforcer to the client. In addition, in those therapies that encourage action, behaviors performed successfully tend to be reinforced, thus aiding the patient's improvement.

Desensitization. Repeated discussion of the client's problems with the therapist allows the client to examine them in a more dispassionate, less personalized, and less anxiety-arousing way. The anxieties get extinguished in the security of the therapeutic environment and with the absence of negative consequences.

Confronting one's problems. The client is confronted be it cognitive-ly or behaviorally, with the anxiety-inducing situation rather than be-ing allowed to continue avoiding it. In doing so, clients discover that there are no truly catastrophic consequences.

Mechanisms of Change: Specific Therapist Techniques

Garfield (1989) points out that the application of common principles does not mean that specific techniques for specific clients or problems may not be useful as well. In addition to the common factors just described, Garfield prescribes therapist activities which he feels are often undervalued both in long-term and brief therapy.

Listening. "The therapist must be a good listener, and particularly in brief therapy must be attuned to what the patient is saying" (p. 35). This includes the patient's references to the therapist or therapy, which should be carefully explored.

Reflection. The therapist should reflect the attitudes of the client in an empathic manner, thereby conveying to clients that he or she is listening carefully and trying to understand the client's attitudes.

Suggestion. Direct suggestions may be offered to clients but they should be delivered in a nonauthoritarian fashion. This will allow for some discussion about the suggestions in a collaborative manner.

Explanation and interpretation. Explanations and interpretations should be offered in a tentative, not a dogmatic or accusatory, way (see Wachtel, 1993; Wile, 1984). This also includes orienting the client to the rationale for the treatment.

Providing information. Therapy should not be made into a question-and-answer process, but the therapist may help clients understand such matters as how AIDS is contracted.

Confrontation. Confrontation should be tried primarily in the con-text of a good therapist-client relationship, says Garfield. Although con-frontation can be nontherapeutic, there are times when a client must be confronted with a self-defeating pattern, such as lateness, evasive-ness, lack of participation in therapy, and so on. The therapist must carefully gauge the client's response to such confrontation.

Reassurance. Reassurance should not be administered routinely or falsely but in a situation where it is justified and needed to sustain the patient.

Homework assignments. Assignments are an activity more typical of the behavioral or cognitive therapist and should be suggested where there is a reasonable chance of success. For example, in treating bulimia, the client may be encouraged to keep a diary of individual food items consumed, the time, the setting, and any related feelings. If this task is not successful, the reasons for noncompliance should be assessed and discussed.

Modeling and role playing. The use of modeling and role playing is an approach most familiar to Gestalt and cognitive-behavioral therapists. For example, if assertiveness is a problem, the client can role play being assertive, with the therapist taking the role of the other, such as a boss or girlfriend, a technique also known as cognitive or behavioral rehearsal. The client may also model some values or attitudes of the therapist and, in fact, there is research indicating that there is some convergence in the beliefs of therapists and clients at the conclusion of therapy (Beutler, Crago, & Arizmendi, 1986).

Questioning. Questions can be employed to elicit information either about factual matters, as is typical in early sessions, or about important aspects of the client's thoughts or feelings. The questioning should not be in the manner of a prosecuting attorney, or with the expectation of a yes or no answer, but formulated to help deepen the client's experience and self-awareness.

Self-disclosure. This should be done infrequently and only with regard to the client's, not the therapist's, needs. It can resemble an empathic response and may also be modeling a means of coping with a problem. Overly personal matters or therapist problems should not be shared.

In his book on brief therapy, Garfield (1989) spells out in detail the requirements of each phase of brief therapy, including the initial interview, the early and middle sessions, and the termination period. He provides case vignettes to guide the therapist and illustrates how the common factors described above are put into practice. The interested reader is referred to his book for a more comprehensive rendering of his common factors brief therapy.

Research on Garfield's Brief Therapy

There has been no research specifically comparing Garfield's form of brief therapy to other therapies or to control groups. To support the utility of his therapy, Garfield cites the general findings on the efficacy of brief therapy, which we reviewed in Chapter 1. Based on a review of the psychotherapy outcome literature (Lambert et al., 1986), Lambert (1992) estimates that, among therapeutic factors, approximately 30% of improvement in psychotherapy patients is a function of common factors. This may be compared to the effect of techniques, which he estimates to account for 15%. He also points out that insofar as eclectic therapies provide treatment that overlaps with traditional methods that have been tested, they rest on a firm empirical base and should prove to be as effective as traditional therapies and certainly more effective than nontreatment controls. To illustrate the kind of findings that lend credence to the common factors approach, we will cite two studies, one based on patient perspectives and the other on therapist perspectives.

In a well-known project comparing brief psychoanalytically oriented therapy to brief behavior therapy (Sloane, Staples, Cristol, Yorkston, & Whipple, 1975), successful patients were asked to respond to a questionnaire to elicit the factors they considered to be responsible for their improvement.

> The following items were each termed "extremely important or "very important" by at least 70 percent of successful patients in both groups:
> 1. The personality of your doctor
> 2. His helping you to understand your problem
> 3. Encouraging you gradually to practice facing the things that bother you.
> 4. Being able to talk to an understanding person.
> 5. Helping you to understand yourself. (p. 206)

In the words of Sloane et al. (1975):

> None of the items regarded as very important by the majority of either group of patients describes techniques specific to one therapy. . . . Most noticeable is the great overlap between the two groups, suggesting that, at least from the patient's point of view, the effectiveness of treatment was due to factors common to both therapies rather than to any particular theoretical orientation or techniques. (p. 207)

Of course, what patients meant by items such as "Helping you to understand yourself" may have been quite different in the two therapies, but there is not enough information available to address that possibility.

In order to study commonalities from the standpoint of the therapist, Grencavage and Norcross (1990) reviewed 50 publications that focused on individual psychotherapy and encompassed at least three therapeutic systems. The most frequent category of common factors

mentioned was change processes (41%), followed by therapist qualities (21%). The most agreed-upon commonalities were the development
of a therapeutic alliance (56% of all authors), the opportunity for catharsis or emotional expression of problems (38%), the acquisition and practice of new behaviors (32%), patients' positive expectancies, such as
hope for change (26%), beneficial therapist qualities, such as the capacity to instill hope, (24%), and the provision of a rationale for the
patient's problems (24%). Grencavage and Norcross emphasized the
difficulty they experienced categorizing the proposed common factors,
in part because of the different technical language employed for what
may (or may not) have been the same construct.

The findings support Goldfried's (1980) proposal that the most
fruitful level of abstraction at which to find common factors is neither
theory nor techniques but therapeutic processes. In addition, there is
considerable overlap between the factors on this list and those enumerated by Garfield, which tend to corroborate his particular list. Note,
however, that these common factors are ones perceived to be such by
the authors of the 50 publications, rather than what researchers found
or patients actually experienced. For reviews of the research related
to common factors in psychotherapy, the reader is directed to chapters by Weinberger (1993), and Lambert (1992).

Critique of the Common Factors Model

There is considerable appeal in the prospect of a therapy that teases
out the factors which contribute to successful outcomes in many or all
therapies. This approach has the virtues of pragmatism and parsim-
ony, as well as being consistent with the general research literature on
psychotherapy outcome. By emphasizing what the psychotherapies
share rather than what separates them, common change principles provide a meeting ground for proponents of different schools, thereby
promoting a more open, less doctrinaire stance.

Regarding the research literature, however, the fact that outcomes
have tended to be similar across therapies can lead to conclusions other
than the presence of common factors. For example, therapies may
achieve similar goals by different routes. Or the problem may lie in
the research instruments employed, which may not be sensitive enough
to pick up real differences in outcome. Studies comparing different
psychotherapies have also been criticized as having too little statistical
power to pick up differential outcomes because of small sample sizes
(Kazdin & Bass, 1989). Furthermore, there is no guarantee that we have
correctly discerned what are the most efficacious common factors and,
therefore, cannot confidently advocate which ones should be empha-

sized. For example, only half of the authors studied by Grencavage and Norcross cited the most popular candidate—the development of the therapeutic alliance. Other factors were only agreed upon by 24% to 38% of the sample.

Thus, the identification of common factors presently has a subjective cast. In fact, there has been practically no research directly comparing an eclectic therapy to standard models, or even research on the process of eclectic therapy (Lambert, 1992; Mahalik, 1990), which points to an obvious need if the claims of the superiority of eclectic models are to be accepted. Even defining a common factor in an agreed-upon way has proven to be problematic. For example, Tichenor and Hill (1989) compared six measures of the working alliance and found only three to be equivalent.

Another problem is the lack of specificity of the common factors. The level of generality in which they are stated may allow initial agreement about their commonality, but on closer inspection they look quite different across therapies. To take the therapeutic relationship as an example, it may be true that a warm, caring, nonjudgmental attitude on the part of the therapist is important in any therapy. But the way in which the relationship is developed and employed differs for each school (Messer, 1988a). The common element, as it gets expressed in psychoanalytic therapy, for example, is referred to as the "real relationship" and the "working alliance." The former is the genuine person-to-person relationship between client and therapist, which can be characterized as appropriate, realistic, objective, and authentic. The working alliance is the cooperative and willing inclination of the client to overcome his or her problems and to achieve the insights that psychoanalytic therapy has to offer.

The transference relationship, by contrast, is the idiosyncratic and fantasied way in which the client experiences the therapist. To foster the latter, the analytic therapist maintains a certain degree of neutrality and ambiguity of presence. The behavioral therapist, having little interest in transference, often emphasizes the role of therapist as teacher, counselor, and environmental arranger. In client-centered therapy, the relationship is viewed at all times as real. Its concept of "congruence" (Rogers, 1957) requires that therapists be accurately aware of their feelings and be willing to share them when appropriate.

Viewing all three therapies together, how can one be simultaneously neutral in the service of transference, didactic in the service of guiding the client, and real and genuine in the service of authenticity when each role interferes to some extent with the other? In this connection, Rice (1988) has pointed out that the emphasis on transference interpretation in psychoanalytic therapy would dilute the power of the real relationship fostered in client-centered therapy.

Thus, even while there is something shared among approaches in the nature of the therapist–client relationship, the broader context in which it occurs gives it quite a different shading and emphasis. The so-called common element is colored by the theoretical frame in which the therapy occurs. Since Garfield states that a focus on transference is unnecessary in his brief therapy, he is freer to take on the role of advice-giver or coach with impunity. But such a stance creates a very different relationship to the client and may be detrimental to the process and goals of a psychoanalytically based brief therapy. From the latter perspective, a didactic stance may lead clients to comply with therapists' suggestions in an effort to please them (Lazarus & Messer, 1988). In Berman's (1985) experience, when psychodynamic therapists set themselves up as actual authorities, patients became less free to verbalize their feelings, especially when the therapist's advice was not followed.

Perhaps Garfield's brief therapy is better characterized as counseling rather than psychotherapy. Psychotherapy, as it is typically understood within psychoanalytic and humanistic frameworks, emphasizes personal awareness of the self and the interpersonal implications of this enhanced awareness. Interpreting transference and linking it to past and present relationships is employed in psychoanalytic therapy as a major way to achieve that end. In this sense, psychotherapy is not just problem solving as Garfield describes it, even if it is related at least indirectly to solving a problem. The psychodynamic therapist does not directly teach a skill, model appropriate behaviors, or overtly reinforce desired behaviors. This would be viewed as too directive, potentially usurping what typically should be the client's reponsibility. What patients should take from a psychoanalytic (or client-centered) therapy is the capacity to be more empathic with themselves and others, just as the therapist is empathically attuned to them. Viewed within a psychoanalytic perspective, more active and direct guidance, counseling, and problem solving, as described in Garfield's therapy, is reserved for the more disturbed client, and is commonly referred to as "case management" or "supportive therapy" (discussed in Chapter 6).

The pivotal role of theory in determining the aims and techniques of therapy apply as well to Goldfried's (1980) common change principles. Drawing upon his examples, we would argue that *offering feedback* about smoking is not the same as giving feedback about a client's defenses or character traits (Messer & Winokur, 1981). *Providing a corrective emotional experience* in response to patients bringing forth warded-off material in the therapy room may be quite different from the experience resulting from direct exposure to an anxiety-eliciting stimulus in the natural environment.

In this connection, Schacht (1984) has pointed out that "salt in one's soup is quite different from salt in one's gas tank. There is a common element (salt) involved, but the vast differences in context destroy any possibilities for easy and straightforward extrapolation or inference from one case to the other" (p. 121). Regarding the role of therapists, Strupp (1986) has argued that one cannot readily disentangle the common (or nonspecific) factor from a technical (or specific) factor because therapists' personal and technical skills are tightly woven into every aspect of the structure and process of their relationship to the patient. A related point is that one cannot put considerations of theory or technique aside when one examines common factors. There is a "trickle-down" effect of theory which guides the therapist along certain technical paths (Safran & Messer, 1995), and these are bound to differ among the therapies, based as they are on quite different theoretical premises.

It is also hard to demonstrate that a common factor, such as the arousal of hope, actually brings about positive outcomes even if it is correlated with outcome. As Arkowitz (1992) has pointed out, it is just as plausible that as the patient improves due to other reasons, hope is aroused, or that a third factor such as a supportive relationship increases both hope and progress. Alternately, the common factor may interact with other variables in a nonlinear manner as a function of phase of therapy or type of psychopathology. Thus, a factor which may be a common change principle for higher functioning patients may not be so for more disturbed patients (e.g., Jones et al., 1988). This leads us to a consideration of technical eclecticism because one of its features is matching patients to therapy.

TECHNICAL ECLECTICISM

Eclectic therapists are prepared to draw on techniques from whatever source when they seem called for in a particular case, rather than relying solely on the techniques of a single system of therapy. Technical eclecticism has also come to mean, in the psychotherapy literature, applying different therapies or techniques to different patient groups as guided by theory, clinical experience, or research.

The emphasis in technical eclecticism is on what works, preferably as determined by empirical research. Theory is accorded less importance. In the past, eclecticism has had somewhat of a shady reputation in psychotherapy circles, since it implied to many a promiscuous approach in which techniques were combined indiscriminately (this notion is the opposite of the original meaning of "eclectic," which is derived from a Greek word meaning "selective"). However, with the advent of systematic, carefully conceived models of eclecticism, and with books, articles, and even a journal devoted to it (*Journal of Psychotherapy Integration*), eclecticism has attained considerable respectability. In addition, surveys have found that a substantial percentage of practitioners identify themselves as eclectic, although there is a certain degree of ambiguity about just what the term might mean to them.

There are two major technically eclectic systems of therapy: one is Lazarus's multimodal therapy, which draws largely on cognitive and behavioral techniques, and the other is Beutler's systematic eclectic psychotherapy. As neither is strongly psychodynamic in thrust, we describe them only briefly in order to illustrate the nature of eclectic psychotherapeutic models.

In Lazarus's (1992) brand of technical eclecticism, a person's problems are assessed across seven modalities: behavior, affect, sensation, imagery, cognition, interpersonal relationships, and drugs/biology (which, together, make up the acronym BASIC ID). Interventions are chosen to target each problem in each modality. Thus, anxiety (in the affective modality) may be countered by deep muscle relaxation and stress inoculation training, and perfectionism (in the cognitive modality) by cognitive restructuring. The two-chair technique adapted from Gestalt therapy may be employed to help a patient rehearse becoming more assertive (the behavioral modality). The approach, although eclectic in practice, is single-minded in its reliance on social learning theory. It is Lazarus's contention that one can incorporate diverse techniques without bringing along pieces of the theoretical framework in which they are embedded (Lazarus & Messer, 1991).

Whereas Lazarus's technical eclecticism combines techniques from different sources in the same therapy, Beutler's (1991) systematic eclectic psychotherapy (s.e.p.) tries to determine the kinds of patient, therapist, and treatment variables that will interact to produce the best results. This can be a very complicated endeavor, as one can generate a very long list under each of these headings. To trim the list, Beutler suggests that the choice of variables be guided both by theory and by the results of empirical research already undertaken. For theory he draws on social influence processes because this is how he views therapy as exerting its effects.

Examples of patient variables are problem complexity, problem severity, reactance or resistance level, and coping style. We shall focus on the latter two here. Reactance or resistance "is the tendency to respond oppositionally to external demands. . . . This trait is related to an individual's acquired sensitivity to perceived interpersonal threats to one's autonomy . . . " (Beutler & Consoli, 1992, pp. 273–274). Thus, the use of directive therapies with high reactance-prone/resistant patients may result in a worsening of their condition. With regard to coping style, *internalizers* are characterized by self-blame and self-devaluation, accompanied by compartmentalization of affect and idealization of others. They tend to attribute their problems to their own lack of skills or abilities. Internalizers with a low reactance potential tend to be intrapunitive and to constrict their emotional responses (avoidant personality disorder), whereas those with a high reactance level are prone to overcontrol their feelings, masking their anger, which periodically gets expressed through explosive outbursts. This may be followed by apologies and guilt (obsessive personality disorder).

By contrast, *externalizers* attribute their discomfort to external factors or to other people. Among externalizers with low resistance, symptoms rather than people may be blamed for their problems, and they feel unable to control what happens to them (passive–aggressive and narcissistic personality disorders). Externalizers with high resistance tend to blame others and to act out, including being oppositional and extrapunitive (paranoid and antisocial personality disorders).

Beutler et al. (1991) designed a study to test the interaction of these two patient variables—resistance potential and coping style—with responsiveness to therapies which differ in their emphasis on insight versus cognitive-behavioral change, and on self-directed versus authority-directed focus. The patients were diagnosed with major depressive disorder. The results were supportive of the hypothesis that there would be an interaction between patient types and therapy types in predicting outcomes. The three therapy types were group cognitive therapy, group experiential therapy (insight oriented but directive) and a supportive, self-directed therapy which was conducted by telephone.

Consistent with most comparative studies, all treatments produced equivalent positive effects. However, as predicted, there was an interaction between the person variables and responsiveness to treatment. Externalizers improved more than internalizers in cognitive therapy, whereas internalizers improved most in self-directed therapy. Conversely, high resistant (or reactive) patients improved more in self-directed therapy than in either experiential therapy or cognitive therapy, whereas low resistant patients improved more in cognitive therapy than in self-directed, supportive therapy. There were no significant changes in these results on 1 year follow-up (Beutler, Machado, Engle, & Mohr, 1993). The studies supported the authors' suggestions of assigning patients with externalizing coping styles and/or low resistance potential to cognitive therapy, and patients with internalizing coping styles and/or high resistance potential to supportive, self-directed therapy.

Regarding prescriptive matching for brief psychodynamic psychotherapy, there is a study (Jones et al., 1988) highly suggestive of its value. Patients diagnosed as suffering from stress response syndromes following a traumatic event or bereavement were treated in Horowitz's brief therapy (described in Chapter 3). Improvement was predicted best by an interaction between patients' pretreatment disturbance level and the nature of therapist interventions. The more highly disturbed patients did best when therapists were didactic, reassuring, gave advice and guidance, and strengthened defenses. The less disturbed patients did better with therapist silences, reference to the interaction, emphasis upon feelings, and drawing connections between the therapeutic relationship and other relationships. In other words, the more disturbed patients, who were looking for a restorative relationship from the therapist, profited from a more supportive, reality- oriented brief therapy, and those who were less disturbed were helped by a more exploratory/interpretive brief therapy. In a sense, this study also supports the selection of less disturbed patients for the purer application of Horowitz's form of BPT, and the necessity to modify it for the more depressed, dependent patients.

In turning to psychoanalytically based, brief, technically eclectic therapy, we should say at the outset that there is none that has been developed systematically in the manner of multimodal therapy or s.e.p. However, in reviewing the brief therapies with a psychodynamic base, we consider two to fall within a technically eclectic tradition: Wolberg's (1980) dynamic short-term therapy and Bellak's brief and emergency psychotherapy, the latter of which we will now describe.

Bellak's Brief and Emergency Psychotherapy

Bellak (1992) dates his interest in brief therapy back to 1946, when he was working for the Veterans Administration and seeing ex-soldiers for three sessions. Later, in trying to serve the mental health needs of the population of the borough of Queens in New York City, Bellak and Small (1965, 1978) developed a way of working with a wide variety of patients in both emergency and brief therapy. As a psychoanalyst, Bellak tried to show how psychoanalytic principles could be harnessed, albeit with modifications, to serve patients falling into many diagnostic categories. It is eclectic both in Lazarus's sense of combining techniques, as well as in Beutler's sense of applying different techniques to different syndromes. In addition to the volumes cited above, Bellak's therapy is described in the *Handbook of Intensive Brief and Emergency Psychotherapy* (Bellak, 1992), that also contains a chapter pertaining to brief therapy with children by Abrams, and one on brief cognitive therapy by Ackermann-Engel.

Bellak enumerates the following principles for his brief and emergency psychotherapy (BEP):

1. The patient is understood within a broadly conceived psycho-analytic framework, which can include cognitive, behavioral, or systems theory.

2. A focus is established which emphasizes why the patient came to the clinic at this time, when the problem started, and when it appeared at other times in the patient's life.

3. There is an attempt to ascertain the continuity between the present and the past, waking and sleeping thought, and what is conscious and unconscious within the context of the biological, social, familial, and physical aspects of the patient's life.

4. Symptoms are viewed as attempts at problem solving and at coping with anxiety, conflict, and deficit.

5. BEP focuses on what has been poorly learned and what needs to be unlearned and relearned. Treatment is an attempt to help the person attain better devices for coping with reality, conflicts, and defective introjects.

6. The therapy lasts five sessions, with a sixth session held one month later. The chosen length is a practical matter as patients often are not willing to remain longer.

7. BEP applies to a very broad array of patients, with the problem being the focus for treatment rather than the patient. Brief therapy is seen as the method of choice, and only if more extensive change is needed or desired should long-term therapy be considered.

8. BEP may be useful for primary prevention: for example, in people at risk, such as those facing surgery or bereavement; for secondary prevention, that is, for those with existing acute conditions; and for tertiary prevention, which, in this case, means dealing with the acute exacerbations of chronic conditions rather than the chronic condition itself.

The Six Sessions of BEP

The assessment conducted in the first session is very broad and includes the chief complaints and their history, a life history, a family history, a dynamic and structural formulation, and an assessment of the transference and the therapeutic alliance. At the end of the session, the therapeutic contract is discussed.

In the second session, the therapist asks how the patient has spent his or her week and inquires specifically about the complaints. Further historical data are gathered to fill out the dynamic picture. Bellak also asks if the patient has had a dream, especially a recurrent dream, and, if so, he takes up the material in the dream in light of the problems as a way of discerning transference and facilitating communication.

Thus, for example, a patient repeatedly dreams of herself as a little girl in her mother's house. This probably expresses her wish to be a little girl again and to be cared for instead of having to be a mother herself and to take care of her own child. Communication of this inference may lay the groundwork for bringing out her oral longing and anger over its frustration, as well as anger directed at her child who demands attention and who may also be an identification figure for the patient's younger sibling who was the original rival. (Bellak & Small, 1978, p. 67)

In the third session, an attempt is made to work further on the problem. If it seems called for, this might be a conjoint or family session, which is one eclectic aspect of this brief therapy. Bellak also starts referring to the impending separation, warning patients that they may feel worse as separation looms.

In the fourth session, insights about the problems are offered, and there is a discussion of separation issues.

In the fifth session, the patient is asked to review the treatment and work is continued on the focus. Bellak strives to terminate with a positive relationship by being more chatty with the patient and more self-revealing in order to decrease the distance between himself and the patient. (If he is preparing the patient for therapy *termination,* one wonders why he wants to *decrease* this distance.) He encourages the patient to try to bear the immediate discomfort of termination. In Bellak's words, he gives a double message: "I am available if you really need me, but try not to need me because it's good for you if you can go it alone rather than be dependent" (Bellak, 1992, p. 33). However, he says to the patient that if further therapy is necessary it will be offered.

In the sixth session, held 1 month later, the therapist assesses the gains and makes dispositions accordingly.

Methods of Intervention in BEP

In addition to relying on standard methods such as interpretation, catharsis, and support, Bellak includes other processes which give his therapy its eclectic form. One such process is *mediate catharsis,* in which he verbalizes feelings or potential actions that the patient may be unwilling to experience or contemplate. In social learning terms, he seems to be modeling certain feelings or actions that the patient needs to learn about. Another is the use of *conjoint sessions or family network therapy,* in which a circumscribed goal is set for the session which includes significant others.

Bellak is not hesitant about *giving advice* where he feels it will prevent a patient from engaging in dangerous activity. He proscribed promiscuity by an adolescent female patient who felt she had to be so in order to be accepted by her peers; he hoped to buy time during which the patient could be strengthened to withstand the pressure (see section below on treating acting out disorders). He *educates* patients where necessary about a medical situation that is contributing to their mental difficulties. To help patients control their anxiety, he will offer a stabilizing explanation to *promote intellectualization* as a coping defense. Similarly, he uses *reassurance* where it is called for. Finally, as another eclectic element, he employs *psychoactive drugs* to help in the control of anxiety, depression, or disturbed thought processes, so that the patient will be able to remain in the community and continue with psychotherapy.

In addition to the eclectic elements just described, Wolberg (1980), in his eclectic model of brief therapy, gives patients relaxation tapes to use between sessions, assigns homework, and applies hypnosis within sessions.

Prescriptive Matching

A particular strength of Bellak's BEP is his separate recommendations for different psychiatric conditions or situations. As such, it illustrates the second meaning of technical eclecticism, which is matching therapy to the patient or syndrome. He discusses, among other conditions, depression, acting out, suicide, acute psychotic states, surgery or physical illness, panic, phobias, and feelings of unreality of the self and the world. To illustrate this specificity, we will describe his different therapeutic recommendations for panic disorder and acting out (Bellak, 1992).

Therapeutic recommendations for *panic disorder:*

1. Establish the unconscious cause of the panic such as fear of loss of impulse control, separation anxiety, severe superego, or moral masochism.
2. Demonstrate clearly to patients the continuity between the panic attack, the precipitating factors, and their life history, which will give them a greater feeling of control.
3. Offer patients an intellectual understanding of the panic reaction which reassures them that they are not crazy.
4. Where the external triggering event is known, it is essential to understand the unconscious meaning that it holds for the patient, as its emotional charge derives from that meaning.
5. Help the patient to get some perspective on the experience of panic and make it ego-alien by pointing out that others have reacted with less anxiety to the same situation. This helps patients to explore the specific meaning the external event has for them.

6. Make yourself very available to the patient since he or she will often feel helpless, defenseless, and alone. Enlist the support of family members who can be supportive when panic strikes.
7. Provide structure, calm, and an assuring sense that the panic can be handled and brought under control.
8. Interpret the denial or repression that typically surround panic attacks.
9. Allow for the expression of emotions and cognitions associated with the panic.

Therapeutic recommendations for *acting out:*

1. Bargain for a delay in acting out, which allows for an opportunity to intervene (as in the case of the promiscuous adolescent mentioned above).
2. Try to make the act ego-alien. Point to the connection between acting out and the patient's life history, so that the patient will understand that he or she is being programed by unconscious factors.
3. Interpret the underlying drive so as to decrease the push from the unconscious: for example, "You want to do that because it makes you feel big and you felt so small when XYZ happened" (p. 60).
4. Sensitize the patient to cues that precipitate the acting out so that he or she can anticipate it and thereby head it off.
5. Explain the negative consequences of acting out both for the patient and others, in an attempt to strengthen the superego.
6. If possible or necessary, have the patient avoid the situation that triggers the acting out.
7. Enlist the help of others to prevent the person from acting out.
8. Use medication to help the patient avoid acting out.
9. Where necessary, consider hospitalization to help the patient get through the most difficult phase of the condition.

As we can see from the preceding examples, there are commonalities in the treatment of both panic and acting out, but also clear differences geared to the nature of the condition. Regarding research, there are no controlled studies that we are aware of specifically on Bellak's model. It rests largely on the considerable experience of Bellak and his colleagues in applying brief therapy in clinical practice with a wide variety of diagnostic conditions under acute, emergency conditions.

Critique of Technical Eclecticism

Technical eclecticism has the virtue of pragmatism, calling on what works regardless of the dictates of a particular theory. It is empirically oriented, paying attention to what has been learned from research or clinical practice even more than from theory. It takes patients' (and, to lesser extent, therapists') individuality seriously by attempting to tailor the therapy to their particular needs. It encourages therapists to think systematically about what kinds of treatments or individual techniques may apply to the patients in their care. Because it is inclusive of a variety of approaches, it is less choosy about patients, thus permitting wider applicability.

What are the problems faced by a technically eclectic approach? To begin with, there is the assumption that a given technique can be imported into a therapy without changing its meaning in the context of the new therapy. For example, in the midst of a psychoanalytic therapy, Frank (1990) introduced a relaxation technique to which the patient responded angrily, saying that it felt like she was submitting or losing herself. Further exploration revealed that her mother had encouraged the patient's dependence on her, only to let her down by not protecting her from her assaultive father. The patient then transferred this interpersonal expectation to the interaction with the therapist, feeling that he, too, was exposing her to danger. The therapist acknowledged that, in taking a more directive role, he seemed to have threatened her feelings of autonomy.

In another example of how context matters in an eclectic therapy, when Lazarus imported a Gestalt two-chair technique into his multimodal therapy, it took on the attributes of behavioral therapy. That is, it was used to help the patient become more assertive rather than being applied towards conflict resolution the purpose to which it is put in Gestalt therapy (Messer, in Lazarus & Messer, 1991).

What we learn from these examples is that when a clinical procedure which is conceptualized and practiced within one therapy is incorporated into another it is important to consider (1) its *conceptual fit* within the different theoretical framework, (2) its *clinical meaning* within the new therapeutic context, and (3) the *empirical validity* of its efficacy, which must be established anew (Messer, in Lazarus & Messer, 1991). The theoretical context of a therapy cannot be ignored. It should also be added that there is very little research on eclectic forms of therapy, including Lazarus's multimodal therapy.

Turning to prescriptive matching, a major difficulty noted by several authors (e.g., Arkowitz, 1992; Barber & Luborsky, 1991; Patterson,

1989) is the number of potential variables that can interact in a variety of ways to produce different outcomes. Systematic eclecticism requires a taxonomy of client problems, therapist qualities, technical interventions, and outcomes, as well as a theory to suggest how they will interact to produce maximal effects. The research demands to fill the cells with enough subjects is daunting. Understandably, with the exception of Beutler's work, there is very little research justifying specific matches among these variables. Nor is this problem confined to research only. From a practical standpoint, how many modalities of therapy can one therapist be expected to master? And how many therapists of different orientation and personality style will be found in any one clinical setting to match the many possible dimensions of relevant client characteristics?

With regard to Bellak's eclectic brief therapy, there seems to be little effort to distinguish between its conception as emergency treatment and as brief psychodynamic therapy. Emergency therapy aims to reestablish patients' equilibrium, that is, to return them to the existing state before the eruption of symptoms. The aims of BPT are more ambitious, namely, to help people resolve conflicts, repair deficits, enhance self-esteem, improve interpersonal relations, and so forth, which is going to require more than five sessions. With only five sessions, one is considering termination just after one has gotten a full history. There would have to be convincing empirical evidence that it does more than help alleviate symptoms or take patients through a crisis. Is there really no difference between a BPT of five or six sessions and one that lasts, say, 20 sessions?

Bellak does not provide a theory to tie together the eclectic practices he advocates nor empirical evidence that it improves upon any alternative such as a pure model. He implicitly acknowledges that BEP is not the same as longer-term therapy, but does not spell out what the differences are.

In addition, there is a much greater reliance on authority, directiveness, and suggestion in BEP than in psychoanalytic therapy, even in its briefer forms. Defense strengthening via intellectualization is a frequent intervention in BEP, which is more akin to purely supportive therapy than to psychoanalytic therapy. One might argue that this is what is needed for a population that may have little tolerance for a reflective, exploratory kind of therapy or for a more neutral therapist, but this is not made explicit.

In brief, there is not much in the way of theory provided to justify how individual, family, and drug therapy may be combined in an eclectic brew to the client's betterment, which brings us to a consideration of theoretical integration.

THEORETICAL INTEGRATION

In this approach to integration, different theories of therapy are brought together with the aim of creating a stronger framework than any one individual theory provides. Such integrative efforts also show how techniques from the separate therapies can complement one another and work together in a synergistic way. When a large sample of clinical psychologists were asked to select the type of eclecticism that best represented their practice, the majority did not choose atheoretical or technical eclecticism but, rather, theoretical integration (Norcross & Prochaska, 1988). A survey of the theoretical preferences of clinical psychologists, psychiatrists, social workers, and marriage and family therapists by Jensen et al. (1990) is also of interest. Sixty-eight percent of the total sample classified themselves as eclectic, followed by 17% who regarded themselves as purely psychodynamic. Among the eclectics, the highest percentage (72%) used a psychodynamic orientation as part of their eclectic approach. (Thus, the authors concluded that "the psychodynamic approach is the single most influential theory in practice today"; p. 129).

Perhaps the best-known example of theoretical integration is Wachtel's (1977) rapprochement of interpersonal psychodynamic therapy and behavior therapy, based on cyclical psychodynamic theory.

In contrast to a technically eclectic approach, which might consist of a hodge-podge of techniques selected probabilistically because they have seemed to work with patients possessing similar characteristics, cyclical psychodynamics seeks to develop a coherent theoretical structure that can guide both clinical decision making and general principles. (Wachtel & McKinney, 1992, p. 335)

As does psychoanalytic theory, this integrative psychodynamic theory emphasizes unconscious motivations, conflicts, anxiety, and defense, and a concern with their roots in childhood. However, wish and fantasy are not considered the primary or causal motivating factors as in classical psychoanalytic theory, but, rather, the interpersonal experiences involving anxiety carry maladaptive reactions forward.

The childhood experiences and relationships which caused anxiety do not live on in an unaltered but repressed manner impervious to new experiences. . . . mental structures and contents are thought to persist only as long as the person's experience and behavior provide continuing input and reinforcement for them (Wachtel & Wachtel, 1986). Old dynamic issues, and the character structures which develop around them, remain potential sources of anxiety because the ways the person lives his or her life, and the responses

to that way of life from others, make change impossible or provide new con-
firmation of the presence of potential losses of security. (Gold & Wachtel,
1993, p. 60)

In other words, cyclical psychodynamics emphasizes the vicious
cycles that are set in motion by earlier fixations and relationships and
the way in which the interpersonal patterns formed along the way continue to persist in the present. Although these patterns are sustained
because of the present reality, it is a reality which the person has helped
to create: both internal reality and external events are crucial. This conceptualization, which derives more from Sullivan, Horney, Alexander,
and Erikson than from Freud, opens the way for the introduction of
behavioral techniques to help people alter current interpersonal patterns or to learn ways to manage their anxiety.

For example, a person may avoid interacting romantically with
members of the opposite sex because of the anxiety it generates, leading to a preoccupation with old wishes and fantasies (rather than causa-
tion being in the other direction only). To help the patient overcome
the anxiety, both behavioral and systemic interventions are permissi-
ble within integrative psychodynamic therapy, which can then bring
about a modification of the maladaptive reactions. This alteration can
lead to further insights, which in turn lead to the motivation to try new
behaviors, and so on through the cycle. Alexander's concept of the corrective emotional experience is central, in that the person has to be
exposed to the fearful stimulus where the expected harmful consequences do not occur, thereby dispelling the anxiety and opening the
possibility of new ways of perceiving, acting, and reacting.

What differentiates this integrative therapy from common factors
or technical eclecticism is that there is an explicit and testable theory
that ties together the use of the different techniques. At present, there
does not exist a psychodynamically based, theoretically integrative therapy that is short term by design. However, there is one that does draw
on concepts from across the psychoanalytic spectrum and assimilates
a systems outlook as well—the brief therapy of James Gustafson.

Gustafson's Brief Therapy

Gustafson developed his approach treating college students at the Brief
Therapy Clinic of the University of Wisconsin. Based on that work and
his review of the writings of many of the leading contributors to the
psychoanalytic theory of therapy, he fashioned a brief therapy that incorporates their perspectives and adds a systems view (Gustafson, 1986).
From the premodern psychoanalytic period, he brings to bear the in-

sights of Ferenczi, Rank, Reich, and Alexander and French; from a modern interpersonal and object relational standpoint, he draws on Sullivan, Winnicott and Balint; and from the current BPT scene, he draws inspiration from the therapies of Malan, Mann, Sifneos, and Davanloo. To this mix, he adds the systemic perspective of Bateson and the Milan group, as well as gleanings from the long-term psychoanalytic work of Gedo and Havens (Messer, 1988b).

The Theory

From traditional psychoanalytic teachings, says Gustafson, we learn about *the clash between sexual and aggressive drives and societal expectations.* In Malan's work, this is expressed as the conflict between people's sense of duty (or what the superego dictates) and their true inclinations. In Sifneos's scheme, it is the struggle between childish regressive behavior and adult responsibility. And, for Davanloo, it is the opposition of walls of resistance and the flow of feelings. These are expressions of the drive/structural model discussed in Chapter 2.

From the revisionist psychoanalysts such as Sullivan and Reich, we learn to appreciate the patients' "constant attitude," that is, *the character style or security operations* that keep them stuck. Patients' tendencies to be passive or agreeable, for example, must be attended to in order to join them on the other side of the wall of resistance.

To do good work in brief therapy, adds Gustafson, we must make ourselves aware of patients' *interpersonal relations* and how and why they are so invested in preserving their maladaptive mode of behavior. We must ask what a person gives up in his or her relations in order to feel secure.

Patients often maintain symptoms or interpersonal modes, he argues, in order to protect the lives of others (particularly family members), as well as to preserve their own distorted relationships to them. This is reminiscent of Weiss and Sampson's concept of how pathological beliefs—that one's actions will do harm to others—may prevent a person from attaining mature goals (see Chapter 3). The therapist's attempt to change such modes of behavior will bring about *systemic resistance.* For example, a woman's insecurity may allow her husband to feel superior and may keep her children hovering close to home. Or, "a daughter had to wreck her body and confidence so her mother could feel herself a successful mother, so the daughter could be friends with the father, so the father could tolerate what was missing in his wife" (p. 263). Because the systemic resistance—including counterattacks by the family—will appear after visits back home by college student patients, it is best that these episodes be weathered while the patient has the therapist available. Systemic resistance can also come from friends, from school, or the work place.

The Therapy: Selection

In a preliminary interview of about 30 minutes, Gustafson determines whether the patient is looking for what the University Brief Therapy Clinic can offer. If the answer is yes, he tries to determine whether the patient has allowed others to be of help in the past, and how the patient felt, thought, and acted when at his or her worst. If all goes well, a trial therapy lasting 2 to 3 hours is offered.

Gustafson recognizes three contraindications to brief therapy: When patients have been hurt too much and thus will not form a therapeutic relationship quickly, when the problems are too complex, and when clients cannot stay focused but constantly drift to more and more tangled difficulties. In assessing these contraindications, there are three questions interviewers should pose to themselves (Gustafson, 1984): Has the patient been able to navigate safely through the worst periods of his or her life? Has the patient been able to have a deep give-and-take relationship with another person? Does the trial therapy bring about an actual breakthrough to deep feeling and the recurrent focal problem of the patient's life? Gustafson reports that about half the student population with whom he works are suitable candidates by these criteria.

The Therapy: Process

Gustafson (1984) tries to put the patient in the driver's seat if possible, but does not fear taking control where necessary. "Nearly always the way through the eye of the needle involves, paradoxically, both rough handling and gentleness" (p. 939). He adopts Havens's (1976) notion of working the opposing currents, always noting what is right with the patient as well as what is wrong. It is indispensable, he advises, to locate the problem in each interview, to find the "loose end," and to maintain a fresh attitude as if each interview were the first.

It is also very important to be able to stay with the patient through his or her deepening distress. In interfering with the patient's defenses, one must be empathic or the patient will not follow along. This is not merely a matter of technique but of an overarching attitude that one conveys. Patients may also try to provoke therapists to hurt them, and if therapists do not fall into this trap (but "pass the test," as Weiss & Sampson would say), patients will become bolder in revealing themselves. To illustrate his approach, following are selected excerpts from the case of a patient treated by Gustafson (1984).

The Therapy: A Case

A young man with an 8-year history of severe migraine headaches was referred to our clinic by his internist, who was making little progress with the severity of the attacks. As I attempted to take a history from the patient of the ups and downs of this dramatic disorder, I found him extremely vague in locating when these attacks occurred. After an hour of close inquiry, I had a laundry list of minor irritations and only the vaguest notion of what actually upset the young man. As I began to call this vagueness and minimizing to his attention, he allowed that his headaches seemed to occur in a realm that had nothing to do with the words of his vague and minimizing history, as if there were a realm of words and a completely separate realm of feelings. I then noticed a grimace on the right side of his face, and I asked him where his migraine attacks began. He put his hand up to the right side of his face.

Now when I confronted him that some events in his life must have been more upsetting than others, he decided that a certain omnibus research assignment had been quite vexing. As I explored his vexation about this, the facial grimacing became more and more frequent, and I continually called this to his attention. He then felt he could not continue the grimacing, which he then began to inhibit consciously. As he did this he became more and more restless and felt hot inside. When I remarked how he suddenly pulled away from me, he said that he felt I was laughing at him. I asked when he had felt that before, and he suddenly put up both hands in front of his face and began to cry in a stifled way. I learned that he had had large glasses and an overbite that was ridiculed by his classmates in school from about age 10. I asked him to tell me what these kids called him all those years. He again put up his hands in front of his face, as if the tormenting children were right before his eyes, and stammered but could not speak. Obviously we had made the transition from the vague, minimizing, grimacing, rigid, pathological structure to the fluidity of the previous pathological interaction. (p. 938)

I was also provoked to lose all patience with this patient, to become annoyed and then angry and then punishing. His vagueness and trivial complaints began to give *me* a headache, which I began to want to take out on him. Here I was provoked to test unconsciously the other side of the negative transference, the laughing cruelty of the children to determine whether I could be different from them as well as different from the indifferent mother. . . . What seemed to matter was that when I was fully tempted to be indifferent or be punishing, I could pull myself out of the ditch and get back on the road. . . . Ranging between the receptive and relentless is going to arouse the patient's longing for the good parents, who must do exactly this all day long with a young child, who must drag him down from climbing on the table, then hold him while he sobs about it. Only someone who can both hate and love the patient will be capable of this, which is what the patient needs. Of course, each patient will have to test the doctor in his own specific ways depending on how he had been failed before. In this sense the patient arouses the unsolved family problem, the very difficulty that the parents could not meet because of their own limitations. (p. 939)

Gustafson interfered with the patient's rigid defenses but did so in an empathic manner. As a result, the patient was willing to face what he could not face on his own. For Gustafson, there must be a breakthrough of the rigid wall of character which plunges the therapist and patient into the depths of developmental disturbance and deficit.

A neurotic problem always does something to the buoyancy of the self and confidence in the environment, locates a place where the patient has not been able to defend himself, and generates extreme tension. . . . The therapy, therefore, must arouse the full tides of feeling, and in this flood tide, the patient must find the missing, bridging capability that will get him through such floods when they arise again in life. . . . Only when he could ride out these floods in his brief psychotherapy with his therapist could he begin to retain his self-confidence, his ability to fight back. (p. 940)

Gustafson says that one needs to be able to imagine not only the taunts, but the patient's vengeful urges, and to be able to enjoy them as the patient must have.

Every focal problem, says Gustafson, implies an unsolved family problem which the family colludes in hiding. The patient's newfound capability will come under attack from the family on visits home as the patient tries to confront them with the problem. This is the systemic resistance, that the therapist must help the patient to confront and weather.

His new capability to defend himself came under counterattack from his family who wanted him to come home to work after college. It set off primitive urges to "knock them for a loop" by staying in graduate school, which he could now enjoy with the help of his therapist, since they were clearly in the service of his doing what mattered to him in his profession. (p. 940)

Not only his family, but his teachers would have to be confronted, since he no longer felt the need to be the all-A student he had always been.

Before long, this will certainly bring on various confrontations with his teachers, which will be very emotional, since he wants them to accept him as he actually is. Whether these counterattacks can be negotiated by him, rendering something unto Caesar, keeping something for himself remains to be seen, but it is certain that these powerful tests of his new bridging capability, these tests of "dynamic change" will come. (p. 941)

In this integrative therapy, we see how Gustafson has conducted a focal inquiry revealing the emotional disturbance and the underlying meaning of the somatic symptom, confronted the resistance while remaining in empathic attunement with the patient, and passed the patient's tests in his way of reacting to the negative transference ("you are laughing at me"). He has helped to rebuild the patient's missing capability (his buoyancy and assertiveness) so that he could confront both his family and other authorities. This process was also associated with the relief of his migraine headaches. An eye is kept on the drives (the patient's rage), the interpersonal field (the patient's view of others as mocking him, and his eliciting their indifference or annoyance), the character style (obsessive/intellectual), and the familial and societal resistance to change (the counterforce of his parents and teachers).

Critique of Theoretical Integration

Among the major forms of eclecticism, theoretical integration holds the potential for the most radical and far-reaching kind of rapprochement among the therapies. As applied to the brief therapies, it could result in a new integrative therapy that is more widely applicable and more efficacious than any single one. Good integrative theories, like those of Wachtel (1977), Prochaska (1995), and Safran and Siegel (1990) open doors to new, testable propositions regarding psychopathology and the process of psychotherapy.

As popular and promising as theoretical integration may be, it, too, comes up against a variety of obstacles. For one thing, any theoretical integration picks and chooses which elements of each school it includes. Inevitably, elements that may be just as important as those embraced are excluded. For example, it was only by deemphasizing drive theory, the role of the past, and therapist neutrality that Wachtel was able to incorporate behavioral interventions in a psychodynamic therapy in a theoretically consistent way. Whether one judges an integrative therapy to be superior to the individual therapies from which it stems will depend on one's view of the importance of the elements included and excluded. It will also depend on the accumulation of clinical experience with, and research on, the new, integrative therapy.

Along similar lines, Kazdin (1984) has pointed out that there are several variants of behavioral and psychoanalytic therapy, some of which are conceptually incompatible with one another. Therefore, one could not ever expect to put them together in one grand synthesis. He also avers that the empirical foundations of each are relatively weak, making integration premature.

Several authors have pointed out that the absence of a common language is a barrier to theoretical integration. A symptom is not just a symptom, nor is it just observable behavior, but the term implies a point of view about the meaning of certain behaviors. Both Franks (1984) and Messer (1992) have argued that an integrated psychotherapy cannot pull terms out of their context and expect them to retain the same meaning: the concept's subtlety and richness can be lost. When one translates from one framework into another, one must keep in mind the cautionary Italian phrase *Traduttori traditori:* Translators are betrayers.

On a metatheoretical level, Messer and Winokur (1984) have referred to the different perspectives and visions of reality that psychoanalytic and behavioral theories encompass, which set limits to their integration. The perspective in traditional behavior therapy, for example, is on the outer world of consensual reality, and the approach to clients is within an objective and external framework. Psychoanalytic therapy, by contrast, views human behavior from a more subjective and introspective angle.

Whereas perspectives suggest a position from which reality is viewed, the visions of reality, as discussed in Chapter 1, constitute assumptions about the very nature and content of human reality. Behavior therapy—in emphasizing the definable, controllable, and predictable aspects of situations and people, in its ameliorative and optimistic spirit, and in its belief in happy endings—falls primarily within the comic vision of reality. Psychoanalytic therapy—in stressing the less definable and predictable aspects of human behavior, the limits to what we know or can know about ourselves, and the difficulties entailed in bringing about even a modicum of change—falls within the tragic vision. When integrative theories are created, a compromise of visions is often necessary, which will satisfy some therapists but not others, whose preference will be for the purity of vision of the original theories (Messer, 1986).

Also at a metatheoretical level, theory integration tends to assume an objectivist stance on the nature of reality in which individual theories are models of a singular, knowable reality. From a constructivist or perspectival viewpoint, in which theories are regarded as narrative constructions, theory integration is an inevitable ongoing process as narratives evolve and change in accordance with social and cultural influences. That is, integrating two theories does not yield a model which is a closer approximation to a fixed reality or truth, but only a third, different model or construction of reality.

To point to one further obstacle to theoretical integration, there is a difference in what is considered acceptable data by cognitive and behavioral therapists, on the one hand, and psychoanalytic and humanistic therapists on the other. The dichotomy can be described as that between the scientific and humanistic outlooks, in which adherents of the scientific view rely on observation, laboratory studies, atomism, and objectivism leading to universal laws, whereas adherents of the humanistic (including psychoanalytic) view prefer case study, holism, and subjectivism, resulting in contextually meaningful, idiographic explanations (Kimble, 1984; Krasner & Houts, 1984). For example, a psychoanalyst might study a subject of interest through the free associations and dreams of a small number of carefully selected cases to assess unconscious or implicit determinants and then place them within a holistic, structural-developmental framework. By contrast, a behaviorist would formulate a hypothesis, construct an experiment, statistically analyze the results, and tie the finding to some form of learning theory (Messer, 1989). As Franks (1984) has pointed out, the behavior therapist will not be prepared to proceed in terms of the more subjective and interpretive style of the psychoanalyst. Thus, an integrative theory has to find some way of bridging the methodological gulf as well.

To return to Gustafson's brief therapy, we see it as an example of "assimilative integration" (Messer, 1992), rather than theoretical integration in the style of Wachtel and others. On the one hand, it is an integrative/analytic model akin to Mann's, insofar as it encompasses several psychoanalytic perspectives. At the same time, it is a type of theoretical integration in its inclusion of systems understanding. By assimilative integration we mean that it incorporates a systems perspective in a way that fits comfortably within a psychoanalytic frame. Note that it does not advocate actual family sessions. This would make it an example either of technical eclecticism or of theoretical integration, if there were a theory that explained how the two approaches could be reconciled.

An assimilative integration is very respectful of the context in which the borrowed technique or intervention is taking place. The reaction of the patient to the intervention must be monitored and understood, just as would be true of traditional interventions. The object is to intervene in such a way that the procedure is woven seamlessly into the fabric of the session (see also Wachtel, 1991). When Gustafson draws the patient's attention to family interactions, he does so in a way that is consistent with a psychoanalytic framework. It is more the attitude or perspective of systems thinking that he assimilates, rather than any technique practiced within that viewpoint.

We expect that if short-term therapy becomes the modal form of psychodynamic practice, new forms of integrative brief psychodynamically based approaches will be developed. For example, one that has been recently described is referred to as an anxiety-reduction modification of short-term dynamic psychotherapy (McCullough, 1993). It is a mixed model, including elements of both integrative/analytic, technically eclectic, and common factors approaches. It is integrative/analytic insofar as it starts with the fundamental components of brief dynamic therapy, to which it adds self psychological techniques. It is technically eclectic in its incorporation of behavioral and Gestalt therapy techniques. And it employs a common factors understanding of the effective ingredients of psychotherapy drawing upon Weinberger's (1993) four-component model (exposure, alliance, mastery, and attribution).

As we discussed above, one of the main advantages of eclectic models is their increased range of applicability. As we turn to the brief treatment of "difficult" or more emotionally disturbed patients, we will see how integrative and eclectic elements are often important in trying to meet their special requirements.

PART IV

Special Topics in Brief Psychodynamic Therapy

CHAPTER 6

Assessing and Treating
the Difficult Patient

DEFINING THE DIFFICULT PATIENT

Referring to some patients as "difficult" suggests that there are other patients who are "easy." All patients in psychotherapy sooner or later present difficulties for the therapist, reflecting intrinsic qualities of being human, particularly in the context of the process of change. The term "difficult" is often used in the clinical literature, however, to refer to a group of patients who present special problems in psychotherapy. These problems can include more severe psychopathology, rigid and intractable defenses, limited motivation for psychotherapy, or other limitations which make the usual forms of psychotherapy inadvisable. It may be argued that patients who are perceived as "difficult" are ones whose problems are not very well addressed by a particular approach to therapy. On the other hand, it does seem to be the case that certain individuals pose a greater challenge than others to a wide range of therapeutic approaches, especially those that requre high levels of focality, therapist activity, and therapeutic engagement.

The authors of the various short-term therapy approaches considered in this volume tend to minimize the problem difficult patients may pose by emphasizing exclusion criteria limiting the range of patients treated. *Thus, for our present purposes, the difficult patient is defined as one who does not fulfill the selection criteria of a given approach to BPT, but who is seen for such treatment anyway, for some reason other than being optimally suitable.* The emphasis here is on the lack of suitability as defined by the particular treatment model. There are patients suitable for BPT who nonethless may prove difficult in some respects, and there are patients not suitable for BPT with whom things may go smoothly as long as the appropriate modifications are made to the treatment model. We are concerned here with the issue of the "fit" between patient and treatment model; difficult patients in this specific sense are those for whom the treatment models must be modified in some ways. These modifications are required by (1) personality dynamics, including rigidity of defenses, intolerance of affects, and instability of object relations, (2) cultural differences, (3) history of trauma, and (4) special problems with loss and separation.

THE BRIEF PSYCHODYNAMIC TREATMENT OF DIFFICULT PATIENTS

Why do we address the problem of time-limited psychotherapy for patients who are admittedly not optimally suited for such treatment? First, there is a great practical necessity. Many patients are seen in settings where there is little flexibility about the forms of treatment available, such as clinics, counseling centers, and other public settings. Such settings frequently have greater demand for services than can be efficiently met without some form of rationing of services. Therefore, many patients are seen in time-limited treatment whether they fit a given model or not. Even in private settings, many patients are not available to pursue a long-term course of treatment. This includes younger patients who are transient by virtue of more rapid developmental shifts and changes; elderly patients who have more limited life expectancy, and others for whom financial resources are limited. These latter include those affected by the dramatic increase in the percentage of health insurance plans that no longer cover psychotherapy except for very short-term approaches. Thus, many more patients are being seen in short-term psychotherapy, whether they are ostensibly suitable or not.

Second, discriminating suitable from nonsuitable patients is not simple or straightforward. Human beings are complex, as are the kinds of problems for which they seek help. Strengths and weaknesses have to be assessed on an individual basis; set rules are rarely of great value in actual clinical practice. One must often make do with a less than perfectly clear clinical picture at the outset, although clinical experience does seem to offer some advantages in this regard. We have found in the course of trying to identify patients suitable for BPT that surprises of all kinds can occur over the course of a time-limited treatment. For example, we have been pleasantly surprised by apparently difficult patients whose strength and resiliency was not clearly manifested at the outset of treatment, but who have shown remarkable improvement in relatively brief courses of treatment. We have also seen individuals whose psychopathology was well masked by a superficial appearance of adequate functioning; it was only in retrospect—as the treatment foundered—that we recognized that our dimly perceived early doubts should not have been set aside.

Third, in the history of psychotherapy much has been learned from patients who were seen as not suitable for a given approach. Freud was the first to make the discrimination between suitable and nonsuitable patients in a modern psychotherapeutic framework, placing the matter in terms of a capacity to form an object transference, or transference neurosis (Freud, 1916–1917/1958). Those patients whose problems reflected a fundamentally narcissistic orientation—that is, whose libido remained cathected to the self, rather than to objects—were viewed as "unanalysable," which in more conservative psychoanalytic circles they remain to this day.

However, as greater numbers of patients with a wider range of psychopathology were seen by psychotherapists, the "scope" of analytic practice expanded (Stone, 1954). In fact, one way of understanding the evolution of psychoanalytic theory is in terms of the continual expansion into the "terra incognita" of patients previously thought of as untreatable. The succession of valuable new clinical constructs reflects the encounter with the previously unknown: Melanie Klein's (1946/1975) concept of the "paranoid–schizoid position," Fairbairn's (1941) understanding of schizoid phenomena, Winnicott's (1960) "false self," Kernberg's (1975) use of the borderline concept, and Kohut's (1977) "narcissistic transferences" are but a few notable examples. Today's difficult patient is tommorow's new conceptual and clinical vista. Each of these theorists made significant contributions to the practice of psychotherapy by bringing attention to new ways of thinking about clinical techniques and the patient-therapist relationship. Their theoretical contributions are linked to modifications in the treatment approach. There are undoubtedly things yet to learn from those patients who do not readily fit our treatment models.

A SAMPLE CASE: MR. C.

The following case is offered to illustrate some of the clinical and theoretical issues which will be raised later in the chapter. We would direct the reader to consider in particular what was *not done* in this treatment that might have been attempted in a more open-ended treatment. On the other hand, we invite the reader to consider how the treatment goals and methods were distinctively psychodynamic, rather than purely supportive or strictly symptom-focused.

Assessment of Suitability

The treatment, conducted by one of the us (CSW), presented difficulties in a number of areas: First, the patient (Mr. C.) was from a cultural background that was not only unsupportive of psychotherapy, but overtly contemptuous of such help seeking, particularly in a man. From the beginning it seemed that this therapy had to be a time-limited treatment, as the patient did not seem likely to accept or tolerate a more prolonged involvement. The patient was not aware of anything in himself that was related to the immediate crisis. He did not seem able to define his problem in psychological terms, but rather viewed the situation as a function of external persons or forces. In addition, it was apparent early on that Mr. C. had a history of trauma, which included severe physical abuse throughout his childhood, raising serious questions about the appropriateness of a short-term model. His motivation was primarily to obtain symptom relief; he did not exhibit curiosity about his inner life or the meaning of the conflicts that had brought him into treatment. It was anticipated that work in the transference would have to be fairly limited; that deep dependency longings could only be superficially acknowledged with little opportunity to address them in any depth; and that homoerotic aspects of the patient's inner life would be too threatening to address in a direct way.

On the other hand, Mr. C. also had a history of significant long-term relationships, had functioned well in his work, and seemed to have been a good father to his three sons. Thus, it seemed reasonable to agree to work with Mr. C. within the context of a delimited or circumscribed focus, with an awareness that important dynamic issues, particularly around early dependency needs and their relation to homosexual feelings, could not be addressed in the present treatment.

Description

Mr. C. was a burly, tough, streetwise man, age 45, who came from an urban blue-collar background and was outwardly quite friendly. He was a detective on the police force of a large city, having been successful in his work as a policeman all his adult life. His father, deceased, had also been a policeman.

Mr. C. came for help during a major life crisis, in which his wife of 25 years had recently left him to be with another man. The other man was a longtime friend of the patient and his family, also being a policeman in the same precinct, and had in fact spent a great deal of time with Mr. C. and his wife and children over the course of many years. This was justified by the patient as having appeared harmless and understandable in view of the other man being single and without any family of his own. Mr. C. did not appear to have had any idea that his marriage was in jeopardy, and was overwhelmed and grief stricken in the wake of this disaster.

The Treatment Contract and Course of Treatment

In part because of his great distress, Mr. C. quickly attached himself to the therapist, able to openly share his grief and sadness. The focus that began to crystallize revolved around what appeared to be his complicity in the undoing of his marriage, that is, his having let this other man into his family to such a degree over many years, and his apparent passivity in the situation. No formal time limit was established, but the treatment contract included the implication that the work would be for a flexible but finite period of time.

He soon turned to talk about his relationship with his father, a brutally sadistic and spiteful man who had tortured the patient throughout his childhood, beating him, abusing him, and humiliating him at every opportunity. The patient had taken the full brunt of his father's destructiveness, apparently shielding his younger brother, who was far less athletic and resilient, as well as protecting a younger sister. Mr. C. wept openly during much of this phase of the treatment as he recalled incidents involving his father. In one such incident, at the age of 10 or 11, he recalled desperately wanting roller skates so that he could play hockey with his friends, but his father refused to buy them. One day he found a pair discarded in the garbage, rusty and damaged. He worked on them for some time, cleaning and repairing them by himself, finally proudly restoring them to a usable state. When his father found the skates he became enraged, and threw them away. The patient recalled with great pain and sorrow the depth of his own rage and despair.

Mr. C. had been an outstanding athlete as a boy and young man, and consistently gained notice and appreciation from his peers and coaches, but his father failed to attend the games in which he played. One day in a fit of rage the father destroyed all his son's trophies, accumulated over years of athletic accomplishment. As the patient described his relationship with his father, his resilience and freedom from bitterness became more and more impressive. Somehow he had been able to protect some part of himself from this abuse, becoming a loving, protective, and involved father to his sons, a good father where he had none. Yet it seemed that the fault line ran from this apparent triumph over his environment to the catastrophic loss of his family that had brought him into treatment.

We made it our task to understand what connection there might be between his long-buried grief and his terrible mishandling of his marriage. A thread of self-destructiveness appeared, echoed by a certain recklessness in his police work. He described taking risks that didn't always seem justified, short cuts in procedures that put him at some greater risk of harm. He arrived for his session one day straight from an attempted bank robbery which he had single-handedly broken up. While he usually came from home, that day he was in his work clothes, sweaty, with his gun and holster strapped to his back. He nonchalantly described the hold up attempt, and his striding up to a perpetrator who was armed with a shotgun, disarming him as easily as if it were a toy. I found myself thrilled with his machismo, straight out of the movies, and was also aware of a heavy homoerotic undertone to the session. It was as though he had brought to me his male power and competence in a strong, concrete, and bodily way. I wondered if he was trying to excite and enthrall his father, to finally obtain his approval and admiration. I also felt the death-dealing side of his father, his destructiveness, contained in Mr. C.'s devil-may-care attitude of boldness and self-neglect. These themes, though noted, could not be taken up adequately in the course of the 20-session treatment.

The theme that we came back to time and again was Mr. C.'s passivity, his inability to assert himself in a variety of situations, which was almost paradoxical in the context of his outward "tough guy" demeanor and macho attitudes. We began to recognize that beneath his apparent lack of anger and effective assertion was a terror of becoming his murderous and destructive father. He had determined to be a good man, and succeeded to a large degree. The price was a lack of an inner sense of entitlement, that is, a healthly demandingness and possessiveness that would have enabled him to better pursue his aims in life. It was interpreted that he had been as passive in relation to his friend as he had been to his father — and to the therapist, though this last could not be fully interpreted to the patient.

There was noticeable progress around this theme. The patient would bring in incidents weekly in which he recognized his interpersonal passivity, and experimented with taking on a more assertive stance. In one incident, disconcerting to patient and therapist alike, Mr. C. described running into his friend at what had been his home while visiting his ex-wife. In what sounded like a forced provocation, he found himself enraged at his friend and struck him, knocking him to the ground. It was the first time he had so openly expressed his anger. To the therapist's relief, it was the only occurrence of actual violence — though I must admit that there seemed to be at least some justice in the act. Mr. C. was relieved by the physical contact, noting that his friend wasn't really injured, and feeling that he had been able to release some anger without killing someone.

Termination

It was at this point in therapy, having worked for some weeks on this issue of self-assertion, being able to use his anger more effectively, that the patient announced his wish to end treatment. His grief and depression were greatly diminished, and he had been able to unburden himself of long-held pain and sadness. The treatment had lasted about 5 months, or about 20 sessions. It may be emphasized that the main vehicle of this work was exploration, clarification, and interpretation. The patient's actions were taken on his own initiative, with no directives, assignments, or specific advice given by the therapist. Interpretation of transference was minimal. Rather, the patient's idealized admiration of the therapist was utilized to enable the patient to reveal his vulnerable aspects, to mobilize him toward more effective action, and to enhance his self-esteem. Although the fault line in Mr. C.'s personality remained, it appeared that he had been able to make an important shift which left him more comfortable and apparently effective in his relations with others, better able to integrate aggressive feelings in appropriate assertiveness. Perhaps his interpersonal successes would reinforce his new, exploratory behavior, which in turn would lead to further shifts in self-perception and self-experience in a positive feedback loop (Wachtel, 1987). Perhaps he would also be able to rely on his increased awareness of the personality tendencies therapy had brought to light and better compensate for them in the future.

Discussion

This case illustrates a number of themes of the present chapter. Mr. C. presented with several contraindications for brief psychodynamic therapy. His history of traumatic abuse raised questions about the appropriateness of a brief approach. His difficulty, while arising in a current crisis, clearly had long-term precipitants and precursors rooted in his basic character structure. Given his limited psychological-mindedness and motivation, these characterological issues would not be addressed in a time-limited framework. Yet the patient was not interested in long-term therapy, nor was he likely to be engaged for that purpose. His motivation for insight-oriented psychotherapy was limited, arising primarily from immediate and pressing distress. His cultural background did not support the development of a prolonged dependent relationship, especially to another man. His willingness to engage was also limited by a basically counter-dependent personality orientation.

While not ideally suited to a time-limited psychodynamic approach, Mr. C. was unlikely to accept a prolonged psychotherapy. Thus, the brief treatment offered seeemed the best possible under the circumstances. The therapeutic focus needed to be narrowed, with little exploration of a number of important areas possible, including his relationship to his mother, his sexuality, masochistic elements of his personality, and identifications with his abusive father. There could be little attention to the transference, particularly in its homosexual aspects, simply because the patient could not tolerate that much direct attention to our relationship in the here-and-now. Nonetheless, the patient made significant gains as a result of psychotherapy, unburdening himself of a lifetime of unexpressed anger and grief, and coming to understand in a meaningful way an aspect of his personality that interfered with his functioning, freeing him to explore different ways of relating to others and gaining access to parts of himself that had been previously unavailable. Perhaps Mr. C. could seek help sooner the next time, averting a crisis or traversing one with less costly consequences.

RELEVANT THEORY OF PERSONALITY

Personality and character structure comprise one dimension of "difficultness" in a patient. For the most part, this is the domain of the difficult patient as understood within the psychoanalytic tradition. There are a variety of theoretical viewpoints within this tradition that are applicable, of which we will mention the most prominent. These viewpoints can be categorized as follows: (1) ego weakness and "borderline" personality organization, (2) problems in separation and attachment, (3) self weakness and problems of narcissism, and (4) sequelae of trauma. (5) The distinction between oedipal and preoedipal psychopathology is also discussed, as it is understood that developmentally earlier pathology is less accessible in short-term treatment.

Structural Theory and Borderline Personality Organization

A structural approach to clinical diagnosis as elaborated by Kernberg (1975, 1976, 1986) is one way to understand the different treatment needs of healthier and more disturbed patients. Kernberg's adaptation of object relations theory places particular emphasis on the strength and adaptability of the ego relative to the instinctual forces of sexuality and aggression. Between the neurotic personality structure, well described in the psychoanalytic literature, and the psychotic personality structure which is deemed more or less untreatable using traditional psychoanalytic technique, a middle range is defined as the borderline level of personality functioning.

Here we find many of the patients only marginally suitable for the systematic approaches to brief therapy. Unlike the psychotic patient, the borderline patient is ordinarily able to differentiate self and other. On the other hand, borderline patients have ego weaknesses not found in healthier patients, relying on "primitive" defense mechanisms such as splitting and projective identification. Transient losses of reality testing occur, and unstable and contradictory experiences of self and others make for difficulties in treatment. The brief psychotherapist cannot rely on a basic, prevailing trust, or therapeutic alliance. The patient at times may not be able to distinguish the transference relationship from reality, fusing past and present objects. Explosive, fluid, and highly charged affect states may be difficult to contain in brief treatments.

Thus, the basic difficulty of the borderline patient is not centered around conflicts in loving and hating between separate and well-defined objects, but rather around problems with ego integration and object constancy. The problem for the brief therapist is that there is not time to enable the patient to develop more cohesive and integrated experiences of self and other — accomplishments which the healthier patient brings into psychotherapy.

Separation–Individuation Theory

Another way to understand more difficult patients is within the framework of *separation and individuation* theory (Blanck & Blanck, 1974; Mahler, Pine, & Bergman, 1975). From this point of view, these patients suffer from significant disruptions in the developmental process, such that the normal differentiation of self and other was not attained. Conflict is over attachment itself, taking place in the arena of differentiation of self and other, rather than being concerned with the qualities of an already differentiated object (Pine, 1985). Such patients are conflicted between the need to maintain contact with the other and the need to maintain a differentiated sense of self and other. Such persons lack stable and cohesive representations of self and other as the result of deficiencies in their maturational environment, leaving them vulnerable to intense anxieties over fragmentation and abandonment.

Patients with problems in attachment and basic trust have difficulty engaging and disengaging rapidly, requirements of a time-limited therapy approach. In addition, such patients, often having traumatic losses in their histories, may not be well suited to treatment approaches which rely so much on termination. They may require a greater degree of control over the therapy relationship and its ending.

Self Psychology

A different approach to patients seen previously as untreatable in psychoanalytic psychotherapy is taken by Kohut's self psychology. In this view the relevant dimension is that of self-esteem, or self-experience along a developmental continuum of narcissism (Kohut, 1971, 1977, 1984). Kohut's work led him to describe the narcissistic transferences of patients viewed as not capable of forming the more familiar object transferences of psychoanalytic theory and practice. These narcissistically disturbed patients, in Kohut's view, form particular kinds of transference organized around the need to maintain adequate, coherent, and continuous self-experience. The therapist functions to "mirror" and "affirm" the patient's need for recognition and appreciation, providing an empathic environment in which responses to earlier environmental failures can be experienced safely and worked through.

Stolorow and Lachman (1980) differentiate between psychopathology as conceptualized from the point of view of dynamic conflict between already structured parts of the psychic apparatus, and from the point of view of developmental arrests and structural deficits in the personality. These latter refer to gaps or deficiencies in the structure of the self arising from the failure of a child's caretakers to provide needed "mirroring" or validation. These gaps then lead to behavior and self-organizations whose purpose is to repair, hold together, or shore up their fragmenting or disintegrating sense of self.

Such patients may be inaccessible to the short-term therapist, blocking real contact with the therapist by offering only a defensive "false self." The narcissistic patient, by definition vulnerable to injuries to self-esteem, may not be able to tolerate the brief therapy contract, feeling it to be a rejection of his or her importance and need. There may be a retreat to omnipotence. The context of safety, so important to the narcissistic patient, cannot be readily assured in the time-limited framework.

Trauma Theory

Yet another group of difficult patients are those whose personalities are organized around severe traumatic experiences, such as physical or sexual abuse at the hands of caretakers. For such patients it is useful to distinguish between reliance on repression as a psychic defense mechanism versus reliance on dissociation of affects, experiences, and whole sectors of self-experience (Fairbairn, 1943/1952; Ferenzci, 1988). Two contemporary theorists describe this difference as follows:

Unlike repression, which is a horizontal division into conscious and unconscious mental contents, dissociation involves a vertical splitting of the ego that results in two or more self states that are more or less organized and independently functioning. These two or more ego states alternate in consciousness and, under different internal and external circumstances, emerge to think, behave, remember, and feel. Such dissociated states are unavailable to the rest of the personality and, as such, cannot be subject to psychic operations of elaboration. (Davies & Frawley, 1994)

These patients may share psychodynamic characteristics with other patients with severe personality disorders and, in fact, the two groups are likely to overlap substantially. For example, recent studies suggest high correlations between borderline personality disorder and a history of severe childhood trauma (Herman, Perry, & van der Volk, 1989; Shearer, Peters, Quaytman, & Ogden, 1990). However, it is clinically useful to recognize the particular treatment needs of these traumatized patients and to understand the ways in which they present a special challenge to the brief dynamic therapist.

It is necessary to recognize the universal human tendency to dissociate unbearable or overwhelming emotional experience that may occur at various points during the developmental process and the structuralization of the ego. Such dissociated experience is typically not organized or symbolized in thought, language, or other abstract forms of representation, but instead is coded in various forms of highly concrete experience. These forms of "direct" expression include bodily sensations, recurrent dream images, inexplicable sexual arousal, repetitive thoughts outside of any apparent context, or ritualized behaviors. Tramautic experience is thus not "experienced," but rather is frozen in split-off fragments of self contained in these concrete representations. It follows from this that the treatment process will be different than for other conflictual or less catastrophic traumatic memories. Fully formed and organized memories of such experience may not appear, as might occur in the instance of repression. Instead, such memories have to be constructed anew and experienced for the first time by a central ego-structure via the mediation of the therapist's containing or ego functions.

Such patients are likely to have difficulty forming an adequate therapeutic alliance under the conditions of brief psychotherapy. They may go undiagnosed, as dissociative disorders often do, in the absence of more sustained inquiry. Time, therapeutic devotion, and sustained commitment are required to establish deep levels of trust necessary to doing therapeutic work with terrifying and profoundly disturbing affect states and memories that arise in the course of treatment with such patients. Individuals with more severe dissociative disorders, including multiple personality disorder, almost certainly cannot be treated adequately in short-term psychodynamic psychotherapy.

Preoedipal Psychopathology

The differentiation of "oedipal" from "preoedipal" is thought to constitute the central defining feature of the difficult patient. Freud laid the groundwork for this distinction in his early discussions of narcissism (Freud, 1914a/1958, 1916–1917/1958). In these papers Freud differentiates libido aimed at others, and libido attached to the ego itself, or narcissistic libido. It was his contention that patients with primarily narcissistic libido, such as schizophrenics, could not be psychoanalyzed, since they could not develop a transference neurosis to the therapist. Some form of this distinction has been made by virtually all significant contributors to psychoanalytic theory. Melanie Klein (1946/1975) distinguished the "paranoid–schizoid position," an early developmental phase, in which the subject's relationship is to part-objects such as the breast, the mother's "inside," or the penis, and the later "depressive position" in which the other is related to as a whole object, with distinctive defenses and modes of relating associated with each of these phases. Following Klein, Fairbairn (1941) and Guntrip (1961) described schizoid phenomena with their associated defense mechanisms as developmentally prior to, and underlying, the oedipal conflicts described in classical Freudian theory. Balint's (1968) notion of the "area of the basic fault" similarly defines a "two-person" region of psychic functioning developmentally prior to the "three-person" region of the oedipal period. Kernberg (1975) follows Klein in distinguishing the "primitive" defense mechanisms of splitting and projective identification, and mature defense mechanisms such as repression in which self and object representations are differentiated and integrated. Along different lines, Stolorow and Lachman (1980) differentiate psychopathology rooted in conflictual personality structures versus that rooted in arrested development and deficient personality structure.

In fact, what unifies these diverse views is the idea that there are conflicts which are either specific to more disturbed individuals or are universal (though often hidden), over basic issues of relatedness, attachment, dependency, and self structure. Such issues are thought of as arising within the early dyadic system of infant and caretaker, rather than within the triadic system of mother, father, and child that characterizes oedipal conflict. The former are usually thought of as developmentally prior, underlying triadic conflicts. They also tend to be thought of as arising from significant external, enviromental failure or early trauma, rather than the later inevitable intrapsychic conflicts over love and aggression of the oedipal phase.

Patients with significant preoedipal pathology are not well suited to time-limited models. They are likely to present difficulties around engaging and disengaging rapidly. Their defenses will not be easily interpreted or confronted, instead tending to rigidify under the pressure of the interpersonal anxiety of connecting or terminating. Because their problem is in experiencing basic trust, they may not succeed in treatment approaches which require such trust as a condition of the treatment.

SUITABILITY AND ASSESSMENT OF THE DIFFICULT PATIENT

We begin this section with a review of the patient characteristics that would delineate the difficult, or nonoptimal, patient. We do not address the obviously unsuitable patient, such as one who was actively psychotic, who would not be considered for any form of brief psychodynamic psychotherapy, but instead focus on a midrange of patients who may be treated in brief therapy but are likely to present special difficulties to the psychotherapist.

Types of Difficult Patients

Significant Preoedipal Psychopathology

These patients often diagnosed as having severe personality disorders such as schizoid, borderline, or narcissistic personality disorders, tend to present global, diffuse complaints rather than a clear focus. They have difficulty attaching themselves to the therapist, and when they do, they have difficulty separating. These patients often exhibit emotional volatility and tend to be unable to form stable representations of self and therapist. Because these patients frequently rely on idealization, splitting, and projective identification, their perception of the therapist tends to shift in contradictory and polarized ways not readily acessible to interpretation. Thus, some active techniques are risky, as the therapist cannot count on the patient's experience of a consistent, more or less benign therapeutic alliance. Such patients can be thought of as having a limited capacity to symbolize their experience, and thus are likely to find language insufficient to communicate what they wish, and the therapist may not be able to rely on this crucial medium of therapeutic change. Impulsivity and extreme affective states make various forms of dangerous or self-destructive behavior a clinical risk.

Traumatic Backgrounds

In this category are patients with a wide range of traumatic life experiences, including alchoholic parents, mentally ill parents, physically or sexually abusive caretakers, or other historical traumas such as political incarceration and torture. Such patients typically have evolved strongly counterdependent personality styles, minimizing or splitting off altogether overwhelming experiences of intrusion, abandonment, and neglect. Such patients often do not present as such; their true complaints may appear only later in the course of treatment. There are powerful resistances against dependency of any kind, including in the therapy situation, and the therapist is often faced with a kind of "caretaker self" who guards and protects a vulnerable and dissociated self. Authentic affective engagement can be difficult to achieve in the brief therapy situation. In more severe instances these splits take on the character of more extreme dissociative disorders, with multiple personality farther along the continuum.

Early Object Loss

The group of patients with early object loss is really a subgroup of traumatized patients. We have in mind those persons who have suffered the loss of a primary object early in life, leaving profound anxiety about dependency and separation. The patient who has suffered the loss of a parent during early development, even if mitigated by other positive circumstances, is likely to require a therapeutic frame which is sensitive to the issue of abandonment anxiety and the need for control and mastery in the therapy relationship, and thus will likely do better in a more open-ended psychotherapy.

Somatic Complaints

Patients who present for treatment with vague, chronic bodily symptoms with no clear physical etiology often prove difficult to treat in brief psychotherapy. The use of the body to communicate and to contain affects and ego states suggests the inability to transform "upward" using the symbolic medium of language (McDougall, 1989). Such symptomatology is often accompanied by rigid character defenses that prove intractable in a time-limited therapy arrangement. There may be difficulty in expressing emotions and making real affective contact with others. The case of Vera (presented in Chapter 2) illustrates some of these problems over the course of a brief psychotherapy. Her presenting symptom, acute stomach cramps with no organic etiology, seemed

to contain a range of meanings, including suppressed anger in relation to her mother and her fiancé, and also was connected in a dream
to a fantasied pregnancy in the context of her relationship with her
father. However, the course of treatment was rocky, with many missed
sessions, including a 2-month hiatus while she repaired her car. Recognizing certain feelings was very hard for Vera, and she was not able
to discuss this difficulty, nor attach any meaning to all her missed
sessions. She remained reality oriented and tended to attribute her
difficulties to external factors such as her living situation and her
finances. She was not able to use interpretations of any kind and was
avoidant and closed even though the therapist modified treatment
toward a more supportive and empathic stance. Vera ended treatment
abruptly around a paranoid concern that her records were not con-
fidential. Thus, in this case the initial symptom of stomach pain indicated more severe psychopathology than was otherwise apparent, linked
as it was to deep concerns about dependency and loss. These concerns
could not be put into words, and Vera's body became the medium of
communication.

Physical Loss or Illness

Goodheart (1989) adds another group of patients to the "difficult"
category: those with physical losses, illness, or disability. Here the
difficulty for the brief therapist arises from the merging of the personality issues that might form a therapeutic focus with ongoing issues
around bodily integrity and rehabilitation: "The challenge to the clinician is to work with the tangled psyche–soma interactions, combined
with the developmental phase of life and underlying personality structure" (Goodheart, 1989, p. 18). Here we would also include patients with
terminal or life-threatening diseases, such as persons with AIDS who
may be in need of psychotherapeutic treatment. Such patients, while
in need of psychodynamic treatment, will also require a variety of forms
of assistance from the therapist, including education, counseling, supportive forms of psychotherapy, and other interventions not usually
considered part of psychoanalytically oriented treatment. Such patients
are not necessarily a challenge to the theory underlying psychodynamic models of brief therapy, but rather to the usual scope of such treatment and its technical application.

Different Cultural Backgrounds

Not all subcultures are equally supportive of the aims or methods of
psychodynamic psychotherapy. Some patients may prove difficult be-

cause their immediate family or community does not sanction a more insight-oriented approach to treatment. Such patients may hold values and ways of understanding life problems that conflict with the therapist's. Resistance to treatment in other members of a family system can undermine individual psychotherapy.

For example, one of us has treated a number of urban Hispanic adolescent girls who were brought in by their mothers, with whom they tended to be enmeshed. The mothers had their own difficulties with absent or unavailable husbands, but focused their attention on their daughters. The result was a kind of stalemate, where the adolescent resisted real involvement in therapy for fear of betraying her mother, while the mother undermined the psychotherapy by demanding quick and dramatic changes in her daughter. In such instances, it is impossible to separate out the identified patient's symptoms from the context of family conflict and ongoing structural dysfunction. We return to this issue in Chapter 7, in a discussion of the brief treatment of children and adolescents.

The case of Mr. C. illustrated another way cultural factors can challenge the psychotherapist. It should be noted, however, that this sort of difficulty is not necessarily exacerbated by the use of time-limited approaches. In fact, such patients may be less likely to agree to long-term treatment than to one with clearly defined objectives and a specified ending point.

Selection and Suitability

The issue of suitability cannot be separated from a particular clinical approach, for each has its own conceptualization of what makes a patient difficult. Different models are more or less selective when it comes to the issue of suitability, and each tends to make different demands on the patient, requiring more or less modification for a given difficult patient.

For example, Sifneos makes quite explicit the requirements for his treatment approach. His patients must be fairly verbal and intelligent, be able to reflect on their own psychological processes, present with a clinical focus that can be framed in oedipal terms, and have sufficient ego strength and flexibility so as to be able to tolerate and utilize his highly active, confrontational approach (Chapter 2). Toward the other end of the spectrum is Mann's time-limited psychotherapy (Chapter 4), which is far less confrontational and stressful to the patient, and which focuses on the issue of loss and the patient's particular adaptations to loss. Mann would appear to accept a much wider range of psychopathology, including patients with more rigid character defenses and less psychological sophistication and articulateness.

Other approaches lie at different points along a dimension of selectivity or exclusiveness. Nonetheless, all have some criteria for exclusion and inclusion. The following criteria apply to all the models discussed.

1. First, all require a *capacity for engagement with the therapist in some emotionally meaningful way*, whether this is understood in terms of response to trial interpretations (Davanloo, 1980) or in terms of a response to the therapist's empathy with the patient's enduring pain (Mann, 1973). Thus, for example, individuals who have a schizoid personality organization, those who are predominantly narcissistic, or those with prominent psychopathic elements will not be able to form the necessary therapeutic relationship within the required time frame. For example, a narcissistic young man presented in a pleasant, cheerful way, but maintained a subtly wary stance, always keeping his distance from real emotional contact. He appeared to be relating to the therapist— but it didn't feel real to him. It was impossible to reach his real pain and anguish in a brief time frame.

Patients in psychotic states also cannot be engaged within the required time frame, as they will remain too disorganzed to form the kind of relationship called for by the various models. Chemically dependent individuals also will be generally unavailable for the quality of relatedness that these brief therapies rely upon.

The necessity for a capacity to engage leads to a corollary requirement: *the capacity to disengage at termination.* Some patients are able to become involved, but have great difficulty with separation and loss, particularly people who have not sufficiently separated from their primary objects or who have suffered severe losses in the area of their primary relationships. Here, the therapist is faced with the dilemma of recapitulating the traumatic loss through the scheduled termination required by the brief therapy process.

2. The second general selection criterion is the *focality of the patient's difficulties.* Each approach requires the early formulation of a clinical focus, which becomes the conceptual structure that organizes the gathering of clinical data and therapeutic interventions. In fact, it is debatable as to whether the presence of a therapeutic focus is more a function of the therapist's theory and clinical approach or characteristics of the patient's personality. Either way, however, if the patient's problems seem vague, diffuse, and unformulated, then any attempt to work briefly is likely to prove difficult.

3. The last general selection criterion is *the patient's capacity to tolerate the emotional requirements of the therapeutic process,* which, as we have mentioned, vary from model to model. Nonetheless, all models make some demands on a patient's ego strength: that is, the patient's reality test-

ing, emotional flexibility, and adaptiveness and flexibility of defenses. Thus, the nonsuitable patient is one who lacks a sufficient degree of any of these characteristics. For example, none of the brief models will attempt the treatment of patients with psychotic illnesses for the reason that such persons are unlikely to have the ego strength to fulfill the requirements of the task.

There are some notable recent attempts to apply brief therapy models to more difficult patients, such as those with personality disorders, though Binder (personal communication, 1995) suggests that such patients have always been treated in short-term therapy, but simply not described using the criteria of the various editions of the *Diagnostic and Statistical Manual of Mental Disorders* (DSM). These approaches represent modifications of existing models, or are models based on evolving clinical theory of personality and psychopathology (Alpert, 1992; Høglend, 1993a; Leibovich, 1981; Perry, 1989; Winston et al., 1991). In most cases, patients with more severe personality disorders are not treated. Discriminations are made *within* diagnostic groups, so DSM diagnoses by themselves are not viewed as a basis for selection. For example, Leibovich (1981) suggests the following characteristics as necessary to briefly treat a patient with borderline personality disorder:

(1) Evidence of sufficient reality testing . . .

(2) Motivation: patients have to manifest the wish for psychological help . . .

(3) Patients must exhibit some degree of intrapsychic and emotional separateness . . . the borderline patient's tendency to psychically enmesh or fuse should not be too strong . . .

(4) . . . There must be evidence of some positive emotional connection with the evaluator . . .

(5) . . . there must be evidence of some warm, positive interactions . . . the ego capacity for having attempted relationships must be present . . .

(6) . . . A positive feature . . . is a basic mood of contentment . . .

(7) Patient's complicated ego function of verbalization must have developed sufficiently . . .

(8) . . . Conflict-free ego capacities like perception, discipline, perseverance, desires for advancement, tenacity, etc. manifested through achievments in occupational, social, political, academic or familial spheres must be evident. . . . (pp. 260–261)

In an early research study, Malan (1976a, 1976b) suggested that the only patient variable predictive of outcome of the many examined in the study was "motivation for insight." Piper et al. (1990) similarly examined patient predictors of psychotherapy outcome across a wide range of DSM-III Axis I and Axis II diagnoses. Their finding was that the two strongest predictors of outcome were patients' quality of object relations (QOR), and "defensive style," both measures derived from psychoanalytic theory and diagnosis, rather than from the categorical approach of DSM. Research by Høglend and his associates in Norway also support the use of psychodynamic criteria for the prediction of outcome (Høglend, 1993b). (For a more complete review of patient predictors of psychotherapy outcome, see Chapter 2.)

It appears that symptomatic description and psychiatric diagnosis are not adequate for the selection of patients even within the narrower range of more difficult patients. Instead it is suggested that, just as for better functioning patients, more difficult patients have to be selected on the basis of interpersonal or object relational dimensions of personality functioning that appear to underlie the process of change in psychotherapy.

Although suitability decisions are usually treated as categorical— that is, the patient is either suitable or not—we suggest that the process of assessment is rarely straightforward. It appears to us that suitability can be thought of as a dimension along which patients may lie, although even this conceptual improvement tends to oversimply the situation by implying the existence of a single underlying variable which is responsible for "difficultness." There are some patients who are quite easy to exclude on the basis of their history or clinical presentation, such as chronic schizophrenics, patients with organicity, those with active chemical dependence, and so on. At the other end of the spectrum there are patients who seem to possess many or all of the characteristics thought of as desireable for psychotherapy, such as the capacity to tolerate unpleasant affects, evidence of mature relationships and other significant emotional commitments, and psychological flexibility and responsiveness. Such patients would likely be viewed as suitable by any therapeutic approach. It is in the gray area between these two groups of patients that the problematic decisions have to be made.

As we have mentioned, practical considerations are an essential part of the suitability question for such patients. What alternatives are there to the treatment that can be offered? Is it brief therapy versus no therapy? Is there a mandate to treat the patient, such as would be the case in many community settings or counseling centers? Is there a third party who will restrict the duration of therapy under any circumstance? Is there an external, environmental factor, such as a patient imminently moving away, which will limit the duration of treatment? These questions have to be kept in mind while the clinical characteristics of the patient are considered. Many patients whom we consider "difficult" are those who are not really suitable for brief treatment but must be seen anyway, for one of these practical reasons. In many such cases, the patient would be difficult for any therapist under more optimal circumstances, but the difficulty is exacerbated by the presence of some time limitation. *In the end, we are required to change our approach with such patients as the question of suitability metamorphoses into the question of how we are to modify our technique.* It is our view that the patients we designate as difficult generally would be treated in more open-ended psychotherapy if that were possible. If the context of the therapeutic setting is not flexible then *we* must be if we are to be of use to such patients.

Of course, this raises the interesting question of one's outlook or worldview insofar as duration of psychotherapy is concerned. We recognize that some clinicians advocate brief therapy as the primary treatment approach for all patients, with long-term treatment only as a treatment of last resort, if at all. That certainly is the position taken by the managed care industry, which is increasingly shaping mental health care policy and psychotherapy practice via the changing scope of third-party reimbursement. Nonetheless, with some notable exceptions, a psychoanalytically informed outlook continues to give weight to time-unlimited treatment in the consideration of more difficult patients, a view supported for the most part by the research literature, as will be surveyed shortly. At present it appears that the assertion that brief psychotherapy—of any kind—is the treatment of choice for more severe psychopathology is motivated more by economic concerns than by clinical or scientific evidence.

THE FORMULATION OF THE FOCUS

If patient selection is one central concern in the practice of brief psychodynamic therapy, another is the issue of the clinical focus. In fact, the ability of the therapist to formulate such a focus is for some a crucial aspect of patient selection (Malan, 1976a; Mann, 1973; Sifneos, 1987; Strupp & Binder, 1984). Although the models we discuss in this volume have distinctly different approaches to the formulation of a clinical focus, all view some form of focus as a necessity in accomplishing psychodynamic goals in a time-limited framework.

Lack of a Dynamic Focus

The inability of the therapist to derive a psychodynamic focus during the early assessment phases of treatment suggests that a time-limited psychotherapy will not be optimal. Such patients might be those with vague chronic complaints or symptoms, those without clear precipitants for the current crisis, and those who shift between several different problem areas with little apparent commitment or capacity to work on any one area.

We may hypothesize that such patients have suffered particularly severe deprivations or traumas, resulting in problems in the structuring of the ego. Thus, problems of relatedness, separation–individuation, and self-cohesiveness are in the fore, rather than more focal conflicts in relation to well-defined others. In fact, the therapist's experience of the patient as diffuse and vague, with the significant others in the patient's life seeming to lack depth and richness, may be a way such impaired object relations in the patient are represented in the mind of therapist. Descriptions of important others or interpersonal situations that are lacking in emotional richness, detail, and complexity suggest impoverishment of object relations. Often the therapist is struck by a quality of unrelatedness which cannot be directly experienced as such, but is instead inferred from what does *not* happen in the therapeutic relationship. With such patients, countertransference may include boredom and "spaceyness," bewilderment, and frustration at what feels like something important missing, physical sensations or unusual bodily experience, or the sense of not being able to keep in mind patients' descriptions of other people in their lives.

Structural Deficits Rather Than Conflict?

In considering patients who seem either to lack a clinical focus or have multiple foci, we have to ask ourselves whether there is actually no focus or whether the focus might take a form different from what a given treatment model would lead us to expect. With our difficult patients, is it the case that a central focus does not exist, or is it that we cannot find a focus, given our clinical and theoretical presuppositions? The notion of a psychotherapeutic focus arises from a more verbally oriented, rational, oedipal, conflict-oriented notion of personality and psychopathology. Therapeutic foci are often framed in terms of insights the patient needs to attain, conflict between different parts of the psychic structure, or structures of interpersonal functioning. An alternative view is that for some individuals deficient internal structuring is the essential psychopathology rather than intrapsychic or interpersonal conflict (Stolorow & Lachman, 1980). In this view, we have difficulty formulating a therapeutic focus because the theory of personality and psychopathology do not adequately represent the nature of the patient's problems. For example, if we expect that psychopathology is related to oedipal conflict, then perhaps our inability to make the psychodynamic formulation in a particular case is because the patient struggles with other dynamic issues, such as separation–individuation (Blanck & Blanck, 1974), basic trust–mistrust (Erikson, 1950; Fairbairn, 1941), or self-coherence and stability of self-structure (Atwood & Stolorow, 1984). Such patients are not adequately understood in terms of a specific clinical focus, and simply do not make use of the kinds of psychotherapeutic interventions that naturally follow from a focus, such as persistent confrontation of resistances, interpretations of trans- ference feelings, or clarification of defenses.

For such patients, the therapeutic endeavor may be better thought of as the provision of a nurturing, maturational environment in which development may progress (Winnicott, 1965), rather than a situation in which insight must be fostered. The focus correspondingly will con- sist of the ongoing recognition of the patient's use of the therapist to regulate internal states and affects. It remains to be seen whether such a process is well suited to short-term psychotherapy. Intuitively, it does not appear so, though some authors are exploring the use of empathic techniques in brief psychotherapy (Alpert, 1992).

Selfobject Transferences and the Therapeutic Focus

One of the most important recent contributions to clinical psychoana- lytic theory is Kohut's recognition of the particular forms of related- ness that occur in the psychotherapy of narcissistically organized patients. In the course of developing psychoanalytic self psychology he describes what he calls the "selfobject transferences," including the "mirroring transference" and the "idealizing transference" (Kohut, 1971, 1977). These forms of transference represent the revival in the psy- chotherapy relationship of developmentally early forms of relatedness characterized by self-centeredness and fantasies of omnipotence. Kohut views such narcissistically organized relationships as necessary to the development of self-cohesiveness and stable self-esteem. Patients who did not have sufficiently empathic, attuned, mirroring responsiveness from primary caretakers require such responsivness in the therapeu- tic situation, which will in turn permit continued development of the self. The internalization of the therapist's affirming, validating stance results eventually in the patient being able to progress toward more mature forms of self-esteem regulation.

It is noteworthy in the present context that these forms of trans- ference were previously overlooked altogether because they did not have the form of the more familiar object transferences of neurotic psychopathology. In Kohut's view, selfobject transferences were not recognized by classical analysts because object relationships had been defined primarily in terms of drives and infantile sexual development. Instead, he emphasizes the needs of the self for validation and affirmation of developmentally appropriate forms of narcissism characteristic of the selfobject transferences. The therapist's provision of selfobject functions is indeed a form of relatedness, in fact, a crucial form that Kohut came to believe underlay all personality development and pathology (Kohut, 1984).

Thus, as Rosegrant (1984) has suggested, it may be more appropriate with some patients viewed as difficult to substitute the provision of a "holding environment" in place of a reliance on a more traditional dynamic focus. Rosegrant applies to brief therapy Winnicott's (1965) concept of the "holding environment," which refers to a quality of the maturational environment in which the infant's vulnerability to impingement by the environment and by internal stimulation such as pain or hunger is cushioned by a primary caretaker. Lazarus (1982) and, more recently, Gardner (1991) also apply self psychology theory to brief psychotherapy with narcissistically organized patients, emphasizing the restoration of self-esteem and self-cohesion as the central therapeutic tasks. Both authors identify the establishment of the self–selfobject bond as the primary agent of therapeutic change. They also emphasize the importance of continued working-through of self-esteem issues after the termination of therapy. Other authors have recently begun to apply self psychology concepts to the practice of brief therapy as well (Baker, 1991).

Another group of workers have evolved a form of brief treatment based on Davanloo's intensive short-term dynamic therapy, which they have called "accelerated empathic therapy" (Alpert, 1992; Foote, 1992; Fosha, 1992). In this treatment model the emphasis shifts from the characteristic confrontation of defenses and resistances of Davanloo's approach to a highly supportive and empathic therapeutic stance, leading to the "melting" of defenses, a high level of reciprocity and collaboration, and the use of the therapist's self to enable the patient to experience and bear highly aversive and painful affects (Alpert, 1992). This time-limited treatment model calls for active techniques, distinguishing it from long-term psychodynamic therapy, but emphasizes empathy and attunement, in contrast to Davanloo's emphasis on confrontation of resistances. Although they did not begin with a self psychological framework, it appears that these clinicians have begun to understand their work in the light of Kohut's contributions (Foote, 1992). In each of these approaches, there is a lessened emphasis on a dynamic focus per se, and a greater attention to patient experience, affects, countertransference feelings, and "staying with the patient," a stance which characterizes more experiential or existential-humanistic approaches to psychotherapy.

TREATMENT ISSUES AND TECHNIQUE

In this section we discuss some of the modifications in a treatment approach required to work successfully with difficult patients in brief psychodynamic therapy. Characteristics of such patients, described in previous sections, have important implications for treatment techniques. These technical problems can be enumerated as follows: First, the therapist must find a way to make contact with patients whose defensive structures require a high degree of emotional distance, or who may rely heavily on dissociation and other forms of emotional cut-off. Second, there is the problem of dealing with the inevitable separation and loss entailed in brief therapy with individuals who have particular anxiety concerning abandonment, and thus cannot readily tolerate the termination phase of brief treatment. Third, there is the challenge of maintaining a "therapeutic alliance" or "working alliance" (Greenson, 1967; Zetzel, 1956). Such an alliance is more difficult to achieve with those patients who struggle with issues of basic trust, and have concerns related to cohesiveness of the self, containment of impulses, and maintenance of interpersonal and intrapsychic boundaries. Such patients fail to differentiate clearly between the transference relationship and the "real" relationship to the therapist. Thus, the therapist may be seen by the patient to be just as abusive as the abusive parent of childhood. Fourth, patients with disturbed object relations tend to have a harder time holding in mind a representation of the therapist as basically "good enough." Reliance on "splitting" results in such persons seeing others as all good or all bad, which in turn leaves them terrified or full of rage as the therapist is perceived in a contradictory and ephemeral light: at one point idealized, and at another moment demonized. Last, there is a cluster of problems pertaining to disruptions of therapeutic boundaries. "Acting out" is the impulsive expression of feelings in non-verbal modalities which threaten to disrupt the therapy situation. These would include self-mutilating behavior, missing sessions, threats of dangerous behavior or suicide, or other attacks on the integrity of the therapeutic frame. Also in this category can be included unintentional boundary disruptions caused by characterological disorganization or transient decompensation to psychotic modes of experience.

Modifications of Technique in Brief Psychotherapy with Difficult Patients

The real question behind the issue of the difficult patient in brief therapy has to be formulated in terms of treatment technique: How do we need to modify our treatment approach to be able to accomplish something of psychodynamic value to this patient? Do we apply an existing model as best we can to a challenging patient? Do we formulate a new approach to accommodate that patient? Implied in these questions are two conflicting aspirations. On the one hand, we would like to be of the greatest use to the patient, and thus as therapeutically ambitious as possible given what constraints there are. On the other hand, we wish to minimize the risk of harming the patient by using a treatment approach that is not appropriate for him or her. Out of the dynamic tension between these two goals we may be able to evolve a treatment strategy which is flexible enough to stay with the patient and to offer the patient what we can.

Supportive Techniques

In general, treating nonsuitable patients in brief psychotherapy will call for a shift from the "expressive" end of the spectrum toward the "supportive" end (see Pinsker, Rosenthal, & McCullough, 1991, for a recent discussion of short-term supportive psychodynamic psychotherapy). This entails an increased emphasis on the therapeutic qualities of the therapy relationship, such as warmth, empathy, emotional availability, and other ego-supportive characteristics of the "real relationship." There is a corresponding decrease in the emphasis on interpretation, confrontation, and the attainment of insight, and less attention to the transference relationship. There is less interpretation of defenses, and more support for the adaptive aspects of defenses. There is an increased reliance on nonpsychodynamic interventions, such as education, counseling, modeling, reframing, and encouragement (see Chapter 5, and Pinsker et al., 1991).

We have already discussed the idea of framing the psychotherapy as a "holding environment" (Rosegrant, 1984). This idea is consistent with the increased use of supportive techniques providing containment, self-esteem enhancement, and anxiety reduction through an empathic, affirming stance. The curative effect here is not primarily through insight but via amelioration of anxiety, internalization of the relatively benign therapist and therapy framework, and mitigation of otherwise intolerable affects through the mediating effects of the therapist's personality in the form of acceptance, empathic understanding, and tolerance for the patient's affect states and the therapist's own reactions.

Modification of the Focus

Since more difficult patients so often present problems in the area of establishing or maintaining a consistent therapeutic focus, it may be necessary to narrow the range of clinical attention to the immediate, here-and-now situation of the patient. This adaptation-oriented approach may result in less psychodynamic change, but may make possible a valuable adjustment in the patient's course of development, permitting further growth and adaptation. Depth-oriented treatment may not always be indicated: The resolution of a developmental snag or of a transitional life situation may be ambitious enough, given a particular patient's (or therapist's) resources. For example, a young woman with a borderline personality disorder comes to a counseling center with symptoms arising in the context of graduating from college. The focus is selected with a limited time-frame in mind, addressing the immediate issue of separation anxiety and the developmental crisis rather than the personality disorder per se. The goal of treatment is to get this patient through a current life crisis so that she might continue to progress on her own. The need for future treatment is probable, but something of dynamic value can be accomplished in the immediate situation. The transference situation is minimized as the focus is shifted for the most part from the therapy relationship to the developmental obstacle and external relationships. It is, however, valuable for the therapist to be aware of the transferential implications of what goes on in therapy, even if these are not interpreted to the patient. The focus may be clearly defined and actively applied, but its scope will be narrower and less ambitious than with more suitable patients.

Extratherapeutic Treatment Modalities and Structure

There are a variety of modifications of a standard framework for BPT that may be employed when necessary. These include additional, supplementary treatment modalities, such as group, couple, or family therapy, which may be integrated with the ongoing or terminating short-term psychotherapy (Goodheart, 1989). Other forms of extratherapeutic structure may include specific injunctions around acting out or dangerous behavior (see Bellak's brief therapy, Chapter 5), the involvement of significant others in the patient's life through phone contacts or conjoint sessions, referal to self-help organizations like Alcoholics Anonymous, and assistance with medical self-monitoring (Goodheart, 1989). These various nonpsychodynamic interventions may be required either to maintain a safe therapeutic structure or to have some additional therapeutic value in addressing a situational disturbance or developmental impasse. Such supplemental interventions should be used with care, as they often have complictating effects on the therapeutic relationship from a psychodynamic point of view. They can create complicated transferences organized around idealization, oppositionalism, or dependency. Nonetheless, such technical modifications may be required within the context of a broadly psychoanalytic approach, providing flexibility and a wider scope of application.

Modifications of the Termination Phase

These modifications of usual brief therapy technique have to do with the impact of termination and its effects on marginally suitable patients. One obvious modification is extension of the original brief therapy contract. This need not be the abandonment of the short-term framework altogether, but may be, instead, a response to a crisis in the therapy process or in the outside life of the patient, such as the death of a family member, making termination along the orignal lines impossible. Such extensions can provide a valuable addition to the termination phase, allowing the therapist and patient to continue to process issues of loss and separation. In other situations it may be appropriate to extend the therapy so as to give the patient a greater sense of control over the treatment process, and to mitigate the experience of abandonment and loss so that it can be mastered.

Another alteration is the tapering off of treatment, or the scheduling of intermittent sessions over some extended period of time (Goodheart, 1989). This can help certain patients with the process of "internalizing" the therapist, that is, enabling the patient to form a stable, internal representation of the therapist as a reliable and consistent other. This process may be of special use for patients who have experienced traumatic losses or who have had insufficient response to their emotional needs. Such special arrangements may give the patient the sense that his or her needs are taken seriously, and that he or she can be responded to as an individual.

Finally, it is sometimes necessary and desirable to modify the termination by referring the patient to long-term therapy. For some patients a successful outcome to a brief therapy would be the recogntion of the importance for them of more in-depth therapeutic work, and some greater sense of optimism about the possibilities for further change.

Countertransference in the Time-Limited Treatment of the Difficult Patient

There are particular emotional reactions in the therapist to the difficult patient who is seen in a short-term context. The interaction of the pressure of the time limit and the relatively greater clinical demands of such patients makes for intense and difficult countertransferences.

Strupp has noted that less suitable patients (defined by poorer psychotherapy outcome) elicit more negative interactions even with experienced psychotherapists (Strupp, 1980a, 1980b, 1980c, 1980d). The interpersonally oriented work of the Vanderbilt group using Benjamin's Structural Assessment of Social Behavior (SASB) scale also strongly supports the notion that interactions with more disturbed or difficult patients tend to be characterized by greater levels of hostility and negativity on the part of both participants (Benjamin, 1974, 1982). Object relations theory, such as Kernberg's (1974), predicts stormy and hostile interactions with others as the result of the persecutory and destructive character of internalized representations of self and others. We wish to emphasize, with Strupp (1980a), that it is the interaction with such patients that is negative, which by necessity involves the therapist and his or her own negative, retaliatory, punitive, and critical feelings. Thus, attention to the countertransference is of the greatest importance with more difficult patients, as unrecognized feelings will be likely acted out with the patient in destructive and countertherapeutic ways.

Working with less suitable patients in brief settings leaves the therapist on the horns of a dilemma. On the one side is therapeutic grandiosity, a "gung-ho" attitude that minimizes conflict and difficulty, relying on an overly optimistic vision of psychotherapy and its possibilities for producing positive change in all of one's patients, regardless of how troubled or entrenched their problems. Such an attitude relies on denial of the full extent of the patient's difficulties and overestimation of the patient's resources. On the other side is therapeutic nihilism, the attitude that it doesn't matter what one does, because the patient is too disturbed to be helped. One gives up on the patient, the technique, and oneself in the face of seemingly insurmountable problems, so as to be spared the pain of partial or inadequate results.

It may be noted that these two reactions are connected by the underlying dimension of the therapist's own need for self-esteem and feelings of effectiveness and competence, all of which are undermined by the more difficult patient. One way out that is available in open-ended psychotherapy is to postpone the pain of limitations into the indefinite future. In time-limited settings there is no such recourse, and the limitations of therapist, therapy, patient, and the human condition are made painfully clear more or less from the outset (cf. the "tragic vision," Chapter 1). Both therapeutic grandiosity and therapeutic nihilism are defensive positions that enable the therapist—and patient—to avoid painful realities. Also avoided, however, are realistic possibilities: the uncomfortable middle ground of partial solutions, compromises, ambiguous outcomes, and, in the end, the real possibility of the patient living with more satisfaction and success. Thus, these two countertransference attitudes, however understandable in light of the patient's limited psychological or financial resources, represent the therapist's flight from therapeutic difficulties into idealized positions that offer the patient little of real value.

One other therapist reaction worth noting are the guilt feelings that may accompany working with the difficult patient in a time-limited setting. This is the natural extension of the typical guilt reaction of the short-term therapist: "Am I offering this patient what he or she needs? Is this enough?" The more difficult the patient, the more likely the answers to these questions will be disquieting to the therapist. Such feelings may intensify as the course of treatment progresses, or appear after termination, when there is time to look back and question the value of the work in retrospect. These concerns are important and represent the therapist's commitment to professional and personal standards in the face of limited treatment resources. Such feelings can be used in different ways. There is the possibility of taking a position of advocacy for the provision of adequate psychotherapy resources within a given community or setting, thus directing these countertransference feelings into realistic political activity. Another solution is to find the value in what is offered, with the recognition that even less suitable patients can obtain something of real value in a brief setting. Yet another solution is to innovate useful modifications of existing treatment approaches. Therapist guilt, like omnipotence and despair, can serve a defensive function against the pain of therapeutic imperfection, through identification with a "perfect" critical ideal.

RELEVANT RESEARCH

There is little systematic research on the modifications of standard short-term therapies in the treatment of nonoptimal patients. This is probably because of the methodogical requirement of holding psychotherapeutic treatments constant across groups of subjects in a research study, as opposed to treating research patients more individually. Nonetheless, a number of research findings are relevant to such questions as what makes a patient difficult, and which treatment approaches appear to be of use with wider ranges of patient problems. We will also review the outcome literature as it pertains to the treatment of more disturbed or difficult patients. (For a review of patient predictors of outcome, see Chapter 2.)

There have been a number of research programs aimed at understanding what makes some patients more difficult to treat in short-term psychotherapy. Strupp (1980a, 1980b, 1980c, 1980d) published a series of papers utilizing side-by-side, qualitative comparisons of pairs of patients, in which one patient was identified as having a successful treatment outcome and the other identified as a treatment failure. Strupp wished to understand how these paired patients differed from one another in terms of initial characteristics and of the rated psychotherapy process. He noted that differences in terms of qualitative diagnostic categories did not appear to be highly relevant. Patients with similar MMPI profiles and similar DSM diagnoses had widely divergent outcomes and therapeutic process. The "difficult" patient in the pair did differ, however, on variables such as focality of difficulties, motivation for treatment, patient activity in therapy, psychological-mindedness, and a more differentiated view of self and others (Strupp, 1980a). Individuals also differed in terms of the responses they elicited from their therapists, with more difficult patients becoming involved in more negative interactions (Strupp, 1980d). Therapists, including experienced clinicians, tended to respond more negatively to such patients, exhibiting more hostility, coldness, and rejection. The management of negative transference is more critical with less suitable patients.

Other studies have also suggested that differential outcome in BPT is a function of initial patient characteristics, with more disturbed patients having less successful outcomes (Høglend, Sørlie, et al., 1993; Husby et al., 1985). This finding is robust, with a review of such literature suggesting that DSM-III Axis II diagnoses (personality disorders) are correlated with poorer response to short-term psychotherapeutic treatment (see also Reich & Green, 1991). Consistent with Strupp's findings, however, measures other than DSM-III diagnoses appear to be more useful in predicting therapy outcome. For example, Høglend (1993b) found that a measure of interpersonal relations was significantly more predictive of a measure of psychodynamic outcome in BPT than DSM-III diagnoses. Another study by Høglend (1993a) suggested that patients with personality disorders showed more psychodynamic improvement when the duration of therapy was longer. In fact, in this latter study, length of treatment was a better predicter of outcome than were other initial patient characteristics. On the basis of his data, Høglend (1993a) asserts that "a brief, focused dynamic treatment approach is insufficient for patients with personality disorders" (p. 179).

However, other studies suggest that brief treatment approaches can be successful with certain groups of more difficult patients. Winston et al. (1991) found that two different brief psychodynamic psychotherapies were equally effective in treating a group of patients with DSM-III Axis II diagnoses (personality disorders) compared to the waiting list control group. This study was repeated with a larger sample, and again it was found that both a Davanloo-type approach (ISTDP), and what the authors call brief adaptive psychotherapy (BAP; Pollack, Flegenheimer, & Winston, 1991) resulted in treatment outcomes significantly better than the waiting list controls, with no significant difference between the two treatment approaches (Winston et al., 1993). The latter treatment, BAP, was designed especially for the treatment of patients with personality disorders. It should be pointed out that in these studies patients with only the less severe forms of personality disorder are treated, such as patients with avoidant, dependent, obsessive–compulsive and passive–aggressive personality disorders. Patients with schizoid, paranoid, narcissistic, and borderline psychopathology were excluded.

Thus, the results of outcome studies with less optimal patients are mixed and difficult to interpret. There are a number of sources of this ambiguity. First, the category of difficult patient, even if narrowed down to Axis II diagnoses (personality disorders) is extremely heterogeneous. In addition, as we have outlined, there are patients who are challenging for reasons other than having personality disorders. Patients are defined differently in various studies. Second, even with current, "manualized" treatment approaches, it is hard to determine what part of the outcome can be attributed to the specific effects of that approach as opposed to nonspecific therapeutic factors.

Finally, it is difficult to generalize the results of the studies conducted so far which attempt to examine a standardized treatment approach. We suggest that, in reality, many of the patients who are deemed difficult are treated in clinic and private settings on a case-by-case basis with highly diverse modifications of existing psychotherapy approaches. In fact, it may be the specificity of treatment modifications that account for the success or failure of a given psychotherapy.

A CRITICAL EVALUATION

In this chapter we have followed an informal nomenclature which makes reference to the "difficult patient," as well as diagnostic categorizations that attempt to define and describe such patients. However, the representation of psychopathology as a quantifiable dimension, with "more" being clinically more difficult than "less," relies on assumptions that can be challenged. Even if reliable discrimination can be made between those with "oedipal" problems and those with "preoedipal" pathology, the temporal sequence implied both by the terminology itself and by the developmental theory underlying these terms has been questioned by developmentalists (Stern, 1985) and psychopathologists

(Sass, 1992; Westen, 1990). The traditional emphasis in psychology on scientific procedures, experimental methodologies, and statistical tools have led to an underappreciation of the larger cultural contexts in which discourse on psychopathology takes place. Forming part of the cultural context in which clinical theory arises and decisions about "suitability" are made is a valuing of the verbal over the nonverbal, insight over relationship, structure over formlessness, independence over dependence, and action over being.

These biases are quite apparent in psychoanalytic developmental theories, which have supported a "one-way arrow" of development from primitive and undifferentiated to higher and differentiated (Mahler, Pine, & Bergman, 1975). Recently, infant researchers such as Stern (1985) and Beebe (1994) have questioned the unidirectionality of such models, suggesting that early psychological life is not so undifferentiated after all, and that development is in its essence multidimensional and nonlinear.

Researchers in psychopathology are also concluding that the notion of a single, underlying dimension does not do justice to the complexity of object relations (Westen, 1990). For example, Westen makes the following statement:

> Rather than treating level of object relations as a unitary dimension on which a person is likely to be globally fixated, we are beginning with the assumptions that individuals differ on many cognitive–affective–motivational dimensions relevant to their interpersonal functioning; that some of these covary and others do not; that some of these are chronically activated and others are less so; that specific processes are activated under certain conditions; and that different sets of processes operate at different levels of consciousness. (p. 47)

Sass (1992) also takes issue with the view that various forms of psychopathology can all be projected back onto a single time line of development, with the more severe disorders rooted in earlier developmental derailment.

> All these schools [of psychology] accept some version of the grand and optimisitic Western narrative of progress toward higher levels of consciousness and self-consciousness, and all presuppose a single, unilinear dimension along which all psychological phenomena can be located. At the very top are the reality-adapted, pragmatic, quasi-scientific modes of consciousness presumably obtained by normal socialized adults in modern culture. And, by what seems an inexorable logic, any deviation from this condition is assumed to correspond to an earlier and lower developmental stage. (p. 21)

Finally, the evolving concept of "intersubjectivity" also raises questions about applying categories to individuals without reference to the surrounding relational context (Stolorow & Atwood, 1992). We use the term "intersubjective" here to refer to those aspects of human psychology that exist only in the context of relationships with human others. They are "subjective" in the sense that the phenomena take place in the realm of mind and are located in an experiencing center of human consciousness, and "inter" in that these subjective structures are constituted within the surrounding psychological milieu. This view can be counterposed to psychologies in which the individual subject is understood to be radically separate from others and is presumed to "contain" essential psychological characteristics apart from any immediate interaction or relationship—existing in a psychological vacuum, as it were.

If we take seriously the notion that all human experience is constituted along a dimension of internal structure–interactional structure, then it becomes logically impossible to make definitive statements about the individual without reference to the psychological context. What we observe will always be a simultaneous function of both internal and stable structures of personality on the one hand and the nature and qualities of the interpersonal and intersubjective context on the other (Beebe, 1994; Skolnick & Warshaw, 1992; Stolorow, Brandschaft, & Atwood, 1987).

In this view, when we describe a patient as difficult we are saying something about ourselves as much as about the patient. Who the patient is, and the kind of therapeutic relationship that can be attained, will inevitably be a function of who the therapist is and how the therapist works. Different therapists find different patients difficult. From the patient's point of view, the problem may be a "difficult therapist," one who does not grasp a needed response, leading to frustration and therapeutic failure.

These varied critiques reinforce the idea that definitions of "difficultness" must take into account the defining context, whether it is a particular clinical model which may not suit a given patient, a prevailing cultural trend that values certain psychological aptitudes more than others, or the personality of the therapist with its own particular subjective structures. By refusing to anchor assertions about psychopathology in universal or naturalistic categories, we create the possiblity of greater openness to individual patients and their particular psychological configurations, which contain strengths as well as weaknesses. Perhaps as we recognize the limits to our own constituting grounds of knowledge, fewer patients will seem to us to be difficult.

CHAPTER 7

Treating Children, Adolescents, and the Elderly: A Lifespan Developmental Approach

It can be no coincidence that so many seminal brief therapists developed their models working with populations of young adults (Mann, 1973; Sifneos, 1972). Late adolescence and early adulthood is characterized by developmental changes in family relationships, sexuality, vocational roles, and often changes in geography. These young people are often not available for more sustained therapeutic relationships, and long-term therapy may not best suit their needs. The issues of separation and individuation are predominant, making the themes of loss, separation from family, and development of autonomous functioning natural therapeutic foci. The developmental context is vitally important in psychotherapeutic work with adolescents and young adults.

This developmental context is even harder to overlook in the psychotherapeutic treatment of children, and has had an important place in the evolution of psychoanalytically oriented theory and practice. Anna Freud (1926), Melanie Klein (1932), Margaret Mahler (1968), Rene Spitz (1945, 1946), among many others, added a developmental dimension to psychoanalytic work grounded in observation and practice with children that was conspicuously absent in the work of Freud and the rest of the first generation of psychoanalysts.

Still, the historical link between psychotherapy and developmental theory is rather tenuous in the practice of brief psychodynamic psychotherapy today. Although a great deal of child therapy is both psychodynamically oriented and time limited, there is a notable absence of research and clinical theory on short-term psychodynamic therapy with children (Clark, 1992). None of the therapies described in other chapters of this book specifically address treatment of children. It would seem that treatment of children is thought of as fundamentally different from the treatment of adults, requiring its own set of theories and clinical procedures. There is no question that much of the treatment of children is in reality time limited, and there is a great need for systematic exploration of this work.

At the other end of the lifespan, the health care needs of the elderly have become a greater concern as the proportion of the population of the United States over the age of 65 has steadily increased (Pollock, 1987). Older patients tend to be lumped in with "adults," blurring aspects of psychotherapeutic work that can address their unique needs. There are two main reasons for addressing the elderly separately in the present chapter. First, there are special difficulties faced by older patients in terms of loss, developmental stresses, and identity issues. Developmental and lifespan theory is necessary to address these issues adequately. Second, the psychotherapeutic process has a different meaning, even different aims, in the later stages of human development. Time has special meaning to older patients, and the idea of time limits has powerful resonances as some patients face their own mortality in new, more immediate ways. If futurity is indeed a constituting dimension of all human relationships and personal experience (Stierlin, 1968), then the relationships of older patients are different in crucial ways from their younger counterparts. Brief forms of psychotherapy may have special contributions to make in understanding and treating elderly patients.

DEVELOPMENTAL AND LIFESPAN THEORY

Developmental models historically have had a close and fruitful relation to psychodynamic theory, but psychoanalytic theory alone has not been sufficient to address important questions of child development and human lifepan development. Other influences have been necessary in the expansion of developmental models, including observation of infants and children in normal and clinical settings (Bowlby, 1969; Mahler, 1968; Spitz, 1945), child therapy (A. Freud, 1926; Klein, 1932), as well as nonexperimental research and experimental developmental research on human capacities and individual differences (see Beebe, 1994, for a review). Some have suggested, in contrast to Freud's emphasis on early development, that significant developmental events continue into adolescence and beyond, in fact spanning the entire human life cycle (Erikson, 1950; White, 1959). Family systems theory has influenced psychodynamic approaches to psychotherapy in recognizing the importance of ongoing familial patterns and interaction structures and the continued and powerful influence of current relationships (Ackerman, 1958; Bowen, 1978; Haley, 1976; Minuchin, 1974; Nichols, 1984). Community approaches to psychological problems have expanded our appreciation of the larger cultural contexts in which problems arise and can be understood. Development takes place within concentric circles of social and psychological influence.

The idea of lifespan development, with particular stage-specific issues and conflicts occurring during the various phases of life, has created another context in which to understand human difficulties and their resolution. But most important for the brief psychodynamic therapist, the developmental context provides a means for understanding and addressing problems in their immediate context, bringing a here-and-now emphasis, a crisis-intervention orientation, and suggesting therapeutic foci that do not require sustained exploration of early life, as is the case with more traditional, open-ended psychodynamic approaches.

Developmental concepts form a basis for understanding the predictable or expectable challenges, crises, or transitions an individual is likely to face at various stages of life. For each population — children, adolescents, and the elderly — there are specific developmental factors that can be taken as the basis for focal treatment: One can treat the person with respect to a particular life stage transition or crisis. In this way the developmental context is a vital part of the clinical assessment process, with problems identified not only in terms of symptoms and longstanding personality structures, but also in terms of a failure to meet developmentally determined challenges. Such a perspective need not supplant psychodynamic theory, buts rather adds another dimension to it, enriching the assessment process.

Budman and Gurman (1988) use the term "developmental dysynchrony" to refer to an aspect of this developmental dimension of psychopathology. By "dysynchrony" they mean the subjective experience the patient has in failing to meet some developmentally defined objective. This is the feeling of being behind one's age cohort in some important psychological respect. For example, a woman in her early 30s has never been involved in a serious intimate relationship, although she has always assumed that she would marry and have children. She presented for treatment at the point where the divergence between her expectations (defined in terms of her peer group and broader cultural norms) and her actual life situation created great subjective distress.

While Budman and Gurman seem to emphasize the subjective

aspect of "developmental dysynchrony," it is easy enough to extend the notion to any violation of expected developmental achievements. For example, clinicians and pediatricians have long used rough ideas of developmental milestones to assess the adequacy of development in children. Similar milestones can be applied to older patients as well, such as adaptive responses (or their absence) to retirement or other expectable losses. In fact, it may be said that psychopathology is always in part a function of expectable developmental challenges, and thus generates markers along the dimension of age.

In each of the following sections, an attempt is made to identify the particular lifespan issues that are likely to arise in each age group and to identify models of brief psychodynamic psychotherapy that are best suited to these developmental paradigms. In each case, the formulation of a therapeutic focus relies on the expectable developmental challenge, which is then understood in the particular context of the individual patient.

In a developmental lifespan approach to psychotherapy, the patient's problem is defined in terms of an adaptive failure, usually in the face of new demands from the patient's total life situation. These demands may be accidental, such as illness or other losses, or they may result from the developmental process itself, such as graduating from high school. The natural emphasis of a developmental framework is on situational factors in psychopathology and emotional crisis, rather than on the intrapsychic structure of personality. The latter, usually central to psychoanalytically construed work, is understood more as a background variable in terms of predispositions and previous efforts at adaptation. Such a crisis intervention model identifies the disparity between adaptive resources and situational demands, with the change process primarily aimed at reducing or eliminating the gap. This may or may not require specific psychodynamic change; other interventions may suffice, such as modifying the environment or simply enabling patients to better utilize their existing psychological resources.

The goal of such an approach is to enable the patient to attain new and stable adaptive structures, which ideally will result in a new and improved ability to manage life stresses. At a minimum, the goal is to foster a return to a level of functioning that existed prior to the crisis. Outcome is defined more in terms of the patient's adaptive functioning than any particular psychodynamic achievement. Thus, the relevant approach is through developmental theory and a theory of change processes seen in systemic terms rather than a psychodynamic theory of personality. In fact, advocates of this approach to treatment greatly deemphasize the importance of stable and enduring personality characteristics, and instead focus on the qualities of the situation and the interaction between patient and environment (Budman & Gurman, 1988).

Although we emphasize the importance of a developmental perspective, we view it as compatible with the theory and practice of psychodynamic psychotherapy. Indeed, much of what we are describing as "developmental theory" in the context of this chapter is an outgrowth of psychoanalytic theory and observation. The approaches discussed here are time-limited psychotherapies for children, elderly, and other populations that specifically rely upon psychoanalytic clinical and theoretical principles. As we shall see, these time-limited psychodynamic models of treatment for special age groups utilize the basic principles of psychoanalytic diagnosis, play therapy, the concepts of transference and resistance, defense mechanisms, and psychoanalytic conceptions of development, including the notions of regression, fixation, and developmental breakdown.

CHILDREN

Studies indicate that children are seen in outpatient psychotherapy for six sessions or less, on the average, in a variety of private and clinic settings (Dulcan & Piercy, 1985; Parad, 1978). Yet, the literature on time-limited psychotherapy with children is remarkably sparse. It would therefore appear that much psychotherapy of children is time-limited by default and not by plan. Children may be available only for a relatively brief period of time because of limited financial resources, minimal family motivation, or because of an institutional mandate. Given these realities, there is a pressing need for the development and application of planned, time-limited psychotherapy to maximize the usefulness of psychotherapeutic intervention.

There are other developmental reasons for the use of time-limited models. Children present with greater plasticity than adults. Important issues of character structure have not yet been settled. Children are much more in the process of becoming who they will be than their adult counterparts. Thus, we have every reason to count on the force of the developmental process itself to be a potential ally of the treatment process. For many children, usually those with the least severe psychopathology, a brief intervention might suffice to remove an obstacle to development, permitting the resumption of the developmental process. Thus, an effective psychotherapeutic intervention at the right time may have a disproportionately large effect on the rapidly developing child.

Research suggests the efficacy of a structured or time-limited psychotherapy with children. Parad and Parad (1968) found that explicit time limits reduced the likelihood of premature termination, pointing to parental motivation as the determining factor. Phillips and Johnston (1954) likewise suggest that a clearly defined therapy structure is a critical variable in the outcome of long-term versus short-term psychotherapy. In a more recent comparison of long-term versus time-limited psychoydynamic psychotherapy, Smyrnios and Kirby (1993) found that children in time-limited psychotherapy showed as much improvement as those treated in long-term psychotherapy. The sparsity of the literature on specifically psychodynamic therapies points to the need for more sustained and systematic exploration.

Formulation of the Therapeutic Focus

The Developmental Approach

Child development is characterized by rapid change through very different transitions and phases. From a developmental point of view, child psychopathology can be understood as a breakdown in the developmental process; the child fails to attain developmental milestones in an expected sequence, or there is some regression to previously attained levels of organization. Such breakdowns or regressions are manifested in the areas of cognitive development, social and emotional development, and the development of self structures forming the bases of identity.

Developmental impasses are understood as the result of the interaction of limitations to structural adaptive capabilities in the child and environmental stressors, such as losses, familial inadequacy, illness, or other psychosocial strains. Symptoms can be understood in terms of the child's unsuccessful efforts to cope with the experience of being overwhelmed by traumatic or chronic stressors. Psychodynamic concepts addressing personality structure, such as "ego strength," "reality testing," "tolerance for frustration," and so on, are seen in the context of the adequacy of external support. Character structure as an independent variable is deemphasized, while the adaptive fit of child and environment becomes the locus of attention.

Thus, the clinical emphasis of brief psychodynamic child psychotherapy, relative to longer-term models of treatment, is on familial and other social factors. Because of the brevity of therapeutic contact, there can be less reliance on the notion of restructuring the child's personality, with interventions aimed instead at modifying the existing balance of forces, both internal and external to the child. The formulation of the clinical focus will likely center on some observable, current stressor or life situation, with the hope being the alleviation of that obstruction, permitting the resumption of adaptive and integrative development in the child.

The goal of enabling a patient to attain insights of dynamic importance, which is characteristic of the brief psychotherapy of adults, is very much diminished. Instead, the focus will lead to a structuring of the child's environment, both in the therapy situation and, to the extent possible, in the child's extended environment, to permit the reactivation of thwarted developmental imperatives.

We are aware that many child psychotherapists of a psychodynamic bent would view these principles as fundamental, regardless of the duration of psychotherapy; we suggest that these differences in therapeutic foci are more a matter of degree than either/or propositions. As treatment becomes more time-limited, the necessity for focused attention increases, although naturally the developmental context would be highly relevant to any modality of psychodynamic therapy.

Separation–Individuation Theory

Having presented a general schema for the development of therapeutic foci, we can turn to a universal developmental issue appearing throughout the child development literature that can form the basis of therapeutic formulations. Attachment and separation–individuation is an underlying dimension of all child development, and constitutes a universal arena of conflict in childhood (Bowlby, 1969; Erikson, 1950; Mahler, 1968; Sarnoff, 1976).

The human capacity for attachment is ubiquitous and universal, apparent from the begining of life (Bowlby, 1969). Infants seek the security of being held close. Toddlers keep track of their mother's whereabouts as they explore the world. Young children seek the necessary ego support and emotional encouragement that their parents provide during the course of growing up. Adolescents continue to seek support and contact even as they struggle to develop newfound capacities for independence and autonomy. The effects of the deprivation of primary attachment objects and its relation to psychopathology in childhood have been well documented (Bowlby, 1951; Spitz, 1945, 1946). Although the specific nature of attachment needs continues to be debated by developmentalists, attachment theory has become the dominant paradigm of social development (Lewis, 1990). The need for close contact with consistent caretakers is a central, defining feature of human life, and appears to be a major motivating force that runs through all of development.

The flip side of attachment is separation. If one primary motivation in life is to seek sameness and contact, the other is to seek autonomy and independence. The impetus toward individuation appears to be hardwired as the force that drives the developmental process. Development is characterized by a tension between the need for safety and affiliation and the need for autonomy, differentiation, and "effectance" (Greenberg, 1991; Mahler, Pine, & Bergman, 1975; Murray, 1938; White, 1959). Erikson's (1950) developmental scheme of different lifespan conflicts is driven by the overarching push toward ego synthesis and integration, leading to new developmental challenges and accomplishments. The work of Mahler and her colleagues established separation–individuation theory as the cornerstone of psychoanalytic developmental theory with detailed observation of child development and its relation to the clinical process (Mahler, 1963, 1968, 1972).

Separation–individuation theory provides a framework in which to approach the formulation of the therapeutic focus in brief child treatment. Developmental impasses can be understood as a function of the vicissitudes of the separation and individuation process. Symptoms represent the child's efforts at maintaining and regulating internal affect states in the context of his or her needs for security and competence. While the objects of these needs are constantly changing during the course of development, the underlying structure of attachment needs and needs for mastery continue in an unbroken line from infancy through adolescence and beyond.

Self-Regulation and Mutual Regulation

Theoretical developments in psychoanalytic theory, in particular the British school of object relations, are helpful in understanding psychopathology as the patient's adaptive efforts at self-regulation in the face of environmental failure. Fairbairn (1941) attempted to reconceptualize a range of psychopathology as the result of the unavailability to the child of contact with a whole, loving other. For Fairbairn, if contact with such an object was not available, the individual would find substitute forms of dependency in the form of relations with part-objects, addictions, perversions, and, in fact, the whole gamut of neurotic symptomatology (Fairbairn, 1941). Winnicott (1960, 1963) also posited a need for full and secure dependency on a relatively constant and attuned other, the absence of which throws the infant or child back onto its own insufficient ego resources in the effort to maintain itself. Here, too, symptoms and maladaptive character structures directly result from the failure of the environment to provide a needed maturational matrix.

Contemporary infant research also points to the relationship of self structure in the child to the qualities of the primary attachment object (Beebe, 1994; Stern, 1985). Beebe describes a dynamic process of mutual, dyadic regulation of the infant in the mother–infant relationship on the one hand, and self-regulating capacities in the infant on the other (Beebe, 1994). Where there is insufficiency in the dyadic regulation of the infant's internal states, the child resorts to forms of self-regulation, often pathological in more extreme or chronic instances of mother–infant misattunement.

From these and other contributions it appears that the very structure of self and identity arises and evolves in a relational context, making variations in the quality of relatedness the locus of health and breakdown in development. Once again, this conceptual framework leads the clinician back to careful assessment of the family context of child problems, and to the development of therapeutic foci which address the child's immediate relational environment.

It can be emphasized that this orientation need not lead to family therapy in every case. We would suggest that individual play therapy or psychotherapy can address these relational issues, though it seems more likely that additional interventions at the family level would be made in an attempt to modify ongoing parental perceptions or behavior that are contributing to or maintaining the child's problem. Sometimes parental behavior can be modified through the child, as changes in the child in turn influence the perceptions and actions of parents. There is no close, one-to-one relationship between the clinical formulation, the selected focus of therapeutic work, and the specific technical approach. Rather, the therapeutic focus may be compatible with a range of approaches, selected to suit a particular case scenario and the predilections of the therapist.

Selection Criteria and Suitability

It is possible to identify children who are likely to benefit from brief psychotherapy based on diagnosis or other clinical criteria. However, while case selection may be essential to research protocols and may be an option for some practitioners, many children are seen in settings in which all comers receive some form of treatment. Thus, as in our discussion of the difficult patient (Chapter 6), the issue of suitability may need to be viewed from the point of view of the adaptation and modification of treatment approaches to fit a particular child.

Selection criteria for existing models of time-limited psychodynamic child psychotherapy are congruent with the treatment models for adults. Lester (1968) notes that most important is the assessment of the child's movement through successive developmental phases without serious impasse or breakdown. Thus, the types of difficulties she views as amenable to brief psychotherapy would be transient regressions, mild exaggerations of otherwise age-appropriate behaviors, acute phobias, and other more circumscribed problems. These are distinguished from difficulties unlikely to be successfully treated briefly, including more longstanding, chronic, characterological difficulties and ego weakness, which she views as the result of early defects in the development of object constancy.

Mackay (1967) similarly emphasizes the absence of chronic, characterological psychopathology as a selection criterion, noting that adaptive responses to crises are most likely to be successfully treated in the brief context. He adds that flexibility and responsiveness to interpretation is a key indicator of suitability. Like other workers, Mackay notes the importance of such parental attributes as motivation, flexibility, and the absence of pathogenic attitudes.

Proskauer (1969, 1971) emphasizes a number of criteria for case selection, such as the child's ability to rapidly engage and develop a working relationship with the therapist, the presence of a focal dynamic issue which can be identified, flexible and adequate defenses, and the presence of sufficient basic trust. The qualities of the child's environment must be supportive enough so that treatment efforts will not be undermined. Like Mackay, Proskauer relies on the child's responsiveness to interpretations as an indicator of suitability.

The following synthesis of suitability criteria is offered. These can be seen as corresponding closely to the selection criteria used by the adult treatment approaches outlined previously (see Chapters 2, 3, 4, and 5). Generally, it appears that children with less severe psychopathology are seen as more responsive to brief psychodynamic therapy than those with chronic, developmental difficulties. The developmental context is critical for this assessment. The more severe the history of object loss, maternal or paternal deprivation, family psychopathology, or history of traumatic abuse, the less optimistic one can be about the value of a brief psychotherapy. As with adults, the presence of psychotic symptoms that are not transient contraindicates brief treatment.

We wish to emphasize that placing a child in a particular diagnostic category does not appear to be as useful in the prediction of treatment process and outcome as the relative presence of the interpersonal, intrapsychic, and object relational capacities required by the tasks of brief therapy. Such qualities as basic trust, ego defenses that are functioning adequately and flexibly, and a capacity to rapidly engage and then disengage from a meaningful relationship—all essential ingredients in a useful brief treatment—are not necessarily correlated with categorical diagnoses. Thus, just as with adult patients, the assessment is most usefully conducted from an interpersonal and psychodynamic point of view, with consideration of those characteristics which are most related to the psychotherapeutic process itself.

Last, the assessment of a child for brief treatment must address the characteristics of the child's social and familial milieu to a greater extent than in the treatment of adults. Since the child remains substantially within the influence of family and community, these variables have a disproportionate impact on the likelihood of treatment success. The parents do not have their effect in the treatment primarily as internalizations, as would be the case with an adult patient, but rather are present in the form of ongoing daily transactions and interactions that powerfully affect the child's functioning and ability to use psychotherapy. Family resources are all the more important since the maintenance of a therapeutic effect will depend to a great extent on the continuing influence of the family; potential therapeutic gains can so easily be undone by family psychopathology.

Modifications of Psychotherapy Techniques

Use of Time Limit

As with models of adult treatment, there is some difference of opinion as to the necessity of relying on an explicit time limit. Proskauer (1969, 1971) advocates the use of a clear termination date to be set in the first treatment session, though the time limit does not seem quite so fixed as in Mann's treatment model (see Chapter 4). However, Proskauer emphasizes the impact and meaning of the time limit, much as Mann (1973) does. It is understood that termination issues are activated from the begining of treatment with the statement of a termination date, and the child's ambivalent responses to the issue of loss and separation are utilized throughout the treatment, though especially in the termination phase. The theoretical emphasis is on the use of the time limit to enable the child to address unresolved issues of loss, separation, and differentiation, as in Mann's 12-session approach. In a similar vein, Turecki (1982) advocates the use of a fixed (and explicit) number of sessions so as to enable meaningful work around the issue of object loss. Like Mann, Turecki (1982) suggests that brief therapy "replicates in a condensed form, the evolution of an important object relationship followed by the harsh reality of object loss" (p. 482).

Others make use of an explicit time limit, but do not emphasize the theoretical centrality of the intertwining of the clinical focus and the time limit. Mackay (1967) suggests the use of an explicit contract for the duration of brief treatment in order to encourage a higher level of engagement and involvement with the therapist.

Still others, such as Lester (1968) do not make use of an explicit time limit, but instead emphasize principles of affective engagement, focused work, and the provision of a corrective experience. Time is not made a central issue, but is utilized by the therapist to organize therapeutic activities and aims.

Many authors emphasize the importance of the child's sense of time, particularly those whose work follows Mann's model of time-limited therapy. These authors tend to emphasize the importance of termination, and the child's capacity to work with the time limit and to resolve the issue of loss of the therapy relationship. It may be that this emphasis is more the result of the adaptation of an adult model of treatment than an actual requirement of child psychotherapy, particularly with younger children. It is questionable whether very young children have a sufficiently developed sense of time to make therapeutic use of time limits or interpretations aimed at termination issues in brief treatments (Clark, 1993).

On the contrary, it may be possible to make use of the timelessness of childhood in exercising therapeutic leverage in brief contact with a child. If the unconscious is "timeless" and children's functioning is marked by a fluid boundary between reality and fantasy, then perhaps even a relationship which is limited in time can have a disproportionate impact, as the therapist becomes part of the child's inner world (see Proskauer, 1969).

Use of an Explicit Therapeutic Focus

All models of brief psychotherapy rely on the formulation of a clinical focus, which organizes therapeutic activity and keeps the therapy on track. Models of psychodynamic child psychotherapy likewise rely on such focusing of the treatment, though they differ as to how this focus is used.

Proskauer (1969) recommends the use of a mutually agreed-upon focus, while in most other approaches the central issue is selected by the therapist (Mackay, 1967; Peterlin & Sloves, 1985; Sloves & Peterlin, 1986; Turecki, 1982). In each case, the central issue is formulated on the basis of the child's presenting symptoms, developmental history, and current family situation. It is presented to the child clearly and directly (even in written form, in some cases) so that the child can understand it and can respond in an affective way. Further interventions are related to the central issue, and, in this way, the clinical work is structured and organized around the central theme. An example of such a central theme is presented by Peterlin and Sloves (1985) from the treatment of an angry and disruptive 10-year-old boy:

What I hear you saying is that since you were 2 years old, your mother has been away a lot and has been working very hard. So, you had to learn how to take care of yourself, protect yourself in a way that most 10-year-olds would not have had to do. But, no matter how smart you are, you cannot possibly be expected to do everything that grown-ups do. When you try acting like a grown-up and try taking care of your own business, you get into fights. You fight to get all the things you need because no grown-up is dependable. But, then something happens: everyone gets mad at you and that makes you mad because you feel they don't understand why you are fighting and protecting yourself. (p. 791)

Because the central issue is presented verbally, it is necessary that the child have sufficient use of language. Proskauer (1969) notes that with younger children the focus need not be explicitly stated. Indeed, brief child therapists appear to struggle with a tension between the necessity to organize their therapeutic activities into a formal, verbally representable structure, while at the same time, for younger children at least, relying on the nonverbal treatment modality of play therapy. The challenge is to understand the child's communications in the modality of play and to translate that understanding into a verbal form that is nonetheless meaningful to the child. We would suggest that while the use of a stated therapeutic focus may be of great value in the time-limited treatment of older children and young adolescents, younger children simply may not possess the cognitive or verbal skills to use a stated central issue. The use of a focus, however, need not be explicit; the therapist can still be guided by a central formulation of the child's dilemma and make interventions accordingly.

Playing and Interpretation

There is a tendency among those writing about brief work with children to overestimate the effects of interpretation and clarification of children's expressions in play. There is an overreliance, in our view, on verbal modalities of therapist intervention and not enough trust in the therapeutic effects of expressive play. Clinical examples of interpretations in the literature (i.e., Peterlin & Sloves, 1985) seem, from the point of view of a child, longwinded and rather intellectualized.

Direct creative expression, the hallmark of healthy play in children, may be therapeutic in and of itself. The capacity to play is impaired in thwarted development, and the creation of a "transitional space" (Winnicott, 1971) in which play can take place may in and of itself permit the resumption of development. In fact, if we rely on Winnicott's conception of the function of play, then the goal of therapy is to create in the child the possibility of creative psychic activity *which is itself the vehicle of development.*

One of us worked for about half a year with a boy of 4 whose mother had recently died. The play therapy was characterized by persisent, varied expressions of rage and anxiety in the form of "blowing up games," in which the therapist was to discover bombs hidden around the consulting room or be blown to smithereens. The boy did not appear angry or anxious; on the contrary, he was quite calm, content, and focused in his persistently destructive activities. The number of bombs invariably multiplied to the point where catastrophe was unavoidable. After many weeks of such play, in many variations, the therapist made the error of trying to encourage verbal expression of the feelings the child was so creatively enacting. When asked what feelings all the bombing was meant to be about, the boy looked confused and said emphatically, "Those *are* my feelings!" adding helpfully a moment later, "My feelings are to blow you up!" We would suggest that the goal of "making the unconscious conscious" needs to be modified in child play therapy, regardless of its duration, to address the therapeutic power of the expression of important emotional themes in play and their *recognition by the therapist*. Perhaps this little boy did not need his activities translated into a verbal form, but rather required the psychic containment of his terror and bewilderment as facilitated by the therapist's acceptance of his meanings. For this child it seemed that what was therapeutic was the presence of the therapist as a container of his feelings so that he could manage his internal traumatic affect states better and more creatively.

Interpretations of children's play activities may not need to be so focused on a verbally expressed central theme, but rather may reflect to the child the therapist's respectful understanding of the child's inner world. This accurate and empathic form of communication may not appear to be highly directed, but nonetheless can make a significant difference in the child's experience of self. Naturally, the older the child, the greater the opportunities for communication in a verbal mode.

The child's sense of being understood in the context of a brief psychotherapy is likely to have an impact. It is not clear in what form such moments of being understood are internalized, and certainly they will not have the same impact as if they continued to occur in the course of an ongoing therapy relationship. Nonetheless, the child may feel great relief even if this occurs in a transient relationship. Here again, the fluidity of the child's sense of time may give an intervention impact disproportionate to its duration. It is possible that such moments of felt contact with a new object can permit lifelong shifts in self-perception and experience.

We are suggesting that it may be a mistake to react to the time limitation by attempting to shift the therapeutic work into a more reality-oriented mode, forgetting that brief therapy with children is still child therapy. There is the danger, always connected with time-limited models, of the therapist imposing his or her agenda on the patient; this seems especially true for child patients. We suggest that there is a need for a clinical theory of play therapy in a time-limited context that remains true to the basic principles of psychoanalytic play therapy and the conceptions of play on which it is based.

Contact with Parents

All models of brief dynamic child therapy address the issue of the involvement of parents. Not only is the family seen as an important variable both in selection and outcome, but parents are often actively engaged in either separate or conjoint therapy sessions. It is worth noting that, among the models reviewed, there is an avoidance of "splitting the treatment" between a child therapist and a family therapist, instead relying on one therapist to work with both parents and child (Clark, 1993).

Parents are typically involved at the outset of treatment both for information gathering and in the development of a therapeutic contract (Lester, 1968; Mackay, 1967; Proskauer, 1969). Regular contact is suggested, most often without the child present (Mackay, 1967; Proskauer, 1969). Mackay emphasizes the importance of helping the parents recognize and resolve their own conflicts, taking a parent education approach. Turecki (1982) also emphasizes the use of educative interventions with parents, providing support, clarification, and direction.

It would be impossible to conceive of a time-limited treatment for children that did not directly involve the family. Most child therapists, including those who do more open-ended treatment, arrange contact with parents, so this is nothing new. However, the active participation of parents would seem to be integral to brief treatment in a way not always advocated by psychodynamic clinicians. Because contact with the child is limited, the family must be counted on to support and maintain treatment goals and accomplishments, and thus the parents have to be recruited as allies in the therapeutic enterprise.

Case Vignette

Jane was brought to treatment by her mother when she was about 3½ years old. Her father, with whom she was especially close by mother's report, had died about 6 months before, after a painful and disturbing illness of about 1 year's duration. The mother was distressed by the girl's disruptive and destructive behavior, which was primarily directed at the mother herself. Jane reportedly singled out possessions of the mother's that were particularly special, and would break them. Mother felt she could not control the child in the house, though others in the girl's life did not experience the same degree of anger or behavioral disturbance. The treatment contract was necessarily time limited as the mother planned to move to another city. Sessions were scheduled twice weekly for approximately 5 months.

The first stage of treatment was characterized by the child's inability to play. Instead, the behaviors reported by the mother immediately appeared in the treatment setting, with sessions consisting of one act of destructiveness after another. The hours were filled with anxiety and wanton omnipotence as the therapist chased the girl around his office attempting to protect things from her assaults. She effectively reduced the therapist to helplessness, as all attempts at verbal discourse failed, leaving only a persistent limit setting as the sole form of interaction possible.

The quality of these assaults on the office (as an extension of the therapist?) had a particularly sadistic quality. For example, one day Jane discovered that wiping her saliva on objects and on the clothes of the therapist had an especially disconcerting effect on him. She would pursue him wildly and with great relish, responding only to extremely firm statements banning spitting. She would also "make messes" by dumping things off shelves, and imperiously refuse to clean them up: "*You* clean them up!" It was not long before the therapist greatly regretted taking on this child, given the absence of a playroom which would be less an object of concern. But the therapist's experience could be understood as his identification with the internal states of the child (projective identification) as her affects were communicated not in words or even in symbolic form, but directly. Ogden (1989) describes this direct communication in an elaboration of Klein's "paranoid–schizoid" position:

> In a paranoid–schizoid mode, there is virtually no space between symbol and symbolized; the two are emotionally equivalent. This mode of symbolization, termed *symbolic equation* (Segal, 1957), generates a two-dimensional form of experience in which everything is what it is. There is almost no interpreting subject mediating between the percept (whether internal or external) and one's thought and feelings about that which one is perceiving. (p. 20)

Jane's situation involved catastrophic anxiety which her immature ego could not bear, and so these feelings had to be projected into the therapist, as she had been projecting them into her mother, thereby making the therapist anxious as well. Thus, in these initial sessions Jane was understood to be making use of the therapist as a container to manage and cope with overwhelming affects.

It was clear that a therapeutic focus would not be something discussed verbally, but rather would take the form of the therapist's recognition of the central developmental obstacle faced by Jane, the loss of her father. This recognition would have to be transformed into a therapeutic stance permitting the child to make use of the therapist in ways that would enable her to resume her thwarted developmental aspirations. Jane's situation was conceptualized as the more or less complete shutdown of developmental momentum in the face of impossible strain, first from losing access to both parents as her mother spent enormous energy pursuing the care and treatment of her critically ill husband, and then losing her father altogether at the age of three. Her entire second year was overshadowed by enormous anxiety and pressure, even as the normal crucial events of "rapprochement" were to be taking place (Mahler, 1972). Her cognitive and emotional development were noticeably delayed by age 3½; for example, she showed no interest in drawing, and little ability to use crayons or markers. Thus, the goal of therapy was to attempt to create a sufficiently safe space that there could be a resumption of developmental integration and reorganization of the ego, and to permit the age-appropriate use of symbolic forms of expression via language and creative play.

The begining of a second stage of the psychotherapy was marked by the initation of a game. Jane found an empty tape spool, and would toss it up onto a file cabinet. The therapist was meant to want the spool to remain on top, but her tosses were designed to cause it to roll off. The therapist was supposed to express dismay and exasperation each time the spool fell off. In the next few sessions Jane came in and began the game. She sat herself on top of the cabinet, and would allow the therapist to begin to show pleasure that the spool would finally stay on top, but she would at the last moment knock it off imperiously, relishing the therapist's expressions of dismay. The spool game continued and was elaborated, while all the disruptive behavior of the intial weeks of treatment evaporated.

Jane's ability to play increased. One day, she came in and wanted to play Cinderella. She was to be Cinderella, and the therapist the wicked stepsisters. She was to be mistreated at first, and then would turn the tables, reducing the stepsisters to pleading for mercy and kindness, which she would offer. This game became the central vehicle of therapeutic interaction, as it evolved and was elaborated over many weeks. Through all its variations, a clear theme emerged. There was to be great injustice and misery imposed upon her—with terrible chores, tasks, "messes" to be cleaned, and so forth, and then there would a reversal of fortune, a comeuppance in which the wicked would be brought down and punished, within the sphere of her omnipotence. She delighted in the therapist's expressions of unhappiness as she "tormented" him within the frame of the game, reminiscent of Anna Freud's "identification with the aggressor" (A. Freud, 1966).

The child's attempt to master trauma could be seen in the repetitive impositions of misery onto the therapist, as she made active her own passively experienced suffering. There was the theme of power and control, as Jane was permitted to experience her own omnipotence, which had been so greatly and prematurely truncated by the death of a parent—an event which overwhelmingly brought into awareness her inability to control her father's presence. The content expressed over and over the idea of justice, of cruelty punished, and goodness rewarded in the end. Jane strived to create a world in which she could live, where reasonable expectations, order, structure, and meaning reigned. Finally, the game represented a shared symbolic space, the possibility of a relationship in which a psychological reality is co-created. In playing, there was the experience of an object relationship permitting the internalization of a shared sense of what it means to be in a relationship with an other. It is useful to reiterate that the content of the game contained the very theme of omnipotence and loss that had been manifested directly in her presenting symptom of destructiveness and in her initial presentation in therapy. What had been expressed only through the projection into the therapist of intolerable affect was now being communicated in symbolic forms.

Jane began to draw, and progressed rapidly through the expected phases of drawing. Anxieties persisted, especially around separation from her mother. On one occasion she drew a "spider" which frightened her so much that the session had to be interrupted so she could see her mother. Regressions also occurred, such as when she was brought to a session by a new babysitter. On that occasion the early behaviors appeared as the symbolic space collapsed, and she again reverted to direct communication of affects, as she scribbled off her paper and onto the floor below. At these moments the "mess" could not be contained by the symbolic form of a scribble-mess, but had to become a "real" mess instead. But these regressions were circumscribed, and her overall progress was apparent. Jane spoke more about outside interests, how she was dressed, fantasy characters, other children, and brought toys to sessions, which she shared and played with. There was a noticeable increase in her maturity, far more than would be expected for a child her age over the course of a 5-month period. In fact, it appeared that she had made considerable progress in resuming a course of development, one that would be forever marred by her terrible loss, but perhaps also one in which she could continue to grow and be better able to deal with the ongoing strains of the developmental process.

There had been no formal time limit, and so termination was raised by the therapist as the family's move approached. It would be hard to imagine Jane fully resolving the problem of terminating therapy given her experience of loss, and perhaps here is the one area where a more sustained treatment would have been of great value. Nonetheless, she did not appear unduly anxious at the idea of ending her sessions; her defenses around this were left largely undisturbed. In the last few sessions she left a number of small possessions in the office, and it was understood that the therapist was to care for them.

A number of aspects of this clinical material should be highlighted. First, the case was formulated from an object relational point of view and conducted within a psychoanalytic frame of reference. We note this particularly because the description of some brief therapies with children appears to be "watered down" theoretically and more eclectic in methods and techniques than when conducted with adults. The present case was conceptualized as play therapy in which the aims of therapy were more focused than would ordinarily be the case. There was an emphasis on facilitating the developmental process; in this way it was hoped that a developmental impasse could be traversed, permitting continued future growth.

A number of qualifying points should be made. This child's resources were relatively great, with a concerned and involved mother and supportive grandparents providing emotional and material resources. Thus, the family could be counted on to continue to foster the child's growth after the termination of therapy. The mother, who was obviously suffering from her own loss and pain, could not provide some of the needed emotional responsiveness Jane required, and so the therapy was viewed as a way to support the mother and give her more space to mourn and reconstruct her own life. Perhaps she needed to come back to her daughter after an emotional pause, and so the therapist could be seen as buffering the mother–child relationship, sharing some of the heat of the child's rage and anxiety. Perhaps that pause would enable the mother to resume her own functions of containing Jane's anxiety and strain. In this sense, though the therapy was seen as an individual treatment, it could be understood as a family intervention as well. Also, although consultations with Jane's mother were not a central aspect of the treatment, regular contact was arranged to discuss events in Jane's life and to share the therapist's observations of her progress. These occasional meetings, more frequent early in the treatment, were also used to help mother acknowledge and recognize her own strain and how she, too, needed support to come through the crisis. Jane's difficult behaviors were normalized and reframed in the context of an understanding of her terrible deprivation and the resulting anger, and the mother was educated as to the nature of children's reactions to major object loss. Interacting with the parent was understood as an essential part of the treatment, helping to provide this child with an environment conducive to continued developmental progress.

In short, this treatment was viewed as a crisis intervention with a psychodynamic focus and the technique of psychoanalytic play therapy. It was guided primarily by psychoanalytic developmental theory and by psychoanalytic clinical theory. Although the therapy was time limited, in some respects it was no more active than an ongoing play therapy might be. The child was encouraged to lead the way and the therapist attempted to follow her lead. The case illustrates the therapist's use of a time limit in conceptualizing and formulating a clinical situation and its therapeutic possibilities, more than suggesting particular technical modifications to shorten treatment or to accomplish more in less time. A belief in an essential developmental thrust makes it possible to imagine long-lasting benefits from brief interventions, especially in children. The expression "putting a Band-Aid" on a problem is often used to belittle purportedly superficial solutions to complicated problems. Yet bandaging is exactly what we do for a wound, protecting the injured part of the body so as to permit the healing process to take place optimally. Casting a broken bone may be a more apt metaphor: It emphasizes the holding, structuring, and protective functions a therapist can provide in a time-limited setting, permitting the child's natural tendencies to lead to equilibrium and further growth.

ADOLESCENTS

Because development continues at a rapid pace into and through adolescence, long-term models of psychotherapy can be problematic in some respects. The "moving target" of child development makes the goals and purposes of child and adolescent treatment different from those of adults. The developmental process is still continuing rapidly, and the formation of personality structure is still in progress. The adolescent is still usually living within his or her family of origin, so much of the clinical material worked with in psychotherapy deals not solely with internalizations of parental objects but also with actual ongoing transactions within a developmental, systemic family context.

Brief models of treatment may be particularly suitable for adolescents for a number of reasons. First, this is a patient population notoriously uncooperative with psychotherapists since they are typically rebellious toward authority figures and thus are likely to be difficult to work with. The therapeutic alliance is difficult to achieve, and challenging resistances are often presented (Meeks, 1971). The use of an explicit time frame may make the adolescent more willing and motivated to engage in the psychotherapeutic process. Second, as a matter of practical necessity, much treatment with adolescents is time-limited, as the ongoing transitions and life changes that we expect to take place between the ages of 14 and 20 may preclude long-term commitments to psychotherapy. Certainly for older adolescents, the central task of leaving home tends to make ongoing psychotherapy difficult to arrange. Finally, the clinical importance of separation and individuation is underscored by the use of a time-limited framework. Short-term work is congruent with the natural tendency of adolescents to "push off" attachment objects and to struggle for autonomy and a separate identity. Furthermore, the use of an explicit time limit has the effect of making time, change, separation, and loss central issues in therapy (Mann, 1973). Thus, the tendency of brief psychotherapy to heighten the clinical focus on separation issues is well suited to the adolescent patient's difficulties in the area of separation and individuation.

Formulation of the Clinical Focus

As with younger children, a developmental, lifespan perspective has particular utility in the formulation of the clinical focus in brief psychotherapeutic approaches with adolescents. Since the duration of treatment is to be limited to a few months, the aim of psychotherapy is not so much the thoroughgoing restructuring of personality, but rather the alleviation of a developmental impasse or crisis. Thus, the therapeutic focus will be framed in terms of the life situation of the adolescent, invariably centered within concentric relationships with family, peers, and the larger community. The formulation of the focus might be accomplished in a variety of ways, with different theoretical and clinical emphases. We suggest two central developmental themes as organizing structures for the creation of a treatment focus — *identity formation* and *separation–individuation*. These two processes are different perspectives on the same, unitary developmental process, but they are teased apart here for didactic purposes. A third task, negotiating issues of *sexuality* and *competitiveness*, is understood as a framework for clinical work with older adolescents.

Identity Formation

Erikson (1968) defines the central developmental task of adolescence in terms of the dichotomy of "identity formation" versus "role confusion." The rapid cognitive development of childhood continues, with increasingly abstract formal operations possible, as the integration of ego functions is organized around changing sexual, familial, and vocational roles. From a drive/structural point of view, intrapsychic change takes place around the reorganization of the drives consequent to puberty (Blos, 1962; A. Freud, 1958; Laufer & Laufer, 1984). There is a partial dismantling of the prior structure of personality, with active reworking of previous modes of relating to others. This process, described as "regression in the service of development" (Erikson, 1968), creates room for new modes of self-experience. Interest is displaced from the nuclear family to people in the larger social world. The peer group becomes increasingly important as a source of identifications, as new and more complex forms of relating unfold.

We might conceptualize the movements and shifts of identity in adolescence in terms of fluidity, or plasticity, rather than as regression. Personality is molded and re-formed in response to the changing requirements both from within the self structures and from the surrounding social world. In fact, psychopathology can be understood in terms of a breakdown in the process of moving back and forth between structure and formlessness so that new forms can emerge and become established. Too much rigidity, and the personality cannot contain the force of development: The change process skips and grinds like gears missing teeth. The adolescent holds on too tightly to previous ways of relating to self and others, and loses contact with the flow of his or her developing peer group. There is likely to be subjective distress, anxiety, and dysphoria as old patterns are clung to and adapation is inadequate.

On the other hand, too much fluidity, and identity breaks down. There is a diffusion of personality, with a failure to develop new commitments and ambitions. Identity fails to crystalize out of the formlessness of the developing self. Here there may be psychosis or other kinds of persisting identity disorganization in the face of the mounting tasks of adolescence.

The Task of Separation

The lifelong process of separation and individuation—which is another way of looking at the task of identity integration—takes on heightened importance during the phases of adolescence. While development is

continuous with childhood in the sense of progressing ever farther outward into the world, there is a radical discontinuity at the point of leaving home. While this is rarely a "one-shot deal," with movements back
and forth between the family of origin and an independent life sometimes taking place over years, the establishment of a separate, autonomous existence both in the realm of human relationships and in that
of work are central tasks facing the adolescent.

The importance of these dual accomplishments of finding oneself
in relation to others, including intimate and sustained relationships,
and establishing vocational goals and ambitions presents a framework
for the clinician to formulate the difficulties of a given adolescent. Attention to loss and separation is the essential characteristic of Mann's
time-limted psychotherapy (Mann, 1973; see also Chapter 4). It can be
no coincidence that his special methods were developed partly in the
context of treating late adolescent college students. The loss of family
support and previous modes of functioning in the face of change is
fraught with anxiety. Such losses are bound to resurrect the unresolved
losses of past epochs of development. Some view adolescence as a reactivation of early separation-individuation issues (Laufer, 1981; Mann,
1973).

Psychopathology can always be framed in terms of some failure
of differentiation from the family of origin. Issues such as fearing failure
or success, competitiveness, and concerns about sexuality can all be
traced to conflicts in relationships with parents in the context of the
separation process. Guilt, shame, depressive feelings, and anxiety, along
with the defenses against them, can be understood as disruptions taking place within the matrix of culture–family–self. Boundaries and structure may be overly firm or overly permeable. Enmeshment, at one
extreme, leaves the adolescent with no clear definition of self, and still
partially absorbed by the family. The other extreme, disengagement,
leaves the adolescent without support, resulting in a premature harden-
ing of boundaries and excessive cynicism.

Can the adolescent turn to others outside the family? Can he or
she form commitments to work, politics, culture, which are not fixed
by the family of origin? Can the adolescent move between recognition
of the other and assertion of the self? What will later be, for the adult
patient, the internalized structures of self in relation to parents, are
still, for the adolescent, live, active interactions in the here-and-now,
the outcome of which is not yet fixed. Thus, the therapeutic focus on
differentiation and separation involves the ongoing interpretation and
modification of the unfolding drama of the adolescent's development
and its internalization in the form of lasting psychic structure. The therapist of the adolescent thus has an opportunity to help rework the sep-

aration–individuation process, perhaps leading to enduring change in personality functioning. Here, the distinction of working with developmental impasses as opposed to aiming at deep character change breaks down. In this sense, time-limited interventions may be thought of as having a disproportionately large impact on the structuring of the adolescent personality.

Sexuality and Competition

Another seminal model of short-term psychodynamic psychotherapy was devised by Sifneos (1972, 1979). His model is characterized by a clinical emphasis on conflict, typically oedipal in origin (see Chapter 2). Such conflicts are understood to be reactivated in adolescence, resulting from the reemergence of sexuality under the sway of puberty, as well as from the pressures to define one's self, interests, goals, and ambitions in relation to one's future work life. Thus, the anxieties and impulses of the oedipal phase erupt and demand new integration in the context of sexual activity and vocational identity.

Separation always involves destruction, and one of the tasks of the adolescent is to destroy the parents symbolically. Thus, oedipal anxieties over aggressive feelings toward both parents are likely to arise, along with defenses against the conscious recognition of these impulses. We may expect symptoms and other inhibitions in relation to ideas of competition, success, and achievement. These may well be focused on academic achievement, career choices, and relation to financial matters.

Along with unresolved aggressive feelings toward the parents, there are likely to be the residual unconscious conflicts over sexual longings for one or the other parent. These are often activated with the onset of puberty and, especially later, with the begining of sexual relationships. Sexual conflicts, and conflicts over love more generally, may tend to have an oedipal cast, as the old triangular drama of child–mother–father is revived and replayed on the stage of the adolescent's contemporary relationships.

Selection Criteria

From the little that has been written about it, it may be concluded that the selection of adolescents for time-limited psychodynamic psychotherapy is largely in keeping with the selection of adults and children. Following Davanloo (1980), Malan (1976a), Mann (1973), and Strupp and Binder (1984), we would emphasize the presence of motivation, the presence of clear precipitants to the current crisis, a capacity for basic trust reflected in the existence of prior relationships of reasonable depth and duration, sufficient ego strength to permit rapid engagement and disengagement, affect tolerance, and at least some sense that the present difficulties can be understood by the patient in a psychological way, located at least in part within the self.

As is the case for all approaches to brief therapy, a basic distinction is made between patients whose problems are milder, more circumscribed, less chronic, and more situational, and those patients whose difficulties are more severe, enduring, characterological, and pervasive. The more readily one can identify a clinical focus, the more likely the patient will benefit from treatment. Adolescents who are psychotic, drug addicted, or sociopathic, or who manifest a failure to establish meaningful relationships are not likely to benefit from time-limited psychotherapy.

It is important to evaluate prior developmental accomplishments, since the presence of a long history of poor adaptation or symptomatic behavior and experience would likely predict a poorer treatment outcome. Further, it is necessary to evaluate the role of the family, particularly in younger adolescents, to determine suitability for this modality of treatment. Parents who are motivated and supportive of treatment efforts will make an important contribution to the outcome of treatment and its lasting effects. On the contrary, severe family pathology can undermine treatment because of resistances by both patient and family to any significant modification of the patient's functioning. In such cases, family interventions may be more effective, addressing the whole family system at once rather than one member alone.

Treatment Issues

While many of the modifications of psychotherapy for the treatment of adolescents are not specific to time-limited or brief treatment, we attempt to specify those treatment issues which are most salient to the practice of time-limited psychotherapy. Adolescents are far from homogeneous as a clinical population, merging at one end of the range with children and at the other end with adults. In fact, some of the most important models for the brief psychodynamic treatment of adults were developed in work with older adolescent populations, such as college students (Mann, 1973; Sifneos, 1979). The literature on the modification of brief psychodynamic psychotherapy for younger adolescents is exceedingly sparse, while discussion of technical issues with older adolescents is not usually differentiated from work with young adults. Nonetheless, we offer the following observations on the brief psychotherapy of adolescents.

Working Alliance

Adolescents can be especially difficult to engage in psychotherapy (Meeks, 1971). They are often counterdependent and oppositional, struggling to develop autonomy and independence from parents. They also may be anxious about losing control, being controlled, or experiencing shame and inadequacy. The idea of revealing one's concerns to an adult is filled with the unconscious dread of infantile regression and loss of a newfound and tenuously held sense of self. Thus, attention needs to be paid to the development of a working therapeutic relationship, in which the adolescent can be helped to feel his or her autonomy will be respected, and that help will be offered without intolerable strings attached (Blos, 1983). This may require a greater level of activity and responsiveness than is usually the case with psychodynamic treatment (Meeks, 1971). There may need to be greater flexibility around the structuring of the psychotherapy situation, and more willingness to exploit positive aspects of the transference.

The age of the patient is a crucial variable in arranging the external structure of the therapy relationship. For example, taking walks during sessions or playing board games such as checkers may be the only way to create a comfortable therapeutic situation with a young adolescent, of, say, 13 years of age. However, such parameters would not typically be necessary in the psychodynamic treatment of a college-age adolescent.

The Treatment Contract

The proposal of a formal treatment arrangement with focus of work, and sometimes a time limit, made explicit is the hallmark of virtually all models of brief psychodynamic psychotherapy (Malan, 1976a; Mann, 1973; Sifneos, 1979; Strupp & Binder, 1984). This may take the form of the "central issue," a statement of the patient's "chronically endured pain," along with a statement of the planned duration of the treatment (Mann, 1972). However, other approaches to short-term psychotherapy do not rely on an explicit or prearranged time limit, but instead use a more open, though still structured, treatment proposal (Malan, 1976a; Strupp & Binder, 1984).

The structured treatment contract, with or without a time limit, may be particularly useful with the adolescent patient. Such an arrangement may alleviate anxiety about dependency, giving the adolescent a clear sense of the nature of the therapy relationship. Unconscious regressive anxieties may thus be reduced, freeing the patient to pursue the therapeutic work more fully. Such a contract is also useful in engaging parents, who can be motivated to take their role in treatment seriously when offered a clearly delineated treatment arrangement.

Involvement of Parents

As with younger children, the role of the adolescent's family must be considered and addressed in brief treatment. How this issue is handled will vary depending on the age of the patient. Since adolescence spans such a large arc of development, it is necessary to keep in mind how different the 12- or 13-year-old is from the 19- or 20-year-old. On the average, parents may need to be involved in a diminishing way across the age span, so that the older adolescent in many respects must be treated like an adult, while the treatment of a younger adolescent will tend more to resemble child treatment in this respect.

Older adolescents will often refer themselves for treatment, particularly in the context of college living. In such instances, direct contact with parents may be neither necessary nor helpful, and the patient's legal right to confidentiality must be considered. Further, as the issue of separation is at its height, it may be clinically counterindicated to involve the parents of an older adolescent. On the other hand, adolescents younger than about 17 will virtually always be referred either by parents or other involved adults, such as school personnel. In such cases, the family needs to be involved for both legal and clinical reasons. More motivated parents may support individual treatment and require only occasional contact, either conjointly with the child or separately. Oftentimes parental psychopathology is a factor in the adolescent's treatment, and may need to be addressed in the form of family sessions, psychoeducational interventions, or referral for other appropriate treatment. In either case, there is a need for contact with the family to maintain support for the adolescent's treatment. Without continued parental support, any treatment effort, regardless of duration, will be doomed.

When the patient is an adult, the issue of motivation for treatment can be addressed directly with the patient via the interpretation of resistances and the creation of a therapeutic alliance. However, when the patient is not the same person as the one who is paying or transporting the patient to therapy, the problem of motivation is complicated. It is not uncommon for an adolescent to be interested and engaged in psychotherapy which is, however, undermined by an unsupportive family.

The use of a time limit may thus be of value in motivating parents, in the context of a clear therapeutic contract, to support the treatment of their child. The time-limited arrangement may make more sense to the parents, and may better address their perception of the family's needs.

Addressing Resistances

In a paper on the time-limited psychodynamic treatment of adolescents, Uribe (1988) attempts to address the problem of initial resistances and their management. Some of his suggestions follow from the establishment of a clear contract and working alliance, as described above. He notes that "in dealing with adolescents the therapist may try to prevent the development or minimize the intensity of resistances by clarifying his role and other pertinent issues during the first interview. Accordingly, he makes it very clear to the adolescent that he is available to work together with him to comprehend and resolve the referral issues" (Uribe, 1988, p. 113). Such initial resistances are addressed actively, though supportively, through educative comments, encouragement to use the treatment available, and interpretation of resistances as they may relate to the adolescent's distrust of authority figures.

With older, college-age adolescents, the handling of resistances may take the same form as they would with adult patients. Thus, resistances may be the object of interpretations, confrontations, or other verbal interventions aimed at their resolution. However, even with more verbal, older adolescents, it appears that there is a need for a supportive, transitional atmosphere, in which the adolescent feels supported and accepted.

Selecting a Treatment Model

It has been suggested that the selection of a brief psychotherapy model can be made on the nature of the "fit" between a given model and the developmental tasks of particular phases of life (Burke, White, & Havens, 1981). While this presentation appears to rely too much on the specificity of particular models, it may be that some approaches to brief treatment are more appropriate for adolescents. For instance, those therapies relying on active and persistent confrontation of resistances (Davanloo, 1980; Sifneos, 1979) would be less appropriate the younger the adolescent. In fact, the treatment of younger adolescents would appear to require a strongly supportive and empathic element, as is most obviously true of Mann's (1973) approach.

Perhaps the rigid adherence to any one model of brief psychodynamic treatment would be problematic in the treatment of adolescents, who developmentally require flexibility and responsiveness. A more eclectic approach, drawing from a variety of models, may give the therapist the greatest flexibility to adapt his or her approach to the needs of a particular young patient.

Case Vignette

The patient was an older adolescent who sought treatment at a local clinic. The treatment, which was audiotaped, was conducted by an experienced psychodynamically oriented clinician in a planned time-limited psychotherapy as part of the Rutgers research project in short-term psychodynamic psychotherapy (e.g., Collins & Messer, 1991; Messer et al., 1992; Tishby & Messer, 1995).

Identifying Information

Karol was 20 years old when she presented for treatment. She was single, attending college full-time and living with other students in an off-campus apartment. She had gone to the clinic previously when her parents divorced a year prior to the current treatment. She was seen for about 3 months at that time, and treatment was terminated because the therapist was leaving the center.

When she came for treatment on this occasion, she reported having "family problems" and "confusion with school" (academically). Her mother had remarried during the previous year, and the patient described having a hard time dealing with the new family, new step-siblings, and her stepfather. She reported feeling left out and neglected by her mother and was troubled by feelings of sadness and anger. At that time she was also doing poorly academically, having had trouble with the first exams of the year. She noted problems concentrating and was not able to read or study as she wished.

Karol has two sisters, 2 and 4 years younger, respectively, who remain in the new home. The patient's father lives in the same state as the patient, and she continues to have irregular contact with him. He is reportedly an alcoholic and has had periods of severely limited functioning in the past.

The case was formulated primarily along the lines of conflict over loss and separation. The precipitants for Karol seeking treatment were, in the first instance, the divorce of her parents, and, in the second, the remarriage of her mother. The theme of loss and separation was understood to include Karol's characteristic defenses against affects associated with loss, which included minimizing and supressing her emotional responses, particularly negative feelings like anger, sadness, and disappointment. She acted as though the expression of such feelings would result in the other being hurt. Thus, she needed to protect both herself and the other from her reactions to interpersonal losses.

The case illustrates well the interrelationship between developmental issues and intrapsychic or object relational structures. While the problem of separation is universal and paramount for a person of Karol's age, in her case it was complicated by a family history of traumatic losses, including the loss of her father (and the parental relationship) to alcoholism, financial losses, and her mother's apparent inability to tolerate Karol's emotional responses to the chaos and disruption that took place. Thus, Karol appeared to be stuck at the point where she needed to be able to develop increased autonomy and self-sufficiency, as she struggled with lifelong feelings of deprivation and guilt.

Course of Treatment

The treatment was 17 sessions long, spanning about 6 months. It included a lengthy break after the 11th session, which was scheduled to be the second-to-last. The patient failed to attend the 12th and last scheduled session, and the therapist then extended the termination by six sessions to process this absence and its meaning.

The first phase of the treatment was characterized by the therapist's gentle and persistent inquiry into Karol's feelings. It is clear that her style was to "sweep things under the rug," and the therapist worked at reframing the patient's story of her life to include more of her affective responses to traumatic events.

THERAPIST: You needed a lot more than you got . . .

PATIENT: My father sees that too, he really does, but he doesn't really know how to give it to me.

THERAPIST: What does he see?

PATIENT: Like, we went to this movie, "Hannah and Her Sisters." Did you see it? OK, do you remember the part where, um, Mia Farrow's husband, you know, says, "Your sisters and I think you have no needs," and she's like, "I have a tremendous amount of need." Do you remember that part? They're like in the bathroom or something? Like they felt that she's so self-sufficient that she doesn't need other people. And she was like, "But I really do, I need." . . . And like — and I just, I started crying, like in the movie theatre, it just hit me like a ton of bricks . . . and my father said, "That's you, isn't it?" And I said, "Yeah, dad." I said, "That's how I feel so much." And he started crying cause he felt bad that he, that he couldn't give it to me, like you know, he was really upset by it. [Session 3]

The therapist proceeded to help the patient to connect her fear of loss and abandonment with conflicts over assertiveness and ambition; this theme of "separation guilt" was also addressed in one of the early sessions in which Karol reports that she is interested in a boy whom her roommate had dated and still liked.

PATIENT: She's a very immature girl . . . she still carries the torch for a guy that really has no interest in her, and she's making me, making me feel like shit because he likes me. She can't be mad at me cause he likes me. I'm not doing it to hurt her!

Although she protests, she cannot escape feeling guilty, as she believes that her pursuing her own aims will hurt the other. She feels she is betraying her girlfriend: "I know it's going to hurt. . . . I can understand how she feels, if it was me I would be upset."

THERAPIST: Your tendency is to give up things that are meaningful to you and to be like a "good girl."

PATIENT: [If I don't pursue him] I will always feel cheated.

Later in the hour the patient summarizes her dilemma:

PATIENT: Things I can really go after and want I sometimes get confused with selfishness. . . . I don't like to be that way. . . . I'm very, I'm ambitious and aggressive and I can pretty well get what I want, but not to hurt anybody that way. . . . I could see myself as selfish in this right now. [Session 4]

Of course, the other side of the guilt is her identification with her mother, who "abandoned" Karol for her second husband. Thus, another aspect of this triangular conflict is the patient's attempt to master the hurt and disappointment of her mother's remarriage through identification with the aggressor by putting her roommate in a similar position.

When she is later jilted by the boy, she is helped to experience the loss and her feelings about it:

PATIENT: . . . But I was kind of sad, cause like I—I—felt like, I felt like I didn't feel anything. It was really strange, like after the fact I—I felt like kind of—I was trying to feel something. I was like, "how should I feel?" Should I feel rejected or hurt or whatever, and I just didn't feel anything.

THERAPIST: I wonder if the "feeling nothing" is really a cover for really having some pretty strong feelings.

PATIENT: That's what I was—that's what I was thinking to myself, too.

I was like am I not letting myself get upset, you know, am I not letting myself deal with it? Because I haven't even let myself think about it, I just kind of brushed it under the rug, like, that I'll just forget it.

THERAPIST: If you brought it out from under the rug what would you be feeling?

PATIENT: . . . Just like, I guess rejected, you know, and — but in a way better, I feel better off though, I feel, that what I've seen of him I think I'm better off without, you know. . . .

The discussion moves to her defense against experiencing strong feelings, and how she is able to avoid feeling certain things:

THERAPIST: Well, where do you think you learned to do that so well?

PATIENT: I don't know. You know, I — I don't know. Um, . . . see I didn't even want to tell you about it because I knew you'd make me think of this and I don't want to even think about it, you know. I knew, I knew I was, you know, pretending that I wasn't upset. I knew it.

THERAPIST: You knew that.

PATIENT: Yeah, I knew it, I did it all week. . . . But that was the only way to forget it and that was the only way for me —

THERAPIST: Well, that's your way, that's been your way.

PATIENT: Right, that's the only way — that's the most painless way I can think of to just forget it and act like I don't care. I can't be — I don't know, I'm very, like I consider myself strong and I don't want anybody else to think I'm annoyed, you know, upset by it either, you know, so that's the way I do it. . . . [Session 5]

As the therapy continued, this clarification of Karol's defensive style gave way to work around her ambivalence about the coming termination. She used the same style to avoid the pain of losing the therapist, and distanced herself emotionally through a kind of "flight into health." This culminated in the failed final session, leading to further exploration of the theme of dependency and loss in the sessions which followed the "last" session, that is, after the break.

THERAPIST: How are you feeling about being here today?

PATIENT: I don't feel good in my chest (*coughs*) [in reference to health]. . . . I didn't want to get out of bed. . . . I feel weird today for some reason.

THERAPIST: I sense you go in and out.

PATIENT: I have to deal with other things, I think I'm distracted with that kind of stuff. I'm also thinking that next week is our last session.

THERAPIST: What thoughts are you having about that?

PATIENT: Um, . . . well, when I was walking over here I was thinking, I really want to talk about [boyfriend], you know, and when I came back, and as far as other things, like my parents and stuff, I feel like I beat that into the ground, and I don't really, um, not that I don't want to go into it again, but I feel like we've explored that a lot, and I was thinking that, thinking what other things I want to talk to you about, and I was thinking that I was pretty much done. . . .

THERAPIST: Your own timing.

PATIENT: Yeah, it was . . .

THERAPIST: Your were getting something from it that was important to you. . . .

PATIENT: I know I have to go . . . for some reason it felt like a hassle coming here today—

THERAPIST: Yeah, I know.

PATIENT: It really felt hassled, it felt inconvenient, and I never felt like that before, I didn't have time to have my coffee, I didn't have time to read my paper . . . I don't know why, though . . .

THERAPIST: You don't want to have to finish, like there's more to be gotten from it . . . so when you sense ahead of time that something's going to be taken away from you or cut off, then you go into this thing in your head, there's a whole lot of rationalization, you know, "It's difficult coming over here, I have other things to do."

PATIENT: I like the way you're accepting of everything I say, kind of, I'm gonna cry . . . (crying) (pause)

THERAPIST: You'll really miss me.

PATIENT: (long pause—patient is openly crying) . . . Well, like, I don't know, just like, a lot of people, sometimes they're there, and sometimes they're not—

THERAPIST: And me—

PATIENT: This is a different type of situation, you know, I know that, but—

THERAPIST: But what about it?

PATIENT: Just like whenever, I feel a lot for somebody, whatever reason, artificial, or, not artificial, but whatever, it's just always taken away, I feel like sometimes, and I think that I don't have control over it, . . . I can't wait to have children, because they'll always be mine, you know, and I'd be there for them, like, I don't have to go anywhere, a husband, or whatever. . . . [Session 13]

The remaining sessions were used to deal with the termination process, and the therapist helps the patient to come to terms with this loss, as well as others she has experienced. By the final session, Karol is able to grieve more openly and freely with her therapist:

PATIENT: I'm not afraid, I'm just, I feel like you're, see this is gonna sound weird, whatever I'm going to say —

THERAPIST: Say whatever.

PATIENT: I feel like you're a sister, almost, but I know that you can't be, but . . .

THERAPIST: But you feel that kind of bond.

PATIENT: Right, I always felt like I connected with you, even though it was one-sided, it was, I don't know, when we have silences I feel like we're still communicating, I'm gonna cry, but I feel like crying 'cause I'm sad (*crying*) and . . . (*long pause—patient is crying*).

THERAPIST: So it feels like a special relationship.

PATIENT: Yeah, definitely, you know, not like any other I've ever had, it's weird, like, in a lot of ways, you just gave me whatever side of people, what could, just like patience, try to see my side for once, instead of, you know, people just tend to see what they see. . . . [Session 17]

Discussion

The case illustrates a number of themes in the treatment of adolescents. First, the patient satisfies various criteria for selection for brief psychotherapy. She engages rapidly and with affect; she has a history of significant relationships; her presenting problem is clearly defined and relatively circumscribed; and a central focus can be identified early in treatment. This focus, centering on the themes of loss and separation along with guilt at self-definition, is characteristic of adolescent patients, in this case reflecting both age-appropriate elements and also aspects of a disturbed family system. The therapist clarifies the way the patient's characteristic defenses of denial, minimization, and supression of affects are linked to her current symptoms in the context of her mother's remarriage. The technique includes extensive clarification of feelings, interpretation of resistances, and interpretation of transference, particularly around the enactment connected to termination. While the patient's family is not involved in the treatment, the psychotherapy includes close exploration of current, ongoing family interactions. Termination is handled with an emphasis on expression of feelings around the loss of the therapy. It is hoped that the open and honest expression of feelings of loss during the termination phase enabled the reworking of defenses against loss, permitting greater freedom and flexibility in Karol's future relationships with others, as well as with herself.

THE ELDERLY

Developmental Issues

Erikson (1950) identified the developmental task of old age as the establishment of Integrity versus Despair and Disgust. The bulk of life is past, social and vocational achievements are largely finished, and we face the present with the abiding question of the value and meaning of our efforts over the course of a lifetime. This existential question, ubiquitous but often in the background for younger adults, is heightened and brought to the fore by the immediacy of the older person's mortality. Fantasies of getting to things later, of new accomplishments in the future, of changing and starting anew, which are sustaining to the younger person and energize creative efforts, are no longer effective in warding off the anxieties and pain of mortality and human limitations. If it is true that suffering results from history, from the accumulation of failures, frustrations, losses, and the irreversible accidents of living, then the older person must come to embrace his or her own personal history with acceptance and serenity or retreat into denial, numbness, senility, or contempt.

Perhaps Erikson was too deterministic when he suggested that ego integration at the level of Integrity versus Despair depended on successful integration of all the previous developmental levels. Religious traditions leave open the possibility of the redemption of life to the last moment of earthly existence. Even at the end, perhaps one can find an opening, a moment of freedom and authentic being in which the spark of one's deepest core can be felt and expressed. The secular tradition of Western culture is cynical about the value and truth of such "deathbed conversions," and yet it is not so easy to find a yardstick to measure the value of such religious experience. What ritual or practice has the modernist (or postmodernist) tradition offered in place of the last rites of the Catholic Church, or of the possibility in Judaism of returning to God at any time in one's life, including old age? Perhaps there is a deep need at the end of life to tell our story, to find the threads of meaning that have run through it, and to own all we have been and have had, and all we have not been and have lost. It may be that the abandonment of a spiritual dimension in living has left old age empty of meaning and hence disrespected, and has thus made it possible for us as a society to relegate the elderly to profoundly alienating institutions.

The abandonment of the elderly has included insufficient attention to the place of psychotherapy with older adults. In the psychoanalytic tradition, there is an explicit bias against the treatment of the elderly, beginning, naturally, with Freud (1905b/1958), who wondered whether there was any point in treating persons so near the end of their lives. He questioned whether the substantial resources of psychoanalysis would not be better applied to the younger person, with more of life ahead and less entrenched psychopathology. Others have pointed out the negative countertransferences therapists tend to have in their work with older patients, including distaste for the physical and cognitive limitations of the elderly, pessimism about the possibilities for change, and the anxieties about one's own mortality stimulated by contact with an older person (Busse & Pfeiffer, 1974; Sparacino, 1978–1979; Zinberg, 1965).

It may be that brief forms of psychotherapy are particularly suited to the older patient. Not only do such models address the pragmatic need for a briefer treatment in the context of aging, but some of these therapies deal explicitly with the issues of time and loss, so important to this developmental epoch. In a sense, the time-limited treatment setting precisely recapitulates the central dilemma of old age—mortality and loss. This may permit a reworking of the story of the patient's life to enable him or her to see life in a new light, to embrace in a new way the sum of his or her existence, to mourn, and to accept.

Formulation of the Therapeutic Focus: Faith and Despair in Aging

As a developmental framework is integrated into a psychodynamic approach, the importance of situational factors is highlighted. While personality dynamics are crucial to the adaptation of the older person, these are seen in the defining context of developmental events and life stressors. It is the dynamic interplay of these two domains that then defines psychopathology as the response to a failed effort to cope with the strains of living. Previously successful characterological defenses rigidify under the pressure of aging and new losses. Loss of social support—the death or illness of friends, spouse, or relatives—leaves the older person vulnerable to the continuing, ordinary strains of daily living. Autonomy is diminished as physical constraints increasingly play a part in the daily life of the elderly. Retirement, a major life event, challenges the individual to develop new outlets for creativity and involvement, and simultaneously leads to important changes in the organization of the family. Lifelong sources of self-esteem, such as physical beauty or abilities, work-related recognition, and long-term relationships are all diminished.

In a culture that has not yet found ways to acknowledge and respect old age, the older person may experience new forms of discrimination and devaluing, and, consequently, feelings of shame. Dormant separation anxieties are revived as loved ones die, children move on in their own lives, and long-established patterns of living are disrupted by moves and changes in the extended community. The older person may experience feelings of helplessness and inadequacy as all these and other difficult changes take place.

Any of the difficulties mentioned here—loss, illness, loneliness, etc.—can be a focus of treatment as they are manifested in the particularities of the older person's problematic functioning. For example, retirement may leave the person with diminished self-esteem which can be discussed in the context of the meaning of the loss of the satisfactions of work and the possibility of substitutive gratifications.

The losses of old age can be balanced by new fulfillments, described by Erikson (1950) as Integrity, as ego integration takes place to accommodate and transform losses. It is a time of life in which deep satisfactions are possible. Creative work can continue and flourish, with the challenges of living nourishing the creative process and bringing it to new heights of maturity and fruition. Perhaps one's greatest work has already been done, but there may be great personal pleasure in the smaller works and in the process of creative work itself. Work can often take place with diminished financial need and without the pressures of building or maintaining a career. Work and play can fuse again, as it was in the beginning, in childhood. The relationship of grandparent and grandchildren is uniquely satisfying, with much of the parents' pleasure of being with children and watching them develop but less of the strain and self-sacrifice of parenthood. Eros can be heightened in its spiritual aspect as the sexual drives diminish, diffusing into tenderness, compassion, and deep appreciation of others and the world around. Time, the enemy, at last also liberates, as one's life becomes free of structure and imposed constraints. One *has* time, finally, as the relentless pressures of living, working, raising a family fall away. One might feel the infinitude of life in moments of repose, reflection, and meditation as time shifts and stretches and its linear structure breaks down. Old age can be a sabbath, a mythic time transcending historical time, connected to every moment and encompassing all moments of one's existence (Eliade, 1954). Thus, the focus for the elderly patient can include not only the patient's enduring pain or core psychodynamic theme, but also the possibilities for new outlets and pursuits in life.

Perhaps the idea suggested by Erikson's schema of a dichotomous outcome, either despair or integrity, is an oversimplification. Surely there are moments of despair for even the best adjusted older individual—let alone the rest of us—as he or she faces extraordinary blows, such as losing a lifelong partner, or suffering from chronic illness and physical losses. Despair and faith coexist, and constitute one another all through life. It must be the balance of faith and despair and the richness and rhythms of the interplay between them that matters the most, as individuals transform their struggles into ever-expanding circles of meaning and creative existence or, conversely, retreat into numbness, hidden beneath calcified layers of once-living psychic structure (see Eigen, 1992).

Selection Criteria

The older patient who comes into treatment is one for whom the strains of living and aging have been too much, and there are likely to be symptoms such as anxiety, depression, somatic complaints, or psychosis. The question of selection is much the same as for all patients evaluated for a brief psychotherapy, but there are a number of additional considerations in the instance of an elderly patient.

Because of the increased likelihood of medical conditions that may cause psychological symptoms, it may be necessary to have a medical evaluation of the patient as part of the clinical assessment for suitability. Various forms of dementia in the elderly can masquerade as depression—and vice versa—making this discrimination valuable in recommending psychotherapy. From the point of view of the psychotherapist, the primary consideration may be whether the patient possesses the capacities required for a primarily verbal approach to treatment, regardless of the etiology of those deficits. Some forms of BPT require relatively greater levels of articulateness and intellectual potential, while others rely more on empathic contact with the patient.

So the question of suitability must also include the choice of treatment approach. Nonetheless, all treatment models require a minimum of reality orientation, facility with language, affective presence, and alertness. Thus, patients with organicity, severe depression, or other medical problems which limit these cognitive and affective functions are not likely to benefit from BPT.

While patients with psychotic levels of disorganization would generally not be selected for brief psychotherapy, we have had experience with a form of psychosis that is more prevalent in the elderly, and which may be treated briefly in conjunction with other forms of treatment. Some older people suffer from transient paranoid episodes, often following a loss or some other psychosocial stressor, such as moving to a new living situation. These paranoid reactions, apparently more common in women, used to be described as "involutional melancholia, " emphasizing the affective origin of the disorder. It is characterized by heightened distrust, suspiciousness, and frank delusions of reference or persecution. While generally requiring pharmacological intervention, such patients may also benefit from a psychotherapeutic approach addressing the losses of trusted others, familiar surroundings, or the effects of physical problems that contribute to this form of depression.

One final consideration in the question of case selection is the tendency of defenses to become more rigid and entrenched with some of the increased emotional and physical challenges associated with aging. Under pressure, previous forms of adaptive psychological mechanisms become more extreme, narrowed, and brittle, as the individual attempts to cope with change. We suggest that it is especially important to assess the quality of defense mechanisms in the older patient, to confirm that there is sufficient flexibility and emotional openness to permit the psychotherapeutic process to have a meaningful impact.

Selected Technical Issues in Brief Psychotherapy with the Elderly

Loss, Separation, and the Use of a Time Limit

Issues of loss tend to predominate in the older patient, so treatment models that address loss directly may be the most appropriate. Mann's (1973) 12-session model revolves around the issues of loss and separation (see Chapter 4) and appears to have particular clinical applicability to the older patient. He sees loss as a universal issue, with particular losses and the adaptations to them as a thread that runs through an individual's life. In Mann's model, a time limit is used to amplify the patient's experience of loss and to permit the recapitulation of both the timeless attachment of earliest life and the ambivalence and anxie-ty at the experience of separation. In his view, defenses against loss are profoundly important in determining the characteristic ways in-dividuals cope with life, with maladaptive coping efforts resulting in psychic suffering. Further, the time limit provides an opportunity for a new kind of experience in the face of loss, a reworking of the losses of the past, and an amelioration of the characteristic forms of adapta-tion, leading to an easing of defenses as they become less needed.

For the older patient, the therapeutic time limit is the external, symbolic expression of the great Time Limit: One's life runs out. If a major task of old age is to come to terms with the meaning of death and the finitude of existence, then the time limit in psychotherapy is a vehicle for the work that must be done. Therapy becomes a micro-cosm, a symbolic space in which, optimally, certain experiences are made possible, and certain affects can be borne. One can face one's death—one even dies, symbolically, as therapy time runs out—and life can continue from that point, transformed and enlightened, expand-ed to contain both the immediate loss and also to better contain all the losses that came before. Patient and therapist may play with the polarity of time and timelessness, shifting into and out of different modes of experience. The timelessness of the inner, aesthetic world is juxtaposed against the relentlessness of measured, external reality; in the tension created between the two it is hoped that something new and useful can be attained.

The patient can suffer at either end of the polarity. At one extreme there is only external time, the time clock which drains all meaning, liveliness, and hope. Life becomes a dreary, effortful expression of ex-ternal aspirations with no inner animation. Here time crushes one's life out, grinds one down, as reality closes in. One turns to stone, all rigid shell and nothing living inside. The other extreme is taking flight from time altogether, living in the past, living in fantasies which are summoned up over and over. Here one lives in an endless summer of dreams, a stuporous state of disconnection, a universe without friction or conflict, as objects slide over each other and never touch. Thought is dispersed so thinly that finally one disappears altogether (Bion, 1962).

Thus, the task of psychotherapy is to create a space in which time and timelessness can both exist. The patient can be encouraged to find freedom within constraints, to tolerate the anguish of living and so be free to experience the fulfillments of mortality, to find faith on the brink of disaster. In the end, the time limit represents the therapist's faith that something of value can happen within the frame, within *this mo-ment,* that time can be lived with and in, that there is a universe in ev-ery grain of sand. Finitude is the reality that tempers our optimism, but is also the instrument through which we may have glimpses of eternality.

Treatment of Bereavement

Old age is a stage of life in which losses are ubiquitous and inevitable. These include loss of occupation, physical abilities, and other sources of self-esteem, in addition to the loss by death of lifelong partners and friends. Thus, treatment models which address grief and bereavement are especially useful in treating the elderly.

Horowitz and his colleagues at the Center for the Study of Neurosis have developed a formal time-limited psychotherapy approach to problems of grief and unresolved grief reactions (Horowitz, 1986; Horowitz, Marmar, Krupnick, et al., 1984; see Chapter 3). Theirs is a phase-oriented treatment model, with specific therapeutic goals and tasks for each stage of the therapy process, corresponding to the different aspects of a grief reaction. The model also relies on an information-processing metaphor to understand the effects of trauma and to generate appropriate interventions. Thus, for the early, "acute stage" of a stress response syndrome, techniques of therapy are aimed at providing support, containment, and suppression of intrusive affect states (Horowitz, 1991). For a "denial" stage they propose expressive techniques such as "dosed re-experiencing," and exploration of the traumatic event. The necessary revision of one's life and one's self is encouraged, as patient and therapist attempt to process the impact of the loss on the patient's self-perception and perception of others.

In Horowitz's model, the patient is viewed as a dynamic system which, under the strain of a major stressor, is in a state of disorganization and some degree of dysfunction. Defenses are extreme and highly rigid, as the system attempts to maintain some sort of equilibrium in the face of the stressor. The therapy is conceptualized as having polar functions, both leading to the restructuring of the intrapsychic system. On the one hand, therapy is seen as a containing vehicle to stabilize and support the patient and so to permit better integration of the life event that has taken place. On the other hand therapy functions to open up and stimulate exploration and to challenge rigid, perseverative defensive operations in order to encourage new adaptive behaviors and modes of experience.

Once again, the psychotherapy is focused around crisis intervention requiring a relatively high level of therapist activity, with shifts between different modes of therapeutic action and rapid adjustments to changing states in the patient. The dynamic focus contains, but is not limited to, the specific loss that has occurred. The immediate loss is understood in the context of long-term characterological adaptation and adjustment, and the reworking of self and other schemas may indeed produce longlasting personality change. In this sense, this brief therapy of stress response syndromes can be thought of as using an emotional crisis as leverage in the psychotherapeutic goal of personal growth, although the more immediate goals are symptom reduction and alleviation of suffering. These latter goals are all the more important in working with elderly patients as the effects of personal growth must be telescoped into the remaining portion of the patient's life. The primary aim of the psychotherapy of grief reactions in the elderly is usually to enable as much of a return to previous functioning as possible.

Validation and Selfobject Functions of the Therapist

The historical emphasis in psychoanalytic theory on separation and autonomy has probably contributed to a view of the older person as self-contained and, in health, fully separate and independent. In fact, it appears that the need for affirmation and mirroring is present throughout life (Kohut, 1984). Such a need is reflected in a basic view of human beings as always requiring the presence of sustaining relationships with others, whether actual persons or internalized ideal others. The therapist's validation, recognition, and appreciation of the older patient may play a special part in the recovery and maintainance of a state of self-cohesion and self-esteem.

One of us was taught a valuable lesson as an undergraduate intern about the relative importance of therapeutic techniques versus empathic attention by an elderly woman hospitalized with depression. The intended treatment was a highly structured assertiveness training program, with specific content and designated role playing for each session. Each week the therapist came in armed with materials to be covered, and specific interventions to be made. And each week the patient proceeded to do what she needed to do, namely, to tell stories about her life. These were very moving stories of herself as a young girl, adolescent, and young woman. They didn't seem to go anywhere in particular, and she seemed only to want to tell them to someone. At first there was a rather comical dance, with the young student earnestly trying to redirect the treatment back "on track," with the far more skillful and persistent patient redirecting things in her needed direction. In the end, the patient won out, and the behavioral program was informally abandoned in favor of what could be described as a client-centered psychotherapy, or even just a supportive human relationship. The patient was able to create the possibility of real contact with another human being and, making up for the lack of skill in her therapist, drew the therapist into what appeared to be a therapeutic relationship.

The psychotherapy of the older patient may need to address the more diffuse and nonlinear aspects of the patient's experience. Perhaps such treatment must be divergent, moving in many directions without clear narrative structure, rather than the more familiar convergent methods of brief therapy, relying on foci, activity, and clear therapeutic direction. Insights may be less important than the structure of the self and, as discussed in Chapter 6, the notion of the selfobject function of the therapist may supplant the reliance on a therapeutic focus.

Case Vignette

The following case illustrates some aspects of time-limited work with an older man whose issues are representative of those likely to be addressed with elderly patients, including medical problems, concurrent somatic treatment, family system issues, and a developmental lifespan context.

Mr. F. referred himself for treatment to address a range of symptoms associated with depression. In his own view, Mr. F. was consumed by doubts and anxieties about his marriage, and had a perseverative fear that he would leave his wife. He did not know why he would do this, but he felt that he suddenly wasn't sure if he loved her. He worried that perhaps he made a mistake when he married her more than 20 years before and that he never loved her as he ought to have. He was consumed with guilt at the idea that he was continuing the marriage under these circumstances. Needless to say, his wife was highly perturbed by these preoccupations and encouraged his seeking treatment.

At the time treatment began Mr. F. was 65 years old. He was recently retired from a lifelong occupation with a branch of the federal government. He suffered from a potentially life-threatening blood disease for which he received treatment from a hematologist as well as a holistic doctor to whom his wife had brought him. The latter had prescribed a fairly strict dietary regimen, forcing Mr. F. to change lifelong eating habits and imposing new daily tasks of food shopping and preparation. Mrs. F. did all of this, even though she was beginning to resume work outside of the home. Mr. F. and his wife were devout Catholics, regularly attending church and living in accordance with religious doctrine. Mrs. F. in particular was quite religious, attending daily church services and involving herself in other church-related activities. In a conjoint meeting, she noted that she had more faith in prayer than in the hematologist, and clearly felt that the holistic doctor had more to offer than the traditional medical specialist.

The first two sessions were conjoint meetings, and Mrs. F. did much of the talking. Mr. F., a small and apparently meek man, deferred to his wife at every opportunity. It appeared that Mrs. F. was controlling and exerted a great deal of authority over her husband, as she described him as the "weak one" and herself as being strong in prayer. He readily admitted to his failings and weaknesses, pointing out guiltily that all these only confirmed his sense that he should spare his wife further suffering and withdraw from the marriage. He presented a variety of symptoms of depression, including some psychomotor slowing, repetitive guilty self-recriminations, and an imperviousness to feedback from others. He reported another symptom, that he was afraid of knives in the kitchen, fearing that he might lose his mind and kill his wife. He could report no conscious anger or dissatisfaction with his wife, noting that she was a saint to put up with all this misery and that he had nothing to be dissatisfied with in his marriage since she was adequate in all regards.

Although there seemed to be a clear marital focus, the couple had come seeking individual treatment for Mr. F.'s symptoms, and therefore an individual treatment was proposed, with the understanding that the focus would have to address the marital problem. It was also recognized that Mrs. F. would have to "bless" the treatment or it would fail, as she had so much of the outward control in the marriage. Interventions were directed at her in the early sessions to convey some empathy for her own need for help and support: "You have been so strong for others. Who has been there for you?" This remark brought her to tears, as she acknowledged that she had always had to take care of herself, quickly pulling herself together and adding, "But we're not here to talk about me!"

Mr. F. was engaged for weekly sessions to address his depression. The tentative formulation was suggested by traditional psychodynamic theory, focusing on what appeared to be enormous anger that had been entirely defended against until the recent appearance of symptoms. Thus, Mr. F.'s depression was understood to be the result of the redirection of anger from his wife to himself in the form of guilty and self-recriminating statements. The developmental framework suggested that the rift in his defenses had appeared around the two major life stresses he was under, namely, his retirement from lifelong full-time employment and his medical problem. The latter included the anxiety of a potentially serious illness along with the additional strains of treatment regimens and a restrictive diet. Retirement also changed his relationship with his wife, as he no longer had anything to occupy him outside of the house and the marriage. He had a notable absence of interests in leisure activities. The early sessions were devoted to a clarification of these strains, and interpretations were offered to Mr. F. to help him make connections between his recent distress and these life stressors.

However, Mr. F. continued to perseverate on his guilt themes and seemed to be unable to process much that was offered verbally. He was referred to a psychiatrist for a medication consultation, with his wife's consent, and it was decided that he be treated with an antidepressant drug. However, the focus of the psychotherapy was sharpened to include his apparent imperviousness to help or influence, which appeared to be a long-standing characteristic with some acute exacerbation. This "deaf ear," as his wife described it, appeared to serve an aggressive function, as he "okayed" people, including the therapist, and then went on to do just as he pleased. When this was pointed out, he agreed readily, asking, "Why do I do this, doctor?"—another "Okay."

A new theme began to evolve around Mr. F.'s passivity and compliance. The issue of control, which had appeared in the early marital sessions, seemed again to be at the heart of Mr. F.'s difficulties, taking the form of extreme self-effacing behavior and a submissive attitude toward the therapist. His remarks were consistently self-denigrating, elevating the therapist to a powerful, all-knowing status. On the other hand, there was something obviously fishy about the therapist's "power," since nothing was changing.

As the treatment progressed, a countertransference reaction began to settle in, including a subtle irritation with Mr. F.'s unremitting questions and self-denigration, as well as an impulse to be helpful by offering suggestions to Mr. F., such as encouraging him to find volunteer or part-time work, do more of the special preparation of food for his diet, and try to take long walks. He requested relaxation training to help with his agitation and anxiety, but failed to do any of the exercises at home. He asked for advice about how to find a piano so he could take up music but took none of the suggestions made. The pattern was that Mr. F. would be thankful and appreciative of the suggestion made, but the following week, nothing would have changed.

The therapist at this point was able to recognize the enactment that had taken place, bringing into the transference the very conflict that had brought the patient into treatment in the first place: It became apparent that Mr. F. needed to take an oppositional stance, without the slightest hint of overt assertiveness or outward conflict. He had become highly controlling of the psychotherapy, as he was with his wife, through noncompliance and passive resistance, even as he asked for the next bit of advice or direction. It was now possible to begin to address this with him, pointing out his need to be in control and validating this need. His reported history began to reflect a lifelong feeling of impotence and inferiority in all areas of his functioning. His oppositionalism was noted, but also was framed in terms of his need to be "his own man," to go his own way, and to be the master of his own destiny. Instead of questioning him as to why he didn't take the therapist's suggestions, it was put to him that he was absolutely right not to do as the therapist said, and that he was asserting himself just as he ought to do. When he protested, saying that he was being "bad" for not listening, the therapist pointed out that, on the contrary, it was he, the therapist, who ought to apologize for not recognizing sooner the patient's need to follow his own course in life.

It was recognized that Mr. F. had been engaged in a life of invisible power struggles arising around his own sense of powerlessness. He had no other way to define himself than by negation of the will of the other: the 2-year-old's "NO!" This was seen as the incipient center of his autonomy and self-direction, and was supported and empathized with in the strongest possible terms.

These interactions had a striking effect. Even though by then he predictably had discontinued taking the antidepressant medication, his perseverative preoccupations diminished, and he spent less and less time talking about worries, and began to interact with the therapist around a shared interest in gardening. His initial symptoms disappeared almost entirely. There was no talk of leaving his wife, and he had begun a part-time job that enabled him to be outdoors. Vegetative symptoms of depression, such as sleep disturbance and loss of appetite, were improved.

It is noteworthly that in this case the termination phase was relatively brief and uncomplicated. No time limit had been set, but as more of the time during sessions was spent discussing his increasing activities outside he began to drop hints about ending the treatment. One day he announced that he would not continue to come to sessions anymore. He brought as a gift for the therapist a small container of seeds that he had taken from flowers he had grown, and noted that he had purchased a secondhand piano. The abruptness of the ending was interpreted as an act of self-affirmation, as it was felt that acknowledging Mr. F.'s autonomy around ending was more important than addressing the conflicts around dependency and attachment that were bypassed. He sent a note about 6 weeks after terminating, indicating that he was feeling well, that his blood condition appeared to be stable, and that he and his wife were doing well together.

We wish to point out that much work was never addressed in the treatment, which consisted of about 25 sessions over a 5-month period. Mr. F.'s basic character structure was not essentially different: He remained a passive and compliant man, unable to tolerate his feelings of anger toward others. The whole area of his sexuality was not addressed, though there was ample evidence of sexual dysfunction in the marriage since its beginning. He had a history of isolation and social inadequacy, and an early history suggesting significant early maternal deprivation, none of which was pursued in any depth.

Nonetheless, the case illustrates precisely how a depth-oriented, time-limited intervention around a developmental crisis can enable an individual to traverse the crisis safely and return to a level of functioning even higher than the "premorbid" level preceding the crisis. Furthermore, symptomatic relief, while central to the purposes of brief therapy, relied in this case on a dynamic understanding of the patient's presenting problem and the surrounding situation. The immediate distress was understood within the overlapping frames of intrapsychic, interpersonal, developmental, and cultural structures. Symptomatic relief relied on a psychoanalytically construed conception of personality and the change process. In this case, an arrested developmental need was identified and recognized, permitting some shift, however small, at a deep level of Mr. F.'s personality, resulting in a good outcome.

A CRITICAL EVALUATION

A survey of the literature on treating special age groups in brief psychodynamic psychotherapy strongly suggests the need for further systematic work, research, and writing. While there is a small body of clinical literature and research on brief psychotherapy with children, there is virtually none pertaining to adolescents and older adults. Thus, many of the conclusions reported are without firm basis in systematic study. This seems unfortunate in light of the increasing pressures on providers to work within new economic constraints. As more therapists are increasingly obliged to work within time limits, there is a clear gap in the development of workable models for training and application.

In particular there is a need for the systematic evaluation of brief psychotherapy process with children, to identify the needed modifications to adult models and time-unlimited models of child treatment. This is especially true for psychoanalytically oriented practitioners, for whom there is a need for theory-based approaches to child treatment which attempt to integrate what is known about child development and therapy with the pragmatics of model-based brief psychotherapy (Clark, 1993). While there appears to be a proliferation of time-limited approaches to psychotherapy, many of these do not satisfy the sensibilities or therapeutic values of psychodynamic practitioners. And while most psychodynamic therapists are willing and able to offer a kind of "seat-of-the-pants" eclectic approach to time-limited work with children, it would appear that systematic work in this area would be of enormous value.

We conclude this chapter with a critical reflection on the use of developmental models and theories in approaches to brief treatment of special age populations.

On the one hand, it appears to us that developmental theories and lifespan models are invaluable tools for the brief therapist. Given time constraints, it is necessary to rapidly derive a working clinical formulation which integrates presenting problems and symptoms with an understanding of the patient's personality dynamics and life situation. We bring our knowledge of universal developmental processes and lifespan issues to each patient we encounter. Schafer (1974) notes in regard to a female patient:

> The psychotherapist never starts from the beginning with any patient. He already knows a great deal about her prior to his acquiring any factual information about her; he knows about the psychological development and existence of human beings in general and of girls and women in particular. (p. 504)

On the other hand, we wish to note some of the potential dangers of relying on such general knowledge. While not specific to brief therapy models, the requirement to quickly develop and maintain clinical foci encourages the reliance on developmental schema and lifespan issues at the expense of a more individualized approach to treatment.

For one thing, our presentation makes it appear that developmental issues are of importance only for "special groups." In fact, the kind of analysis applied here to children and the elderly could as easily and usefully be applied to young or middle-aged adults. Lifespan development implies particular challenges and transitions across the whole range of development. Our emphasis on children and the elderly is a corrective to the tendency to generalize from adult populations. The same problem of generalizing is true for differences of gender and race, for example, which are often overlooked in existing clinical and research approaches to psychotherapy. In fact, the problem of generalizing from limited samples appears to be a function of the predominant nomothetic methods of research, which emphasize groups and group differences when evaluating effects and processes. Demographic variables such as age are often averaged, controlled for statistically, or simply set aside as theoretically irrelevant. It is difficult to specify in advance all possible variables of relevance, and, in any case, it would be impossible for researchers to test all possible interactions between all sets of variables. Given limited resources, the special or unique qualities—and needs—of less statistically central populations tend to be overlooked, as more "average" samples ("adults," "college students," "clinic patients") tend to be the focus of study.

We would caution that there is always a danger of assuming we know more than we do when we refer to groupings of people such as "children" or "elderly." These categories, like those of gender, race, or sexual preference, tend to make us feel we understand an individual better than we really do on the basis of their belonging to one or another group. The psychotherapeutic encounter is idiographic and personal, involving distinctive human beings and the unique relationship they meet to form. Our theories and models need to encompass this level, or risk wiping out what is most human and perhaps what is most therapeutic by recourse to categories that paradoxically refer to "people" of whom no actual person is an adequate example.

In a similar fashion, a developmental, sociological approach tends to assume a prototypical, unitary, linear course of development through reasonably well-demarcated phases of life. In fact, we know that there are endless individual differences in the course of life at all stages, and normative notions of development are likely to minimize the idiosyncratic, creative, novel, or unpredictable aspects of a person's life history. It would seem that our task is to balance our understanding of people in their collectivity with the necessity to encounter the other in some immediate and direct way, without preconception.

CHAPTER 8

Epilogue: Whither (Wither?) Psychotherapy?

As we learned earlier in this volume, the advent of brief psychodynamic therapy has substantially advanced the study of psychodynamic psychotherapy by providing an important vehicle for detailed investigation of the psychotherapy process and outcome. Because BPT manuals typically emphasize a time limit, researchers have been better able to standardize treatment approaches. In this way, brief models of treatment have made it possible to collect a manageable volume of data and to examine a wide range of clinically relevant variables.

Brief models also provide an excellent framework for teaching psychotherapy to clinicians-in-training by giving them rapid exposure to a large number of patients and a wide range of clinical phenomena. Training in the use of models has become necessary because all the trainees work in time-limited settings such as year-long practica, residencies, and clinical internships. Brief psychotherapy has also become an important part of private practice.

Based on our experience with patients and supervisees, we are impressed by the substantial gains that brief psychotherapy can bring about. Clinically significant work can take place, under the right circumstances, even in relatively short treatment episodes. For these reasons, among others, we are confident in the enduring value and important place of BPT in the psychotherapeutic repertoire.

Nevertheless, we wish to express a number of concerns and caveats in the face of the current trend toward corporatization of psychotherapeutic practice and the large-scale deployment of time-limited psychotherapy models as the only available therapeutic option. We will close this volume by raising some troubling questions regarding possible misuse of this modality of treatment.

We view models of BPT as expressions of a highly evolved system

329

of thought and practice, and as the outcome of a century of psychological discourse, clinical experience, and scientific research. These models
are difficult to master and require that the practitioner be well trained
and versed in a wide range of developmental models, clinical theories,
and psychoanalytic systems of psychopathology. Many managed care
models of treatment appear to have little in common with what we call
brief psychodynamic therapy, overlapping in the single respect of having a finite duration. This observation is supported by the trend of
managed care and insurance companies to refer to their services as
"behavioral health care," dropping use of the term "psychotherapy" altogether. Limiting clinical services to five or even ten sessions does not
in itself mean that brief psychotherapy models are necessarily applicable or relevant. As such, we suggest that it is in the public interest to
understand what consititutes psychotherapy and what does not, and
to be clearly informed about exactly what services are being made available to the public through managed care.

As third-party payors and managed care personnel increasingly dic-
tate the content and length of psychotherapeutic treatment, a number
of difficult ethical, clinical, and political questions arise. Do brief
models, applied inappropriately, promote a fundamentally flawed attitude toward the role of psychotherapy in our society? Does the
proliferation of brief treatment models provide a rationale to eliminate
a variety of needed treatments? Is accommodation by practioners to
economic interests a self-defeating practice — cutting back on services
rather than advocating more adequate resources? These questions are
even more acute considering the brevity of treatment offered a considerable number of patients whom we deem not entirely suitable for
the models applied. Such questions raise yet others about the place of
psychotherapy in our culture and our priorities as a society.

The kernel of the dilemma is that clinical necessity is being pitted
against non-clinical issues, such as economic factors and administra-
tive convenience. Both sides of the issues make pressing claims on the
practice of psychotherapy, and yet these competing claims exist on
different levels of discourse. The human context of clinical practice
cannot be so easily translated into the pragmatic language of social tech-
nology and health care economics without the loss of the essential meaning of the term "psychotherapy."

This language barrier is further amplified by certain prevalent
ideas surrounding the theory and practice of brief therapy. One example is an attitude that can be described as "making a virtue of necessity." In this connection, we find book authors, practitioners, and third
party payors who advocate brief therapy as *the* treatment of choice, even
for more disturbed or needy patients. These proponents of a brief ther-

apy "ideology" have found great support—and financial reward—in the prevailing environment of cost-containment. In essence, their argument is that intensive, ongoing treatment is unnecessary, the result of obsolete theories and techniques, and that new technologies of change produce the same or better results in far shorter time frames. The idea here is that you get the same—or more—for less, which has obvious economic appeal.

Such advocates of brief therapies are not necessarily opportunistic or motivated by mercenary considerations. Rather, this overly optimistic point of view often seems to represent a comic vision of reality which leads to a devaluing of longer-term treatment. Therapists of different stripes are not looking at the same clinical phenomena nor using the same categories when they think about the nature of human problems and their solutions (see Chapter 1, section on *Visions of Reality*). In many ways, there are different universes of clinical and therapeutic discourse that rest on fundamentally different assumptions. From this vantage point, it appears that attitudes toward short-term versus long-term psychotherapy represent the clash of different paradigms, each with its own set of rules about what constitutes relevant clinical data.

The resolution of these differences will not be accomplished through scientific means alone, but they will be mediated by social and political processes. We are concerned that the industrialization of psychotherapy is taking place outside the traditional arenas of scholarship, research, and reasoned clinical discourse. The managed care movement in the field of psychotherapy has been based largely on presumed financial necessity rather than on systematic psychological theories of personality, psychopathology, and human development. As the evaluation of psychotherapy efficacy and outcome is increasingly conducted by profit-seeking, privately owned entities, we fear a substantial deterioration of the scientific rigor and impartial scholarship required for an informed, democratic, decision-making process regarding psychotherapeutic treatments.

Given the importance of sociopolitical processes in determining psychotherapeutic practice, we propose an examination of the underlying assumptions of various points of view. We believe that the more optimistic brief therapists—those for whom even more disturbed patients can be treated successfully by brief therapeutic techniques—operate under the influence of two powerful forces. One is a cultural variation of the countertransference phenomenon, described earlier (Chapter 6) as a retreat to grandiosity. At both the individual and the social level there is a longing for the experience of competence, effectiveness, efficiency, and control. The idea that every problem has a rational solution, with its origins in the Enlightenment, has come to full fruition in the contemporary United States. It seems that our culture has great difficulty accepting those aspects of human existence that are beyond our control, and that point to human limitation, in accordance with the tragic vision (Chapter 1). There seems to be little place in our culture for the humble—though foundational—experiences of helplessness, weakness, and dependency.

The second source of therapeutic over-optimism (the flip side of the first) is a need to deny the more painful and unpleasant aspects of human experience by minimizing emotional suffering. There is a prevalent notion, exploited by the burgeoning managed care industry, that people needlessly seek open-ended psychotherapy because it is gratifying and enjoyable rather than because they truly need help. At a cultural level we seem to distance ourselves from emotional pain and despair by trivializing the depth and extent of subjective suffering. It is all too easy to accept our patients' superficial solutions to life's difficulties because it makes our job easier. In fact, our patients undoubtedly pick up on the ways in which we cannot hear about or tolerate their pain, and accommodate us through pathological reenactments of their early relationships with caretakers who could not contain or tolerate their feelings. As psychotherapists we will only hear that which we are prepared to bear. We suspect that some brief therapists may never hear the full extent of their patients' suffering.

Having raised these concerns, we nevertheless maintain the position that the brief psychodynamic therapies occupy an important place in the psychotherapeutic treatment of human problems. The majority of patients who are seen in psychotherapy, regardless of the setting, elect to work briefly, and this will no doubt continue to be the norm. There always will be settings in which resources are limited and where brief treatment is the only therapy that can be offered. Because time-limited techniques remain the one form of psychotherapy available to many who require treatment, this in itself is sufficient justification for the continued development and application of these methods.

References

Ackerman, N. W. (1958). *The psychodynamics of family life.* New York: Basic Books.

Alexander, F. (1956). *Psychoanalysis and psychotherapy.* New York: Norton.

Alexander, F. (1965). Psychoanalytic contributions to short-term psychothera-py. In L. R. Wolberg (Ed.), *Short-term psychotherapy* (pp. 84–126). New York: Grune & Stratton.

Alexander, F., & French, T. M. (1946). *Psychoanalytic therapy: Principles and application.* New York: Ronald Press.

Alpert, M. (1992). Accelerated empathic therapy: A new short-term dynamic psychotherapy. *International Journal of Short-Term Psychotherapy, 7,* 133–156.

Appelbaum, S. A. (1988). Psychoanalytic therapy: A subset of healing. *Psychotherapy, 25,* 201–208.

Arkowitz, H. (1992). Integrative theories of therapy. In D. K. Freedheim, H. J. Freudenberg, J. W. Kessler, S. B. Messer, D. R. Peterson, H. H. Strupp, & P. L. Wachtel (Eds.), *History of psychotherapy: A century of change* (pp. 261–303). Washington, DC: American Psychological Association.

Arlow, J. A., & Brenner, C. (1964). *Psychoanalytic concepts and the structural theory.* New York: International Universities Press.

Aron, L. (1990). One-person and two-person psychologies and the method of psychoanalysis. *Psychoanalytic Psychology, 7,* 475–495.

Atwood, G. E., & Stolorow, R. D. (1984). *Structures of subjectivity.* Hillsdale, NJ: Analytic Press.

Baker, E. L. (1985). Psychoanalysis and psychoanalytic psychotherapy. In S. J. Lynn & J. P. Garske (Eds.), *Contemporary psychotherapies: Models and methods* (pp. 19–68) Columbus, OH: Charles E. Merrill.

Baker, H. S. (1991). Shorter-term psychotherapy: A self psychological approach. In P. Crits-Christoph & J. P. Barber (Eds.), *Handbook of short-term dynamic psychotherapy,* (pp. 287–322). New York: Basic Books.

Balint, M. (1968). *The basic fault.* London: Tavistock.

Balint, M., Ornstein, P., & Balint, E. (1972). *Focal psychotherapy.* London: Tavistock.

Barber, J. P. (1994). Efficacy of short-term dynamic psychotherapy. *Journal of Psychotherapy Practice and Research, 3,* 108–121.

Barber, J. P., & Crits-Christoph, P. (1993). Advances in measures of psychodynamic formulations. *Journal of Consulting and Clinical Psychology, 61,* 574–585.

Barber, J. P., & Luborsky, L. (1991). A psychodynamic view of simple phobias and prescriptive matching: A commentary. *Psychotherapy, 28,* 469–472.

Barth, K., Nielsen, G., Havik, O. E., Haver, B., Molstad, E., Rogge, H., Skatun, M., Heiberg, A. N., & Ursin, H. (1988). Assessment for three different forms of short-term dynamic psychotherapy. *Psychotherapy and Psychosomatics, 49*, 153–159.

Bauer, G. P., & Kobos, J. C. (1987). *Brief therapy: Short-term psychodynamic intervention.* Northvale, NJ: Jason Aronson.

Beebe, B. (1994). Representation and internalization: Three principles of salience. *Psychoanalytic Psychology, 11*, 127–165.

Beitman, B. D., Goldfried, M. R., & Norcross, J. C. (1989). The movement toward integrating the psychotherapies: An overview. *American Journal of Psychiatry, 146*(2), 138–147.

Belar, C. D. (1995). Collaboration in capitated care: Challenges for psychology. *Professional Psychology: Research and Practice, 26*, 139–146.

Bellak, L. (1992). *Handbook of intensive brief and emergency psychotherapy* (2nd ed.). Larchmont, NY: C. P. S.

Bellak, L., & Small, L. (1965). *Emergency psychotherapy and brief psychotherapy.* New York: Grune & Stratton.

Bellak, L., & Small, L. (1978). *Emergency psychotherapy and brief psychotherapy* (2nd ed.). New York: Grune & Stratton.

Benjamin, L. S. (1974). The structural analysis of behavior. *Psychological Review, 81*, 392–425.

Benjamin, L. S. (1982). Use of Structural Analysis of Social Behavior (SASB) to guide intervention in psychotherapy. In J. C. Anchin & D. J. Kiesler (Eds.), *Handbook of interpersonal psychotherapy* (pp. 190–212). New York: Pergamon Press.

Bergler, E., & Roheim, G. (1946). Psychology of time perception. *Psychoanalytic Quarterly, 26*, 190–206.

Bergson, H. (1937/1956). Laughter: The comic in character. In W. Sypher (Ed.), *Comedy* (pp. 61–190) Garden City, NY: Doubleday Anchor Books.

Berman, E. (1985). Eclecticism and its discontents. *Israel Journal of Psychiatry and Related Sciences, 22*, 51–60.

Bernard, H. S., Schwartz, A.J., Oclatio, K. A., & Stiner, A. (1980). Relationship between patients' in-process evaluations of therapy and psychotherapy outcome. *Journal of Clinical Psychology, 36*, 259–264.

Beutler, L. E. (1991). Have all won and must all have prizes? Revisiting Luborsky et al.'s verdict. *Journal of Consulting and Clinical Psychology, 59*, 226–232.

Beutler, L. E. & Consoli, A. J. (1992). Systematic eclectic psychotherapy. In J. C. Norcross & M. R. Goldfried (Eds.), *Handbook of psychotherapy integration* (pp. 264–299). New York: Basic Books.

Beutler, L. E., Crago, M., & Arizmendi, T. G. (1986). Therapist variables in psychotherapy process and outcome. In S. L. Garfield & A. E. Bergin (Eds.), *Handbook of psychotherapy and behavior change* (3rd ed., pp. 257–310). New York: Wiley.

Beutler, L. E., Eagle, D., Mohr, D., Daldruh, R. J., Bergan, J., Meredith, K., & Merry, W. (1991). Predictors of differential and self-directed psychotherapeutic procedures. *Journal of Consulting and Clinical Psychology, 59*, 333–340.

Beutler, L. E., Machado, P. P., Engle, D., & Mohr, D. (1993). Differential patient

× treatment maintenance among cognitive, experiential, and self-directed psychotherapies. *Journal of Psychotherapy Integration, 3,* 15–31.

Bibring, E. (1954). Psychoanalysis and the dynamic psychotherapies. *Journal of the American Psychoanalytic Association, 2,* 745–770.

Binder, J. L. (1993). Observations on the training of therapists in time-limited dynamic psychotherapy. *Psychotherapy, 30,* 592–598.

Binder, J. L., & Strupp, H. H. (1991). The Vanderbilt approach to time-limited dynamic psychotherapy. In P. Crits-Christoph & J. P. Barber (Eds.), *Handbook of short-term dynamic psychotherapy* (pp. 137–165). New York: Basic Books.

Binder, J. L., & Strupp, H. H. (1993). Recommendations for improving psychotherapy training based on experiences with manual-guided training and research. *Psychotherapy, 30,* 571–572.

Bion, W. R. (1962/1967). A theory of thinking. In *Second thoughts* (pp. 110–119). Northvale, NJ: Jason Aronson.

Bion, W. R. (1970). *Attention and interpretation.* New York: Jason Aronson.

Blanck, G. & Blanck, R. (1974). *Ego psychology: Theory and practice.* New York: Columbia University Press.

Blos, P. (1962). *On adolescence: A psychoanalytic interpretation.* New York: Free Press.

Blos, P. (1983). The contribution of psychoanalysis to the psychotherapy of adolescents. *Psychoanalytic Study of the Child, 38,* 577–600.

Bolter, K., Levenson, H., & Alvarez, W. (1990). Differences in values between short-term and long-term therapists. *Professional Psychology: Research and Practice, 21,* 285–290.

Bonaparte, M. (1940). Time and the unconscious. *International Journal of Psycho-Analysis, 21,* 427–468.

Bowen, M. (1978). *Family therapy in clinical practice.* New York: Jason Aronson.

Bowlby, J. (1951). *Maternal care and mental health.* New York: Columbia University Press.

Bowlby, J. (1969). *Attachment and loss: Vol. 1. Attachment.* New York: Basic Books.

Brenner, C. (1973). *An elementary textbook of psychoanalysis* (rev. ed.). New York: International Universities Press.

Brenner, C. (1976). *Psychoanalytic technique and psychic conflict.* New York: International Universities Press.

Breuer, J., & Freud, S. (1895/1955). Studies on hysteria. *Standard Edition, 2,* 1–305.

Broskowski, A. (1991). Current mental health care environments: Why managed care is necessary. *Professional Psychology: Research and Practice, 22,* 6–14.

Broskowski, A. T. (1995). The evolution of health care: Implications for the training and careers of psychologists. *Professional Psychology: Research and Practice, 26,* 156–162.

Brown, B. S. (1983). The impact of political and economic changes upon mental health. *American Journal of Orthopsychiatry, 53,* 583–592.

Budman, S. H. (1981). Introduction. In S. H. Budman (Ed.), *Forms of brief therapy* (pp. 1–5). New York: Guilford Press.

Budman, S. H., Demby, A., & Randall, J. (1982). Psychotherapeutic outcome and reduction in medical utilization: A cautionary tale. *Professional Psychology: Research and Practice, 13,* 200–207.

Budman, S. H. & Gurman, A. S. (1988). *Theory and practice of brief therapy.* New York: Guilford Press.

Burke, J. D., White, H. S., & Havens, L. L. (1981). Which short-term therapy? Matching patient and method. *Archives of General Psychiatry, 36,* 177–186.

Burlingame, G. M., & Behrman, J. A. (1987). Clinician attitudes toward time-limited and time-unlimited therapy. *Professional Psychology: Research and Practice, 18,* 61–65.

Burlingame, G. M., Fuhriman, A., Paul, S., & Ogles, B. M. (1989). Implementing a time-limited therapy program: Differential effects of training and experience. *Psychotherapy, 26,* 303–313.

Busse, E. W., & Pfeiffer, E. (1972). Mental disorders in later life. In E. W. Busse & E. Pfeiffer (Eds.), *Mental illness in later life* (pp. 107–144). Washington, DC: American Psychiatric Association.

Clark, B. E. (1993). *Towards an integrated model of time-limited psychodynamic therapy with children* (Doctoral dissertation, Rutgers—The State University, 1992). *Dissertation Abstracts International, 54,* 1659-B.

Cohen, B. D., & Epstein, Y. (1981). Empathic communication in process groups. *Psychotherapy, 18,* 493–500.

Cohen, P., & Cohen, J. (1984). The clinician's illusion. *Archives of General Psychiatry, 41,* 1178–1182.

Collins, W. D., & Messer, S. B. (1991). Extending the plan formulation method to an object relations perspective: Reliability, stability, and adaptability. *Psychological Assessment: A Journal of Consulting and Clinical Psychology, 3,* 75–81.

Crits-Christoph, P. (1992). The efficacy of brief dynamic psychotherapy: A meta-analysis. *American Journal of Psychiatry, 149,* 151–158.

Crits-Christoph, P. (1993). Response to Svartberg. *American Journal of Psychiatry, 150,* 684–685.

Crits-Christoph, P., Barber, J. P., & Kurcias, J. S. (1993). The accuracy of therapists' interpretations and the development of the therapeutic alliance. *Psychotherapy Research, 3,* 25–35.

Crits-Christoph, P., Cooper, A., & Luborsky, L. (1988). The accuracy of therapists' interpretations and the outcome of dynamic psychotherapy. *Journal of Consulting and Clinical Psychology, 56,* 490–495.

Crits-Christoph, P., & Luborsky, L. (1990). Changes in CCRT pervasiveness during psychotherapy. In L. Luborsky & P. Crits-Christoph, *Understanding transference: The CCRT method* (pp. 133–146). New York: Basic Books.

Crits-Christoph, P., Luborsky, L., Dahl, L., Popp, C., Mellon, J., & Mark, D. (1988). Clinicians can agree in assessing relationship patterns in psychotherapy. *Archives of General Psychiatry, 45,* 1001–1004.

Crits-Christoph, P., Luborsky, L., Popp, C., Mellon, J., & Mark, D. (1990). The reliability of choice of narratives and of the CCRT measure. In L. Luborsky & P. Crits-Christoph, *Understanding transference: The CCRT method* (pp. 93–101). New York: Basic Books.

Cross, D. G., Sheehan, P. W., & Khan, J. A. (1982). Short and long term follow-up of clients receiving insight-oriented and behavior therapy. *Journal of Consulting and Clinical Psychology, 50,* 103–112.

Cummings, N. A. (1988). Emergence of the mental health complex: Adaptive and maladaptive responses. *Professional Psychology: Research and Practice, 19,* 308–315.

Curtis, J. T., & Silberschatz, G. (1986). Clinical implications of research on brief dynamic psychotherapy. I. Formulating the patient's problems and goals. *Psychoanalytic Psychology, 3,* 13–26.

Curtis, J. T., & Silberschatz, G., Sampson, H., & Weiss, J. (1994). The plan formulation method. *Psychotherapy Research, 4,* 197–207.

Curtis, J. T., & Silberschatz, G., Sampson, H., Weiss, J, & Rosenberg, S. E. (1988). Developing reliable psychodynamic case formulation: An illustration of the plan diagnosis method. *Psychotherapy, 25,* 256–265.

Dasberg, H., & Winokur, M. (1984). Teaching and learning short-term dynamic psychotherapy: Parallel processes. *Psychotherapy, 21,* 184–188.

Davanloo, H. (Ed.) (1978). *Basic principles and techniques in short-term dynamic psychotherapy.* New York: Spectrum Publications.

Davanloo, H. (Ed.) (1980). *Short-term dynamic psychotherapy.* New York: Jason Aronson.

Davanloo, H. (1988). The technique of unlocking of the unconscious. Part I. *International Journal of Short-Term Psychotherapy, 3,* 99–121.

Davies, J. M. & Frawley, M. G. (1994). *Treating the adult survivor of childhood sexual abuse: A psychoanalytic perspective.* New York: Basic Books.

DeLeon, P. H., VandenBos, G. R., & Bulatao, E. Q. (1991). Manged mental health care: A history of the federal policy initiative. *Professional Psychology: Research and Practice, 22,* 15–25.

Diguer, L., Luborsky, L., Singer, B., Luborsky, E., Dickter, D., & Schmidt, K. A. (1993, June). *The efficacy of dynamic psychotherapy versus other psychotherapies: A meta-analysis.* Paper presented at the meeting of the Society for Psychotherapy Research, Pittsburgh, PA.

Dobson, K. S., & Shaw, B. F. (1993). The training of cognitive therapists: What have we learned from treatment manuals? *Psychotherapy, 30,* 573–577.

Dulcan, M. & Piercy, P. (1985). A model for teaching and evaluating brief psychotherapy with children and their families. *Professional Psychology: Research and Practice, 16,* 689–700.

Eckert, P. A. (1993). Acceleration of change: Catalysts in brief therapy. *Clinical Psychology Review, 13,* 241–253.

Edelson, M. (1975). *Language and interpretation in psychoanalysis.* New Haven: Yale University Press.

Edelson, M. (1977). Psychoanalysis as science. *Journal of Nervous and Mental Disease, 165,* 1–28.

Eigen, M. (1992). *Coming through the whirlwind.* Wilmette, IL: Chiron Publications.

Eisdorfer, L. (1989). *The development, implementation, and evaluation of a training seminar in brief dynamic psychotherapy in a community mental health center* (Doctoral dissertation, Rutgers—The State University, 1988). *Dissertation Abstracts International, 50,* 1105-B.

Eliade, M. (1954). *The myth of the eternal return, or Cosmos and history.* Princeton, NJ: Princeton University Press.

Elkin, I., Shea, M. T., Watkins, J. T., Imber, S. D., Sotsky, S. M., Collins, J. F., Glass, D. R., Pilkonis, P. A., Leber, W. R., Docherty, J. P., Flester, S. J., & Parloff, M. B. (1989). National Institute of Mental Health Treatment of Depression Collaborative Research Study. *Archives of General Psychiatry, 46,* 971–982.

Elliott, R., Stiles, W. B., & Shapiro, D. A. (1993). Are some psychotherapies more equivalent than others? In T. R. Giles (Ed.), *Handbook of effective psychothera-py* (pp. 455–477). New York: Plenum.

Erikson, E. H. (1950). *Childhood and society.* New York: Norton.

Erikson, E. H. (1968). *Identity: Youth and crisis.* New York: Norton.

Eysenck, H. J. (1952). The effects of psychotherapy: An evaluation. *Journal of Consulting Psychology, 16,* 319–324.

Fairbairn, W. R. (1941). A revised psychopathology of the psychoses and psy-choneuroses. *International Journal of Psycho-Analysis, 22,* 250–279.

Fairbairn, W. R. D. (1943/1952). The repression and return of bad objects. In *Psychoanalytic studies of the personality* (pp. 59–81). London: Routledge/Tavi-stock.

Fairbairn, W. R. D. (1952). *Psychoanalytic studies of the personality.* London: Rout-ledge/Tavistock.

Fenichel, O. (1944/1954). Brief psychotherapy. In H. Fenichel & D. Rapa-port (Eds.), *The collected papers of Otto Fenichel* (pp. 243–259). New York: Norton.

Ferenczi, S. (1921/1980). The further development of an active therapy in psy-choanalysis. In J. Suttie (Ed.), *Further contributions to the theory and technique of psychoanalysis* (pp. 189–197). London: Karnac Books.

Ferenczi, S. (1926/1980). Contraindications to the active psychoanalytic tech-nique. In J. Richman (Ed.), *Further contributions to the theory and technique of psycho-analysis* (pp. 217–230). London: Karnac Books.

Ferenczi, S. (1988). *The clinical diary of Sandor Ferenczi* (J. Dupont, Ed; M. Balint & N. Z. Jackson, Trans.) Cambridge, MA: Harvard University Press.

Ferenczi, S., & Rank, O. (1925/1986). *The development of psychoanalysis.* Madison, CT: International Universities Press.

Flegenheimer, W. V. (1982). *Techniques of brief psychotherapy.* New York: Jason Aronson.

Flegenheimer, W. (1985). History of brief psychotherapy. In A. J. Horner (Ed.), *Treating the oedipal patient in brief psychotherapy* (pp. 7–24). New York: Jason Aronson.

Foote, B. (1992). Accelerated empathic therapy: the First self-psychological brief therapy? *International Journal of Short-Term Psychotherapy, 7,* 177–191.

Foreman, S. A., & Marmar, C. R. (1985). Therapist actions that address initially poor therapeutic alliances in psychotherapy. *American Journal of Psychiatry, 142,* 922–926.

Fosha, D. (1992). The interrelatedness of theory, technique and therapeutic stance: A comparative look at intensive short-term dynamic psychother-apy and accelerated empathic therapy. *International Journal of Short-Term Psychotherapy, 7,* 157–176.

Frank, J. D. (1974). Psychotherapy: The restoration of morale. *American Journal of Psychiatry, 131,* 271–274.

Frank, J. D. (1982). Therapeutic components shared by all psychotherapies. In J. H. Harvey & M. M. Parks (Eds.), *The Master Lecture series: Vol. 1. Psychother-apy research and behavior change* (pp. 73–122). Washington, DC: American Psychological Association.

Frank, J. D. (1987). Psychotherapy, rhetoric, and hermeneutics: Implications for practice and research. *Psychotherapy, 24,* 293–302.

Frank, J. D., & Frank, J. B. (1991). *Persuasion and healing* (3rd ed.). Baltimore: Johns Hopkins University Press.

Frank, K. A. (1990). Action techniques in psychoanalysis. *Contemporary Psychoanalysis, 26,* 732–756.

Franks, C. (1984). On conceptual and technical integrity in psychoanalysis and behavior therapy: Two fundamentally incompatible systems. In H. Arkowitz & S. B. Messer (Eds.), *Psychoanalytic therapy and behavior therapy: Is integration possible?* (pp. 223–247). New York: Plenum.

Freud, A. (1926). *The psychoanalytic treatment of children.* London: Imago.

Freud, A. (1958). Adolescence. *Psychoanalytic Study of the Child, 13,* 255–278.

Freud, A. (1966). *The ego and the mechanisms of defense.* New York: International Universities Press.

Freud, S. (1905a/1958). Three essays on the theory of sexuality. *Standard Edition, 7,* 135–243.

Freud, S. (1905b/1958). On psychotherapy. *Standard Edition, 7,* 257–268.

Freud, S. (1911–1915/1958). Papers on technique. *Standard Edition, 12,* 85–156.

Freud, S. (1912a/1958). The dynamics of transference. *Standard Edition, 12,* 97–108.

Freud, S. (1912b/1958). Recommendations to physicians practising psychoanalysis. *Standard Edition, 12,* 109–120.

Freud, S. (1914a/1958). On narcissism: An introduction. *Standard Edition, 14,* 73–102.

Freud, S. (1914b/1958). Remembering, repeating, and working through. *Standard Edition, 12,* 145–156.

Freud, S. (1916-1917/1958). Introductory lectures on psycho-analysis. *Standard Edition, 16,* 243–496.

Freud, S. (1917/1958). Mourning and melancholia. *Standard Edition, 14,* 243–258.

Freud, S. (1917/1963). Introductory lectures on psychoanalysis. *Standard Edition, 15–16,* 3–496.

Freud, S. (1919/1959). Lines of advance in psycho-analytic therapy. *Standard Edition, 17,* 157–168.

Freud, S. (1924/1958). The economic problem of masochism. *Standard Edition, 19,* 159–170.

Freud, S. (1924/1961). The dissolution of the oedipus complex. *Standard Edition, 19,* 173–179.

Freud, S. (1926/1958). Inhibitions, symptoms and anxiety. *Standard Edition, 20,* 87–156.

Freud, S. (1931/1964). Female sexuality. *Standard Edition, 21,* 221–243.

Freud, S. (1933/1964). New introductory lectures on psychoanalysis. *Standard Edition, 22,* 3–182.

Fried, D., Crits-Christoph, P., & Luborsky, L. (1990). The parallel of the CCRT for the therapist with the CCRT for other people. In L. Luborsky & P. Crits-Christoph, *Understanding transference: The CCRT method* (pp. 147–157). New York: Basic Books.

Frieswyk, S. H., Allen, J. G., Colson, D. B., Coyne, L., Gabbard, G. O., Horwitz, L, & Newsom, G. (1986). Therapeutic alliance: Its place as a process and outcome variable in dynamic psychotherapy research. *Journal of Consulting and Clinical Psychology, 54,* 32–38.

Frieswyk, S. H., Colson, D. B., & Allen, J. G. (1984). Conceptualizing the alliance from a psychoanalytic perspective. *Psychotherapy, 27*, 460–464.

Fromm, E. (1944). Individual and social origins of neurosis. *American Sociological Review, 9*, 380–384.

Fromm, E. (1947). *Man for himself.* Greenwich, CT: Fawcett.

Frye, N. (1957). *Anatomy of criticism.* New York: Atheneum.

Frye, N. (1965). *A natural perspective: The development of Shakespearean comedy and romance.* New York: Columbia University Press.

Gardner, J. R. (1991). The application of self psychology to brief psychotherapy. *Psychoanalytic Psychology, 8*, 477–500.

Garfield, S. L. (1986). Research on client variables in psychotherapy. In S. L. Garfield & A. E. Bergin (Eds.), *Handbook of psychotherapy and behavior change* (3rd ed., pp. 213–256). New York: Wiley.

Garfield, S. L. (1989). *The practice of brief therapy.* New York: Pergamon Press.

Geller, J. (1987). The process of psychotherapy: Separation and the complex interplay among empathy, insight, and internalization. In J. Bloom-Feshbach & S. Bloom-Feshbach (Eds.), *The psychology of separation and loss* (pp. 459–514). San Francisco: Jossey-Bass.

Gelso, C. J. (1992). Realities and emerging myths about brief therapy. *The Counseling Psychologist, 20*, 464–471.

Gelso, C. J., & Johnson, D. H. (1983). *Explorations in time-limited counseling and psychotherapy.* New York: Teachers College Press.

Gelso, C. J., Spiegel, S. B., & Mills, D. H. (1983). Clients' and counselors' reactions to time-limited and time-unlimited counseling. In C. J. Gelso & D. H. Johnson (Eds.), *Explorations in time-limited counseling and psychotherapy* (pp. 114–162). New York: Teachers College Press.

Giles, T. R. (Ed.) (1993). *Handbook of effective psychotherapy* (pp. 114–162). New York: Plenum.

Gill, M. M. (1979). The analysis of the transference. *Journal of the American Psychoanalytic Association, 27*, 263–288.

Gill, M. M. (1982). *Analysis of transference: Vol. I. Theory and technique.* New York: International Universities Press.

Glover, E. (1931). The therapeutic effect of inexact interpretation: A contribution to the theory of suggestion. *International Journal of Psycho-Analysis, 12*, 397–411.

Gold, J. R. (1993). The sociohistorical context of psychotherapy integration. In G. Stricker & J. R. Gold (Eds.), *Comprehensive handbook of psychotherapy integration* (pp. 3–8). New York: Plenum.

Gold, J. R., & Wachtel, P. L. (1993). Cyclical psychodynamics. In G. Stricker & J. R. Gold (Eds.), *Comprehensive handbook of psychotherapy integration* (pp. 59–72). New York: Plenum.

Goldberg, A. (1975). Narcissism and the readiness for psychotherapy termination. *Archives of General Psychiatry, 32*, 695–699.

Goldfried, M. R. (1980). Toward the delineation of therapeutic change principles. *American Psychologist, 35*, 991–999.

Gomez-Schwartz, B. (1978). Effective ingredients in psychotherapy: Prediction of outcome from process variables. *Journal of Consulting and Clinical Psychology, 46*, 1023–1035.

Goodheart, C. D. (1989). Short-term dynamic psychotherapy with difficult clients. In P.A. Keller & S.R. Heyman (Eds.), *Innovations in clinical practice: A source book* (Vol. 8. pp. 15–26). Sarasota, FL: Professional Resource Exchange.

Grand, S., Rechetnick, J., Podrug, D., & Schwager, E. (1985). *Transference in brief psychotherapy.* Hillsdale, NJ: Analytic Press.

Greenberg, J. (1991). *Oedipus and beyond.* Cambridge, MA: Harvard University Press.

Greenberg, J. R., & Mitchell, S. A. (1983). *Object relations in psychoanalytic theory.* Cambridge, MA: Harvard University Press.

Greenson, R. R. (1967). *The technique and practice of psychoanalysis.* New York: International Universities Press.

Grencavage, L. M. & Norcross, J. C. (1990). Where are the commonalities among the therapeutic common factors? *Professional Psychology, 21,* 372–378.

Grünbaum, A. (1984). *The foundations of psychoanalysis: A philosophical critique.* Berkeley: University of California Press.

Guntrip, H. (1961). *Personality structure and human interaction.* London: Hogarth.

Gustafson, J. P. (1984). An integration of brief dynamic psychotherapy. *American Journal of Psychiatry, 141,* 935–944.

Gustafson, J. P. (1986). *The complex secret of brief psychotherapy.* New York: Norton.

Haas, L. J., & Cummings, N. A. (1991). Managed outpatient mental health plans: Clinical, ethical, and practical guidelines for participation. *Professional Psychology: Research and Practice, 22,* 45–51.

Habermas, J. (1971). *Knowledge and human interests.* Boston: Beacon Press.

Haley, J. (1976). *Problem-solving therapy.* San Fransisco: Jossey-Bass.

Hamovitch, G. (1985). *An evaluation of competency-based training in short-term dynamic psychotherapy* (Doctoral dissertation, Rutgers—The State University, 1984). *Dissertation Abstracts International, 45,* 3071-B.

Hanly, C. (1992). *The problem of truth in applied psychoanalysis.* New York: Guilford Press.

Hartley, D. E., & Strupp, H. H. (1983). The therapeutic alliance: Its relationship to outcome in brief psychotherapy. In J. Masling (Ed.), *Empirical studies of psychoanalytical theories* (Vol. 1, pp. 1–37). Hillsdale, NJ: Analytic Press.

Hartmann, H. (1939). *Ego psychology and the problem of adaptation.* New York: International Universities Press.

Havens. L. (1976). *Participant observation.* New York: Jason Aronson.

Heiberg, A. (1981). Training in short-term psychotherapy. *Psychotherapy and Psychosomatics, 35,* 112–120.

Henry, W. P., Strupp, H. H., Butler, S. F., Schacht, T. E., & Binder, J. L. (1993). Effects of training in time-limited dynamic psychotherapy: Changes in therapist behavior. *Journal of Consulting and Clinical Psychology, 61,* 434–440.

Henry, W. P., Schacht, T. E., Strupp, H. H., Butler, S. F., & Binder, J. L. (1993). Effects of training in time-limited dynamic psychotherapy: Mediators of therapists' responses to training. *Journal of Consulting and Clinical Psychology, 61,* 441–447.

Herman, J. L., Perry C. C., & van der Volk, B. A. (1989). Childhood trauma in borderline personality disorder. *American Journal of Psychiatry, 146,* 490–495.

Hirsch, I. (1985). The rediscovery of the advantages of the participant-observation model. *Psychoanalysis and Contemporary Thought, 8,* 441–459.

Hoffman, I. Z. (1983). The patient as interpreter of the analyst's experience. *Contemporary Psychoanalysis, 19,* 389–422.

Hoffman, I. Z. (1992). Some practical implications for a social-constructivist view of the psychoanalytic situation. *Psychoanalytic Dialogues, 2,* 287–316.

Høglend, P. (1988). Brief dynamic psychotherapy for less well-adjusted patients. *Psychotherapy and Psychosomatics, 49,* 197–204.

Høglend, P. (1993a). Personality disorders and long-term outcome after brief psychodynamic psychotherapy. *Journal of Personality Disorders, 7,* 168–181.

Høglend, P. (1993b). Suitability for brief dynamic psychotherapy: Psychodynamic variables as predictors of outcome. *Acta Psychiatrica Scandinavica, 88,* 104–110.

Høglend, P. (1993c). Transference interpretations and long-term change after dynamic psychotherapy of brief to moderate length. *American Journal of Psychotherapy, 47,* 494–507.

Høglend, P., Engelstad, V., Sørbye, Ø., Heyerdahl, O., & Amlo, S. (1994). The role of insight in exploratory psychodynamic therapy. *British Journal of Medical Psychology, 67,* 305–317.

Høglend, P., Heyerdahl, O., Amlo, S., Engelstad, V., Fossum, A., Sørbye, Ø., & Sørlie, T. (1993). Interpretations of the patient–therapist relationship in brief dynamic psychotherapy: Effects on long-term mode specific change. *Journal of Psychotherapy Practice and Research, 2,* 296–306.

Høglend, P., Sørlie, T., Heyerdahl, O., Sørbye, Ø., & Amlo, S. (1993). Brief dynamic psychotherapy: Patient suitablity, treatment length, and outcome. *Journal of Psychotherapy Practice and Research, 2,* 230–241.

Holt, R. R. (1976). Drive or wish? A reconsideration of the psychoanalytic theory of motivation. In M. M. Gill & P. S. Holzman (Eds.), *Psychology versus metapsychology: Essays in memory of George S. Klein* (pp. 158–197). New York: International Universities Press.

Horney, K. (1950). *Neurosis and human growth.* New York: Norton.

Horowitz, L. M., Rosenberg, S. E., Baer, B. A., Ureño, G., & Villaseñor, V. S. (1988). Inventory of interpersonal problems: Psychometric properties and clinical applications. *Journal of Consulting and Clinical Psychology, 56,* 885–892.

Horowitz, L. M., Rosenberg, S. E., & Bartholomew, K. (1993). Interpersonal problems, attachment styles, and outcome in brief dynamic psychotherapy. *Journal of Consulting and Clinical Psychology, 61,* 549–560.

Horowitz, L. M., Rosenberg, S. E., Ureño, G., Kalehzan, M., & O'Halloran, P. (1989). Psychodynamic formulation, consensual response method, and interpersonal problems. *Journal of Consulting and Clinical Psychology, 57,* 599–606.

Horowitz, M. J. (1986). *Stress response syndromes* (2nd ed.). Northvale, NJ: Jason Aronson.

Horowitz, M. (1988). *Introduction to psychodynamics: A new synthesis.* New York: Basic Books.

Horowitz, M. (1991). Short-term dynamic therapy of stress response syndromes. In P. Crits-Christoph & J. P. Barber (Eds.), *Handbook of short-term dynamic psychotherapy* (pp. 166–198). New York: Basic Books.

Horowitz, M. J., Krupnick, J., Kalteider, N., Wilner, N., Leong, A., & Marmar,

C. (1981). Initial psychological response to parental death. *Archives of General Psychiatry, 38,* 316–323.

Horowitz, M., Marmar, C., Krupnick, J., Kaltreider, N., Wallerstein, R., & Wilner, N. (1984). *Personality styles and brief psychotherapy.* New York: Basic Books.

Horowitz, M. J., Marmar, C., Weiss, D. S. DeWitt, K. N., & Rosenbaum, R. (1984). Brief psychotherapy of bereavement reactions: The relation of process to outcome. *Archives of General Psychiatry, 41,* 438–448.

Horvath, A., Gaston, L., & Luborsky, L. (1993). The therapeutic alliance and its measures. In N. Miller, L. Luborsky, J. Barber, & J. Docherty (Eds.), *Psychodynamic treatment research* (pp. 247–273). New York: Basic Books.

Hougardy, G., & Luminet, D. (1980). Training in brief psychotherapies. *Psychotherapy and Psychosomatics, 34,* 256–260.

Howard, G. S. (1991). Culture tales: A narrative approach to thinking, cross-cultural psychology, and psychotherapy. *American Psychologist, 46,* 187–197.

Howard, K. I., Davidson, C. V., O'Mahoney, M. T., Orlinsky, D. E., & Brown, K. P. (1991). Patterns of psychotherapy utilization. *American Journal of Psychiatry, 146,* 775–778.

Howard, K. I., Kopta, S. M., Krause, M. S., & Orlinsky, D. E. (1986). The dose-effect relationship in psychotherapy. *American Psychologist, 41,* 159–164.

Howard, K. I., Lueger, R. J., Maling, M. S., & Martinovich, Z. (1993). A phase model of psychotherapy outcome: Causal mediation of change. *Journal of Consulting and Clinical Psychology, 61,* 678–685.

Hoyt, M. F. (1985). Therapist resistances to short-term dynamic psychotherapy. *Journal of the American Academy of Psychoanalysis, 13,* 93–112.

Husby, R., Dahl, A. A., Dahl, C., Heiberg, A. N., Olafsen, O. M., & Wisaeth, L. (1985). Short-term dynamic psychotherapy: Prognostic value of characteristics of patients studied by a 2-year follow-up of 39 neurotic patients. *Psychotherapy and Psychosomatics, 43,* 8–16.

Jacobsen, E. (1964). *Self and the object world.* New York: International Universities Press.

Jensen, J. P., Bergin, A. E., & Greaves, D. W. (1990). The meaning of eclecticism: New survey and analysis of components. *Professional Psychology: Research and Practice, 21,* 124–130.

Johnson, D. H., & Gelso, C. J. (1980). The effectiveness of time limits in counseling and psychotherapy: A critical review. *The Counseling Psychologist, 9,* 70–83.

Jones, E. (1957). *The life and work of Sigmund Freud.* New York: Basic Books.

Jones, E. E., Cumming, J. D., & Horowitz, M. J. (1988). Another look at the nonspecific hypothesis of therapeutic effectiveness. *Journal of Consulting and Clinical Psychology, 56,* 48–55.

Joyce, A. S., & Piper, W. E. (1990). An examination of Mann's model of time-limited psychotherapy. *Canadian Journal of Psychiatry, 35,* 41–49.

Kalpin, A. (1992). [Review of *Handbook of short-term psychotherapy*]. *International Journal of Short-Term Psychotherapy, 7,* 243–248.

Karasu, T. B. (1986). The specificity versus nonspecificity dilemma: Toward identifying therapeutic change agents. *American Journal of Psychiatry, 143,* 687–695.

Kazdin, A. (1984). Integration of psychodynamic and behavioral psychotherapies: Conceptual versus empirical syntheses. In H. Arkowitz & S. B. Messer (Eds.), *Psychoanalytic therapy and behavior therapy: Is integration possible?* (pp. 139–170). New York: Plenum.

Kazdin, A. E., & Bass, D. (1989). Power to detect differences between alternative treatments in comparative psychotherapy outcome research. *Journal of Consulting and Clinical Psychology, 57,* 138–147.

Kernberg, O. F. (1975). *Borderline conditions and pathological narcissism.* Northvale, NJ: Jason Aronson.

Kernberg, O. F. (1976). *Object relations theory and clinical psychoanalysis.* Northvale, NJ: Jason Aronson.

Kernberg, O. F. (1986). *Severe personality disorders.* New Haven: Yale University Press.

Kernberg, O., Burstein, E., Coyne, L., Appelbaum, A., Horowitz, L., & Voth, H. (1972). Psychotherapy and psychanalysis: Final report of the Menninger Foundation's psychotherapy research project. *Bulletin of the Menninger Foundation, 36,* 1–275.

Kiesler, C., & Morton, T. (1988). Psychology and public policy in the "health care revolution." *American Psychologist, 43,* 993–1003.

Kimble, G. A. (1984). Psychology's two cultures. *American Psychologist, 39,* 833–839.

Klein, M. (1932). *The psycho-analysis of children.* London: Hogarth.

Klein, M. (1946/1975). Notes on some schizoid mechanisms. In *Envy and gratitude and other works* (Vol. 3, pp. 1–24). London: Hogarth.

Klein, M. (1950). *Contributions to psychoanalysis.* London: Hogarth.

Klein, M. (1952/1975). The origins of transference. In *Envy and gratitude and other works* (pp. 48–56). London: Hogarth Press.

Kohut, H. (1971). *The analysis of the self.* New York: International Universities Press.

Kohut, H. (1977). *The restoration of the self.* New York: International Unversities Press.

Kohut, H. (1984). *How does analysis cure?* Chicago: University of Chicago Press.

Kopta, S. M., Howard, K. I., Lowry, J. L., & Beutler, L. E. (1994). Patterns of symptomatic recovery in psychotherapy. *Journal of Consulting and Clinical Psychology, 62,* 1009–1016.

Koss, M. P. (1979). Length of psychotherapy for clients seen in private practice. *Journal of Consulting and Clinical Psychology, 47,* 210–212.

Koss, M. P., & Butcher, J. N. (1986). Research on brief psychotherapy. In S. L. Garfield & A. E. Bergin (Eds.), *Handbook of psychotherapy and behavior change* (3rd ed., pp. 627–670). New York: Wiley.

Koss, M. P., Butcher, J. N., & Strupp, H. H. (1986). Brief psychotherapy methods in clinical research. *Journal of Consulting and Clinical Psychology, 54,* 60–67.

Koss, M. P., & Shiang, J. (1994). Research on brief psychotherapy. In A. E. Bergin & S. L. Garfield (Eds.), *Handbook of psychotherapy and behavior change* (4th ed., pp. 664–700). New York: Wiley.

Krasner, L., & Houts, A. C. (1984). A study of the "value" systems of behavioral scientists. *American Psychologist, 39,* 840–850.

Kuhn, T. S. (1970). *The structure of scientific revolutions.* Chicago: University of Chicago Press.

Kupers, T. A. (1986). The dual potential of brief psychotherapy. *Free Associations, 6,* 80–99.

Laikin, M., Winston, A., & McCullough, L. (1991). Intensive short-term dynamic psychotherapy. In P. Crits-Christoph & J. P. Barber (Eds.), *Handbook of short-term dynamic psychotherapy* (pp. 80–109). New York: Basic Books.

Lambert, M. J. (1992). Psychotherapy outcome research: Implications for integrative and eclectic therapists. In J. C. Norcross & M. R. Goldfried (Eds.), *Handbook of psychotherapy integration* (pp. 94–129). New York: Basic Books.

Lambert, M. J., & Bergin, A. E. (1994). The effectiveness of psychotherapy. In A. E. Bergin & S. L. Garfield (Eds.), *Handbook of psychotherapy and behavior change* (4th ed., pp. 143–189). New York: Wiley.

Lambert, M. J., Shapiro, D. A., & Bergin, A. E. (1986). The effectiveness of psychotherapy. In S. L. Garfield & A. E. Bergin (Eds.), *Handbook of psychotherapy and behavior change* (3rd ed., pp. 452–481). New York: Wiley.

Landman, J. T., & Dawes, R. M. (1982). Psychotherapy outcome: Smith and Glass conclusions stand up under scrutiny. *American Psychologist, 37,* 504–516.

Langsley, D. G. (1978). Comparing clinic and private practice of psychiatry. *American Journal of Psychiatry, 135,* 702–706.

Laufer, M. (1981). Adolescent breakdown and the transference neurosis. *International Journal of Psycho-Analysis, 62,* 51–59.

Laufer, M., & Laufer, M. E. (1984). *Adolescence and developmental breakdown: A psychoanalytic view.* New Haven: Yale University Press.

Lazarus, A. A. (1992). Multimodal therapy: Technical eclecticism with minimal integration. In J. C. Norcross & M R. Goldfried (Eds.), *Handbook of psychotherapy integration* (pp. 231–263). New York: Basic Books.

Lazarus, A. A., & Messer, S. B. (1988). Clinical choice points: Behavioral versus psychoanalytic interventions. *Psychotherapy, 25,* 59–70.

Lazarus, A. A., & Messer, S. B. (1991). Does chaos prevail? An exchange on technical eclecticism and assimilative integration. *Journal of Psychotherapy Integration, 1,* 143–158.

Lazarus, L. W. (1982). Brief psychotherapy of narcissistic disturbances. *Psychotherapy, 19,* 228–236.

Leibovich, M. A. (1981). Short-term psychotherapy for the borderline personality disorder. *Psychotherapy and Psychosomatics, 35,* 257–264.

Lester, E. (1968). Brief psychotherapy in child psychiatry. *Canadian Psychiatric Association Journal, 13,* 301–309.

Levene, H., Breger, L., & Patterson, V. (1972). A training and research program in brief psychotherapy. *American Journal of Psychotherapy, 26,* 90–100.

Levenson, E. A. (1982). Language and healing. In S. Slipp (Ed.), *Curative factors in dynamic psychotherapy.* New York: McGraw-Hill.

Levenson, H. (1995). *Time-limited dynamic psychotherapy.* New York: Basic Books.

Levenson, H., & Bolter, K. (1988, August). *Short-term psychotherapy values and attitudes: Changes with training.* Paper presented at the meeting of the American Psychological Association, Atlanta, GA.

Levenson, H., Speed, J., & Budman, S. H. (1995). Therapists' experience, training, and skill in brief therapy: A bicoastal survey. *American Journal of Psychotherapy, 49,* 95–117.

Lewis, M. (1990). Self-knowledge and social development in early life. In L. A. Pervin (Ed.), *Handbook of personality: Theory and research* (pp. 277–300). New York: Guilford.

Loftus, E. F., & Ketcham, K. (1991). *Witness for the defense.* New York: St. Martin's Press.

Lorr, M., McNair, D. M., Michaux, W. W., & Raskin, A. (1964). Frequency of treatment and change. *Journal of Abnormal and Social Psychology, 64,* 281–292.

Lowman, R. L. (1991). Mental health claims experience: Analysis and benefit redesign. *Professional Psychology: Research and Practice, 22,* 36–44.

Luborsky, L. (1984). *Principles of psychoanalytic psychotherapy: A manual for supportive-expressive treatment.* New York: Basic Books.

Luborsky, L. (1990). The everyday clinical uses of the CCRT. In L. Luborsky & P. Crits-Christoph, *Understanding transference: The CCRT method* (pp. 211–221). New York: Basic Books.

Luborsky, L. (1993). Recommendations for training therapists based on manuals for psychotherapy research. *Psychotherapy, 30,* 578–580.

Luborsky, L., Chandler, M., Auerbach, A. H., Cohen, J., & Bachrach, H. M. (1971). Factors influencing the outcome of psychotherapy: A review of quantitative research. *Psychological Bulletin, 75,* 145–185.

Luborsky, L., & Crits-Christoph, P. (1990). *Understanding transference: The CCRT method.* New York: Basic Books.

Luborsky, L., Crits-Christoph, P., Mintz, J., & Auerbach, A. (1988). *Who will benefit from psychotherapy? Predicting therapeutic outcomes.* New York: Basic Books.

Luborsky, L. & Mark, D. (1991). Short-term supportive–expressive psychoanalytic psychotherapy. In P. Crits-Christoph & J. P. Barber (Eds.), *Handbook of short-term dynamic psychotherapy* (pp. 110–136). Basic Books.

Luborsky, L., McClellan, A. T., Woody, G. E., O'Brien, C. P., & Auerbach, A. (1985). Therapist success and its determinants. *Archives of General Psychiatry, 42,* 602–611.

Luborsky, L., Mintz, J., Auerbach, A., Christoph, P, Bachrach, H., Todd, T., Johnson, M., Cohen, M., & O'Brien, C. P. (1980). Predicting the outcome of psychotherapy: Findings of the Penn Psychotherapy Project. *Archives of General Psychiatry, 37,* 471–481.

Luborsky, L. & Schaffler, P. (1990). Illustrations of the CCRT Scoring Guide. In L. Luborsky & P. Crits-Christoph, *Understanding transference: The CCRT method* (pp. 51–81). New York: Basic Books.

Luborsky, L., Singer, B., & Luborsky, L. (1975). Comparative studies of psychotherapies. *Archives of General Psychiatry, 32,* 995–1008.

Lueger, R. J., & Howard, K. I. (1994). The work functioning of psychotherapy patients. Manuscript submitted for publication.

Mackay, J. (1967). The use of brief psychotherapy with children. *Canadian Journal of Psychiatry, 12,* 269–278.

Magnavita, J. J. (1993). The evolution of short-term dynamic psychotherapy: Treatment of the future? *Professional Psychology: Research and Practice, 24,* 360–365.

Mahalik, J. R. (1990). Systematic eclectic models. *The Counseling Psychologist, 18,* 655–679.

Mahler, M. S. (1963). Thoughts about development and individuation. *Psychoanalytic Study of the Child, 7,* 286–305.

Mahler, M. S. (1968). *On human symbiosis and the vicissitudes of individuation.* New York: International Universities Press.

Mahler, M. S. (1972). On the first three subphases of the separation–individuation process. *International Journal of Psycho-Analysis, 53,* 333–338.

Mahler, M. S., Pine, F., & Bergman, A. (1975). *The psychological birth of the human infant.* New York: Basic Books.

Mahoney, M. J., & Craine, M. H. (1991). The changing beliefs of psychotherapy experts. *Journal of Psychotherapy Integration, 1,* 207–221.

Malan, D. H. (1963). *A study of brief psychotherapy.* New York: Plenum.

Malan, D. H. (1976a). *The frontier of brief psychotherapy.* New York: Plenum.

Malan, D. H. (1976b). *Toward the validation of dynamic psychotherapy: A replication.* New York: Plenum.

Malan, D. H. (1980). Criteria for selection. In H. Davanloo (Ed.), *Short-term dynamic psychotherapy* (pp. 169–189). New York: Jason Aronson.

Malan, D. H. (1986a) Beyond interpretation: Initial evaluation and technique in short-term dynamic psychotherapy. Part I. *International Journal of Short-Term Psychotherapy, 1,* 59–82.

Malan, D. H. (1986b). Beyond interpretation: Initial evaluation and technique in short-term dynamic psychotherapy. Part II. *International Journal of Short-Term Psychotherapy, 1,* 83–106.

Malan, D. H., & Osimo, F. (1992). *Psychodynamics, training, and outcome in brief psychotherapy.* Oxford: Butterworth–Heinemann.

Maling, M. S., Gurtman, M. B., & Howard, K. I. (1995). The response of interpersonal problems to varying doses of psychotherapy. *Psychotherapy Research, 5,* 63–75.

Mann, J. (1973). *Time-limited psychotherapy.* Cambridge, MA: Harvard University Press.

Mann, J. (1991). Time limited psychotherapy. In P. Crits-Christoph & J. P. Barber (Eds.), *Handbook of short-term dynamic psychotherapy* (pp. 17–44). New York: Basic Books.

Mann, J., & Goldman, R. (1982). *A casebook in time-limited psychotherapy.* New York: McGraw Hill.

Marmor, J. (1986). The corrective emotional experience revisited. *International Journal of Short-Term Psychotherapy, 1,* 43–47.

Marx, J. A., & Gelso, C. J. (1987). Termination of individual counseling in a university counseling center. *Journal of Counseling Psychology, 34,* 3–9.

Marziali, E. (1984). Prediction of outcome of brief psychotherapy from therapist interpretive interventions. *Archives of General Psychiatry, 41,* 301–304.

Marziali, E., Marmar, C., & Krupnick, J. (1981). Therapeutic alliance scales: Development and relationship to therapeutic outcome. *American Journal of Psychiatry, 138,* 361–364.

McAdams, D. P. (1993). *The stories we live by: Personal myths and the making of the self.* New York: Morrow.

McCullough, L. (1993). An anxiety-reduction modification of short-term dynamic psychotherapy (STDP): A theoretical "melting pot" of treatment techniques. In G. Stricker & J. R. Gold (Eds.), *Comprehensive handbook of psychotherapy integration* (pp. 139–149). New York: Plenum.

McCullough, L., Farber, B. A., Winston, A., Porter, F., Pollack, J., Vingiano,

W., Laikin, M., & Trujillo, M. (1991). The relationship of patient–therapist interaction to outcome in brief psychotherapy. *Psychotherapy, 28,* 525–533.

McDougall, J. (1989). *Theatres of the body: A psychoanalytic approach to psychosomatic illness.* New York: Norton.

McWilliams, N. (1987). The grandiose self and the interminable analysis. *Current Issues in Psychoanalytic Practice, 4,* 93–107.

Meeks, J. E. (1971). *The fragile alliance.* Baltimore: Williams & Wilkins.

Menninger, K., & Holzman, P. S. (1973). *The theory of psychoanalytic techniques* (2nd ed.). New York: Basic Books.

Messer, S. B. (1986). Behavioral and psychoanalytic perspectives at therapeutic choice points. *American Psychologist, 41,* 1261–1272.

Messer, S. B. (1988a). Psychoanalytic perspectives on the therapist-client relationship. *Journal of Integrative and Eclectic Psychotherapy, 7,* 268–277.

Messer, S. B. (1988b). [Review of *The complex secret of brief psychotherapy*]. *Journal of Integrative and Eclectic Psychotherapy, 7,* 222–225.

Messer, S. B. (1989). Integration and eclecticism in counselling and psychotherapy: Cautionary notes. *British Journal of Guidance and Counselling, 17,* 274–285.

Messer, S. B. (1992). A critical examination of belief structures in integrative and eclectic psychotherapy. In J. C. Norcross & M. R. Goldfried (Eds.), *Handbook of psychotherapy integration* (pp. 130–165). New York: Basic Books.

Messer, S. B., Sass, L. A., & Woolfolk, R. L. (Eds.) (1988). *Hermeneutics and psychological theory: Interpretive perspectives on personality, psychotherapy, and psychopathology.* New Brunswick, NJ: Rutgers University Press.

Messer, S. B., Tishby, O., & Spillman, A. (1992). Taking context seriously in psychotherapy research: Relating therapist interventions to patient progress in brief psychodynamic therapy. *Journal of Consulting and Clinical Psychology, 60,* 678–688.

Messer, S. B., & Warren, S. (1990). Personality change and psychotherapy. In L. A. Pervin (Ed.), *Handbook of personality: Theory and research* (pp. 371–398). New York: Guilford Press.

Messer, S. B., & Winokur, M. (1980). Some limits to the integration of psychoanalytic and behavior therapy. *American Psychologist, 35,* 818–827.

Messer, S. B., & Winokur, M. (1981). What about the question of integration? A reply to Apfelbaum and to Ellis. *American Psychologist, 36,* 800–802.

Messer, S. B., & Winokur, M. (1984). Ways of knowing and visions of reality in psychoanalytic therapy and behavior therapy. In H. Arkowitz & S. B. Messer (Eds.), *Psychoanalytic therapy and behavior therapy: Is integration possible?* (pp. 63–100). New York: Plenum.

Messer, S. B., & Winokur, M. (1986). Eclecticism and the shifting visions of reality in three systems of psychotherapy. *International Journal of Eclectic Psychotherapy, 5,* 115–124.

Migone, P. (1985). Short-term dynamic psychotherapy from a psychoanalytic viewpoint. *Psychoanalytic Review, 4,* 615–634.

Minuchin, S. (1974). *Families and family therapy.* Cambridge, MA: Harvard University Press.

Mitchell, S. A. (1988). *Relational concepts in psychoanalysis: An integration.* Cambridge, MA: Harvard University Press.

Moras, K. (1993). The use of treatment manuals to train psychotherapists: Observations and recommendations. *Psychotherapy, 30,* 581–586.

Moss, D. (1985). What you see is what you get: Empiricism, psychoanalytic theory, and brief therapy. *PsychCritique, 1,* 21–34.

Mujeeb-ur-Rahman, M. (1990). *The psychological quest: From Socrates to Freud* (rev. ed.). North York, Ontario: Captus University Publications.

Mumford, E., Schlesinger, H., Glass, G. V., Patrick, C., & Cuerdon, B. A. (1984). A new look at evidence about reduced cost of medical utilization following mental health treatment. *American Journal of Psychiatry, 141,* 1145–1158.

Murray, H. A. (1938). *Explorations in personality.* New York: Oxford University Press.

Nichols, M. (1984). *Family therapy: Concepts and methods.* New York: Gardner Press.

Nicholson, R. A., & Berman, J. S. (1983). Is follow-up necessary in evaluating psychotherapy? *Psychological Bulletin, 93,* 261–278.

Nielsen, G., & Barth, K. (1991). Short-term anxiety-provoking psychotherapy. In P. Crits-Christoph & J. P. Barber (Eds.), *Handbook of short-term dynamic psychotherapy* (pp. 45–79). New York: Basic Books.

Norcross, J. C., & Prochaska, J. O. (1982). A national survey of clinical psychologists: Views on training, career choice, and APA. *The Clinical Psychologist, 35*(1), 3–6.

Norcross, J. C., & Prochaska, J. O. (1988). A study of eclectic (and integrative) views revisited. *Professional Psychology: Research and Practice, 19,* 170–174.

Novey, R. (1983). Otto Rank: Beginnings, endings, and current experience. *Journal of the American Psychoanalytic Association, 31,* 985–1002.

O'Dowd, W. T. (1986). Otto Rank and time-limited psychotherapy. *Psychotherapy, 23,* 140–149.

Ogden, T. H. (1989). *The primitive edge of experience.* Northvale, NJ: Jason Aronson.

Olfson, M., & Pincus, H. A. (1994). Outpatient psychotherapy in the United States: II. Patterns of utilization. *American Journal of Psychiatry, 151,* 1289–1294.

O'Malley, S. S., Suh, C. S., & Strupp, H. H. (1983). The Vanderbilt Psychotherapy Process Scale: A report on the scale development and a process–outcome study. *Journal of Consulting and Clinical Psychology, 51,* 581–586.

Omer, H. (1993). The narrative approach to psychotherapy and the rise of the life-sketch. *Psychotherapy, 30,* 668–673.

Orlinsky, D. E., & Howard, K. I. (1986). Process and outcome in psychotherapy. In S. L. Garfield & A. E. Bergin (Eds.), *Handbook of psychotherapy and behavior change* (3rd Ed., pp. 311–381). New York: Wiley.

Palermo, D. S. (1978). *Psychology of language.* Glenview, IL: Scott Foresman.

Parad, L. (1970). Short-term treatment: An overview of historical trends, issues and potentials. *Smith College Studies in Social Work, 41,* 119–146.

Parad, L., & Parad, H. (1968). A study of crisis-oriented planned short-term treatment, Part I. *Social Casework, 49,* 346–355.

Patterson, C. H. (1989). Eclecticism in psychotherapy: Is integration possible? *Psychotherapy, 26,* 157–161.

Patterson, V., Levene, H., & Breger, L. (1971). Treatment and training outcomes with two time-limited therapies. *Archives of General Psychiatry, 25,* 161–167.

Pekarik, G., & Wierzbicki, M. (1986). The relationship between clients' expected and actual treatment duration. *Psychotherapy, 23,* 532–534.

Pepe, M. M., & Wu, J. (1988). The economics of mental health care. *Psychotherapy, 25,* 352–355.

Perry, S. (1989). Treatment time and the borderline patient: An underappreciated strategy. *Journal of Personality Disorders, 3,* 230–239.

Peterfreund, E. (1983). *The process of psychoanalytic therapy: Models and strategies.* Hillsdale, NJ: Analytic Press.

Peterlin, K., & Sloves, R. (1985). Time-limited psychotherapy with children: Central theme and time as major tools. *Journal of the American Academy of Child and Adolescent Psychiatry, 24,* 785–792.

Phillips, E. L. (1985). *Psychotherapy revised: New frontiers in research and practice.* Hillsdale, NJ: Erlbaum.

Phillips, L., & Johnston, M. (1954). Theoretical and clinical aspects of short-term parent-child psychotherapy. *Psychiatry, 17,* 267–275.

Pine, F. (1985). *Developmental theory and clinical process.* New Haven: Yale University Press.

Pine, F. (1988). The four psychologies of psychoanalysis and their place in clinical work. *Journal of the American Psychoanalytic Association, 36,* 571–596.

Pine, F. (1989). Motivation, personality organization, and the four psychologies of psychoanalysis. *Journal of the American Psychoanalytic Association, 37,* 31–64.

Pine, F. (1990). *Drive, ego, object, and self.* New York: Basic Books.

Pinsker, H., Rosenthal, R., & McCullough, L. (1991). Dynamic supportive psychotherapy. In P. Crits-Christoph & J. P. Barber (Eds.), *Handbook of short-term dynamic psychotherapy* (pp. 220–247). New York: Basic Books.

Piper, W. E. (1988). Psychotherapy research in the 1980s: Defining areas of consensus and controversy. *Hospital and Community Psychiatry, 39,* 1055–1063.

Piper, W. E., Azim, H. F. A., Joyce, A. S., & McCallum, M. (1991). Transference interpretations, therapeutic alliance, and outcome in short-term individual psychotherapy. *Archives of General Psychiatry, 48,* 946–953.

Piper, W. E., Azim, H. F. A., Joyce, A. S., McCallum, M., Nixon, G. W. H., & Segal, P. S. (1991). Quality of object relations versus interpersonal functioning as predictors of therapeutic alliance and psychotherapy outcome. *Journal of Nervous and Mental Disease, 179,* 432–438.

Piper, W. E., Azim, H. F. A., McCallum, M., & Joyce, A. S. (1990). Patient suitability and outcome in short-term individual psychotherapy. *Journal of Consulting and Clinical Psychology, 58,* 475–481.

Piper, W. E., de Carufel, F. L., & Szkrumelak, N. (1985). Patient predictors of process and outcome in short-term individual psychotherapy. *Journal of Nervous and Mental Disease, 173,* 726–733.

Piper, W. E., Debbane, E. G., Bienvenu, J. P., de Carufel, F., & Garant, J. (1986). Relationships between the object focus of therapist interpretations and outcome in short-term individual psychotherapy. *British Journal of Medical Psychology, 59,* 1–11.

Piper, W. E., Debbane, E. G., Bienvenu, J. P., & Garant, J. (1984). A comparative study of four forms of psychotherapy. *Journal of Clinical and Consulting Psychology, 52,* 268–279.

Piper, W. E., Joyce, A. S., McCallum, M., & Azim, H. F. A. (1993). Concentration and correspondence of transference interpretation in short-term pscyhotherapy. *Journal of Consulting and Clinical Psychology, 61,* 586–610,

Pollock, G. (1987). The mourning-liberation process: Ideas on the inner life of the older adult. In J. Sadavoy & M. Leszcz (Eds.), *Treating the elderly with psychotherapy* (pp. 3–29). Madison, CT: International Universities Press.

Pollack, J., Flegenheimer, W., & Winston, A. (1991). Brief adaptive psychotherapy. In P. Crits-Christoph & J. P. Barber (Eds.), *Handbook of short-term dynamic psychotherapy* (pp. 199–219). New York: Basic Books.

Popp, C., Luborsky, L., & Crits-Christoph, P. (1990). The parallel of the CCRT from therapy narratives with the CCRT from dreams. In L. Luborsky & P. Crits-Christoph, *Understanding transference: The CCRT method* (pp. 158–172). New York: Basic Books.

Prochaska, J. (1995). An eclectic and integrative approach: Transtheoretical therapy. In A. S. Gurman & S. B. Messer (Eds.), *Essential psychotherapies: Theory and practice* (pp. 403–440). New York: Guilford Press.

Proskauer, S. (1969). Some technical issues in time-limited psychotherapy with children. *Journal of the American Academy of Child and Adolescent Psychiatry, 8,* 154–169.

Proskauer, S. (1971). Focused time-limited psychotherapy with children. *Journal of the American Academy of Child and Adolescent Psychiatry, 10,* 619–639.

Quintana, S. M. (1993). Toward an expanded and updated conceptualization of termination: Implications for short-term, individual psychotherapy. *Professional Psychology: Research and Practice, 24,* 426–432.

Quintana, S. M., & Meara, N. M. (1990). Internalization of therapeutic relationships in short-term psychotherapy. *Professional Psychology: Research and Practice, 37,* 123–130.

Rachman, S., & Wilson, G. T. (1980). *The effects of psychological therapy.* Oxford: Pergamon Press.

Rank, O. (1929/1978). *Will therapy.* New York: Norton.

Rapaport, D., & Gill, M. M. (1959). The points of view and assumptions of metapsychology. *International Journal of Psycho-Analysis, 40,* 153–162.

Rasmussen, A., & Messer, S. B. (1986). A comparison and critique of Mann's time-limited psychotherapy and Davanloo's short-term dynamic psychotherapy. *Bulletin of the Menninger Clinic, 50,* 163–184.

Reich, J. H., & Green, A. J. (1991). Effect of personality disorders on outcome of treatment. *Journal of Nervous and Mental Disease, 179,* 74–82.

Reich, W. (1933). *Character analysis.* New York: Farrar, Straus, & Giroux.

Rice, L. (1988). Integration and the client-centered relationship. *Journal of Integrative and Eclectic Psychotherapy, 7,* 291–302.

Richardson, L. M., & Austad, C. S. (1991). Realities of mental health practice in managed-care settings. *Professional Psychology: Research and Practice, 22,* 52–59.

Robbins, S. B., & Zinni, V. R. (1988). Implementing a time-limited treatment model: Issues and solutions. *Professional Psychology: Research and Practice, 19,* 53–57.

Rogers, C. (1957). The necessary and sufficient conditions of therapeutic personality change. *Journal of Consulting Psychology, 21,* 95–103.

Rogers, C. R. (1951). *Client-centered therapy.* Boston: Houghton Mifflin.

Rosegrant, J. (1984). Brief dynamic psychotherapy in community mental health settings: Providing a holding environment on a short-term basis. *Psychoanalytic Psychology, 2,* 157–164.

Rosenberg, S. E., Silberschatz, G., Curtis, J. T., Sampson, H., & Weiss, J. (1986). A method for establishing reliability of statements from psychodynamic case formulation. *American Journal of Psychiatry, 143,* 1454–1456.

Safran, J. D., & Messer, S. B. (1995). *Psychotherapy integration: A postmodern critique.* Manuscript submitted for publication.

Safran, J. D., & Segal, Z. V. (1990). *Interpersonal process in cognitive therapy.* New York: Basic Books.

Said, T. (1988). Overview: Trial therapy in intensive short-term dynamic psychotherapy. *International Journal of Short-Term Psychotherapy, 3,* 25–45.

Salerno, M., Farber, B., McCullough, L., Winston, A., & Trujillo, M. (1992). The effects of confrontation and clarification on patient affective and defensive responding. *Psychotherapy Research, 2,* 181–192.

Sampson, H. (1992) The role of "real" experience in psychopathology and treatment. *Psychoanalytic Dialogues, 2,* 509–528.

Sandler, J., & Sandler, A. M. (1978). On the development of object relationships and affects. *International Journal of Psycho-Analysis, 59,* 285–296.

Sarbin, T. R. (1986). The narrative as a root metaphor for psychology. In T. R. Sarbin (Ed.), *Narrative psychology: The storied nature of human conduct* (pp. 3–21). New York: Praeger.

Sarnoff, C. (1976). *Latency.* New York: Jason Aronson.

Sass, L. A. (1992). *Madness and modernism.* New York: Basic Books.

Schacht, T. E. (1984). The varieties of integrative experience. In H. Arkowitz & S. B. Messer (Eds.), *Psychoanalytic therapy and behavior therapy: Is integration possible?* (pp. 107–131). New York: Plenum.

Schafer, R. (1970). The psychoanalytic vision of reality. *International Journal of Psycho-Analysis, 51,* 279–297.

Schafer, R. (1973). The termination of brief psychoanalytic psychotherapy. *International Journal of Psychoanalytic Psychotherapy, 2,* 135–148.

Schafer, R. (1974). Talking to patients in psychotherapy. *Bulletin of the Menninger Clinic, 38,* 503–515.

Schafer, R. (1976). *A new language for psychoanalysis.* New Haven: Yale University Press.

Schafer, R. (1978). *Language and insight.* New Haven: Yale University Press.

Schafer, R. (1981). *Narrative actions in psychoanalysis.* Worcester, MA: Clark University Press.

Schneider, W. J., & Pinkerton, R. S. (1986). Short-term psychotherapy and graduate training in psychology. *Professional Psychology: Research and Practice, 17,* 574–579.

Schwartz, A. J., & Bernard, H. S. (1981). Comparison of patient and therapist evaluations of time-limited psychotherapy. *Psychotherapy, 18,* 101–108.

Segal, H. (1957). Notes on symbol formation. *International Journal of Psycho-Analysis, 38,* 391–397.

Shadish, W. R. (1992). *Mediators and moderators in psychotherapy meta-analysis.* Paper presented at the meeting of the American Psychological Association, Washington, DC.

Shadish, W. R., & Sweeney, R. B. (1991). Mediators and moderators in meta-analysis: There's a reason we don't let dodo birds tell us which psychotherapies should have prizes. *Journal of Consulting and Clinical Psychology, 59*, 883–893.

Shapiro, D., Barkham, M., Rees, A., Hardy, G. E., Reynolds, S., & Startup, M. (1994). Effects of treatment duration and severity of depression on the effectiveness of cognitive-behavioral and psychodynamic–interpersonal psychotherapy. *Journal of Consulting and Clinical Psychology, 62*, 522–534.

Shapiro, D. A., & Shapiro, D. (1982). Meta-analysis of comparative therapy outcome studies. *Psychological Bulletin, 92*, 581–604.

Shearer, S. L., Peters, C. P., Quaytman, M. S., & Ogden, R. L. (1990). Frequency and correlates of childhood sexual and physical abuse in adult female borderline in-patients. *American Journal of Psychiatry, 147*, 214–216.

Shefler, G., Dasberg, H., & Ben-Shakhar, G. (in press). A randomized controlled outcome and follow-up study of Mann's time-limited psychotherapy. *Journal of Consulting and Clinical Psychology.*

Sifneos, P. E. (1968). Learning to solve emotional problems: A controlled study of short-term anxiety-provoking psychotherapy. In R. Porter (Ed.), *The role of learning in psychotherapy* (pp. 87–96). Boston: Little, Brown.

Sifneos, P. E. (1972). *Short-term psychotherapy and emotional crisis.* Cambridge, MA: Harvard University Press.

Sifneos, P. E. (1978). Teaching and supervision of short-term anxiety provoking psychotherapy. In H. Davanloo (Ed.), *Basic principles and techniques of short-term dynamic psychotherapy* (pp. 491–499). New York: Spectrum.

Sifneos, P. E. (1979). *Short-term dynamic psychotherapy: Evaluation and technique.* New York: Plenum.

Sifneos, P. E. (1987). *Short-term dynamic psychotherapy: Evaluation and technique* (2nd ed.). New York: Plenum.

Sifneos, P. E. (1992). *Short-term anxiety-provoking psychotherapy.* New York: Basic Books.

Sifneos, P. E., Apfel, R. J., Bassuk, E., Fishman, G., & Gill, A. (1980). Ongoing outcome research on short-term dynamic psychotherapy. *Psychotherapy and Psychosomatics, 33*, 233–241.

Silberschatz, G., & Curtis, J. T. (1986). Clinical implications of research on brief dynamic psychotherapy. II. How the therapist helps or hinders therapeutic progress. *Psychoanalytic Psychology, 3*, 27–38.

Silberschatz, G., & Curtis, J. T. (1993). Measuring the therapist's impact on the patient's therapeutic progress. *Journal of Consulting and Clinical Psychology, 61*, 403–411.

Silberschatz, G., Curtis, J. T., & Nathan, S. (1989). Using the patient's plan to assess progress in psychotherapy. *Psychotherapy, 26*, 40–46.

Silberschatz, G., Fretter, P. B., & Curtis, J. T. (1986). How do interpretations influence the process of psychotherapy? *Journal of Consulting and Clinical Psychology, 54*, 646–652.

Singer, J. A., & Singer, J. L. (1992). Transference in psychotherapy and daily life: Implications of current memory and social cognition research. In J. W. Barron, M. N. Eagle, & D. L. Wolitzky (Eds.), *Interface of psychoanalysis and psychology* (pp. 516–538). Washington, DC: American Psychological Association.

Skolnick, N. J., & Warshaw, S. C. (1992). Introduction. In N. J. Skolnick & S. C. Warshaw (Eds.), *Relational perspectives in psychoanalysis* (pp. xxiii–xxix). Hillsdale, NJ: The Analytic Press.

Sledge, W. H., Moras, K., Hartley, D., & Levine, M. (1990). Effect of time-limited psychotherapy on patient dropout rates. *American Journal of Psychiatry, 147,* 1341–1347.

Sloane, R. B., Staples, F. R., Cristol, A. H., Yorkston, N. J., & Whipple, K. (1975). Short-term analytically oriented psychotherapy versus behavior therapy. *American Journal of Psychiatry, 132,* 373–377.

Sloves, R., & Peterlin, K. (1986). The process of time-limited psychotherapy with latency-aged children. *Journal of the American Academy of Child and Adolescent Psychiatry, 25,* 1341–1347.

Smith, M. L., Glass, G. V., & Miller, T. I. (1980). *The benefits of psychotherapy.* Baltimore: Johns Hopkins Press.

Smyrnios, K. X., & Kirby, R. J. (1993). Long-term comparison of brief versus unlimited psychodynamic treatments with children and their families. *Journal of Consulting and Clinical Psychology, 61,* 1020–1027.

Sogg, S., & Messer, S. B. (1995). *Assessing session-by-session outcome in brief psychodynamic therapy.* Manuscript submitted for publication.

Sparacino, J. (1978–1979). Psychotherapy with the aged. *International Journal of Aging and Human Development, 9,* 197–220.

Spence, D. (1982). *Narrative and historical truth.* New York: Norton.

Spitz, R. A. (1945). Hospitalism: An inquiry into the genesis of psychiatric conditions in early childhood. *Psychoanalytic Study of the Child, 2,* 53–73.

Spitz, R. A. (1946). Anaclitic depression: An inquiry into the genesis of psychiatric conditions in early childhood, II. *Psychoanalytic Study of the Child, 2,* 313–342.

Steenbarger, B. N. (1994). Duration and outcome in psychotherapy: An integrative review. *Professional Psychology: Research and Practice, 25,* 111–119.

Stein, M. H. (1985). Irony in psychoanalysis. *Journal of the American Psychoanalytic Association, 33,* 35–57.

Stern, D. (1985). *The interpersonal world of the infant.* New York: Basic Books.

Stierlin, H. (1968). Short-term versus long-term psychotherapy in the light of a general theory of human relationships. *British Journal of Medical Psychology, 41,* 357–366.

Stiles, W. B., Shapiro, D. A., & Elliot, R. (1986). Are all psychotherapies equivalent? *American Psychologist, 41,* 165–180.

Stolorow, R. D., & Atwood, G. E. (1992). *Contexts of being: The intersubjective foundations of psychological life.* Hillsdale, NJ: Analytic Press.

Stolorow, R. D., Brandschaft, B., & Atwood, G. E. (1987). *Psychoanalytic treatment: An intersubjective view.* Hillsdale, NJ: Analytic Press.

Stolorow, R. D., & Lachman, F. M. (1980). *The psychoanalysis of developmental arrests: Theory and practice.* New York: International Universities Press.

Stone, L. (1954). The widening scope of indications for psychoanalysis. *Journal of the American Psychoanalytic Association, 2,* 567–594.

Stone, L. (1961). *The psychoanalytic situation.* New York: International Universities Press.

Strachey, J. (1934). The nature of the therapeutic action of psycho-analysis. *International Journal of Psycho-Analysis, 15,* 127–159.

Strenger, C. (1989). The classic and the romantic vision in psychoanalysis. *International Journal of Psycho-Analysis, 70,* 593–610.

Strupp, H. H. (1980a). Success and failure in time-limited psychotherapy: A systematic comparison of two cases (Comparison 1). *Archives of General Psychiatry, 37,* 595–603.

Strupp, H. H. (1980b). Success and failure in time-limited psychotherapy: A systematic comparison of two cases (Comparison 2). *Archives of General Psychiatry, 37,* 708–716.

Strupp, H. H. (1980c). Success and failure in time-limited psychotherapy: A systematic comparison of two cases (Comparison 3). *Archives of General Psychiatry, 37,* 831–841.

Strupp, H. H. (1980d). Success and failure in time-limited psychotherapy: A systematic comparison of two cases (Comparison 4). *Archives of General Psychiatry, 37,* 947–954.

Strupp, H. H. (1986). The nonspecific hypothesis of therapeutic effectiveness. *American Journal of Orthopsychiatry, 56,* 513–520.

Strupp, H. H., & Binder, J. L. (1984). *Psychotherapy in a new key: A guide to time-limited dynamic psychotherapy.* New York: Basic Books.

Strupp, H. H., Butler, S. F., & Rosser, C. L. (1988). Training in psychodynamic therapy. *Journal of Consulting and Clinical Psychology, 56,* 689–669.

Strupp, H. H., & Hadley, S. W. (1979). Specific versus nonspecific factors in psychotherapy. *Archives of General Psychiatry, 36,* 1125–1136.

Sullivan, H. S. (1953). *Interpersonal theory of psychiatry.* New York: Norton.

Sullivan, H. S. (1954). *The psychiatric interview.* New York: Norton.

Svartberg, M., Seltzer, M. H., & Stiles, T. C. (1993). Intrapsychic growth during and after short-term dynamic psychotherapy: An explorative study. Manuscript in preparation.

Svartberg, M., Seltzer, M. H., Stiles, T. C. & Khoo, S. T. (1995). Symptom improvement and its temporal course in short-term dynamic psychotherapy: A curve growth analysis. *Journal of Nervous and Mental Disease, 183,* 242–248.

Svartberg, M., & Stiles, T. C. (1991). Comparative effects of short-term psychodynamic psychotherapy: A meta-analysis. *Journal of Consulting and Clinical Psychology, 59,* 704–714.

Svartberg, M., & Stiles, T. C. (1992). Predicting patient change from therapist competence and patient-therapist complementarity in short-term anxiety-provoking psychotherapy: A pilot study. *Journal of Consulting and Clinical Psychology, 60,* 304–307.

Svartberg, M., & Stiles, T. C. (1993). Efficacy of brief dynamic psychotherapy [letter]. *American Journal of Psychiatry, 150,* 684.

Svartberg, M., & Stiles, T. C. (1994). Therapeutic alliance, therapist competence, and client change in short-term anxiety-provoking psychotherapy. *Psychotherapy Research, 4,* 20–33.

Sved, S. (1983). *Training in short-term dynamic psychotherapy: A review of the literature and of the experience of sixteen psychology graduate student trainees.* Unpublished manuscript, Rutgers—The State University.

Taube, C. A., Kessler, L., & Feuerberg, M. (1984). *Utilization and expenditures for ambulatory mental health care during 1980* (Data Report 5). Washington, DC: U.S. Department of Health and Human Services.

Taurke, E., Flegenheimer, W., McCullough, L., Winston, A., & Pollack, J. (1990). Change in patient affect defense ratio from early to late sessions in brief psychotherapy. *Journal of Clinical Psychology, 46,* 657–668.

Thompson, B. J., Gallagher, D., & Breckenridge, J. (1987). Comparative effectiveness of psychotherapies for depressed elders. *Journal of Consulting and Clinical Psychology, 55,* 385–390.

Tichenor, V., & Hill, C. E. (1989). A comparison of six measures of working alliance. *Psychotherapy, 26,* 195–199.

Tishby, O., & Messer, S. B. (1995). The relationship between plan compatibility of therapist interventions and patient progress: A comparison of two plan formulations. *Psychotherapy Research, 5,* 76–88.

Turecki, S. (1982). Elective brief psychotherapy with children. *American Journal of Psychiatry, 36,* 479–488.

Tuttman, S. (1982). Regression: Curative factor or impediment in dynamic psychotherapy? In S. Slipp (Ed.), *Curative factors in dynamic psychotherapy* (pp. 177–198). New York: McGraw-Hill.

Uribe, V. M. (1988). Short-term pscyhotherapy for adolescents: Management of initial resistance. *Journal of the American Academy of Psychoanlysis, 16,* 107–116.

Ursano, R. J., & Dressler, D. M. (1977). Brief versus long-term psychotherapy: Clinician attitudes and organizational design. *Comprehensive Psychiatry, 18,* 55–60.

Vaillant, G. E. (1971). Theoretical hierarchy of adaptive ego mechanisms. *Archives of General Psychiatry, 24,* 107–118.

Wachtel, E. F., & Wachtel, P. L. (1986). *Family dynamics in individual psychotherapy.* New York: Guilford Press.

Wachtel, P. (1977). *Psychoanalysis and behavior therapy: Toward an integration.* New York: Basic Books.

Wachtel, P. L. (1987). *Action and insight.* New York: Guilford Press.

Wachtel, P. L. (1991). From eclectism to synthesis: Toward a more seamless psychotherapeutic integration. *Journal of Psychotherapy Integration, 1,* 43–54.

Wachtel, P. L. (1993). *Therapeutic communication: Principles and effective practice.* New York: Guilford Press.

Wachtel, P. L., & McKinney, M. K. (1992). Cyclical psychodynamics and integrative psychodynamic therapy. In J. C. Norcross & M. R. Goldfried (Eds.), *Handbook of psychotherapy integration* (pp. 335–370). New York: Basic Books.

Wallerstein, R. S. (1986). *Forty-two lives in treatment: A study of psychoanalysis and psychotherapy.* New York: Guilford Press.

Weddington, W. W. J., & Cavenar, J. O. J. (1979). Termination initiated by the therapist: A countertransference storm. *American Journal of Psychiatry, 136,* 1302–1305.

Weinberger, J. (1993). Common factors in psychotherapy. In G. Stricker & J. R. Gold (Eds.), *Comprehensive handbook of psychotherapy integration* (pp. 43–56). New York: Plenum.

Weiss, D. S., & Marmar, C. R. (1993). Teaching time-limited dynamic psychotherapy for post-traumatic stress disorder and pathological grief. *Psychotherapy, 30,* 587–591.

Weiss, J. (1990). Unconscious mental functioning. *Scientific American, 262,* 103–109.

Weiss, J., Sampson, J., & the Mount Zion Psychotherapy Research Group. (1986). *The psychoanalytic process: Theory, clinical observations, and empirical research.* New York: Guilford Press.

Westen, D. (1986). What changes in short-term psychodynamic psychotherapy? *Psychotherapy, 23,* 501–512.

Westen, D. (1988). Transference and information processing. *Clinical Psychology Review, 8,* 161–179.

Westen, D. (1990). Psychoanalytic approaches to personality. In L. A. Pervin (Ed.), *Handbook of personality: Theory and research* (pp. 21–65). New York: Guilford Press.

White, H. (1973). *Metahistory.* Baltimore, MD: Johns Hopkins University Press.

White, R. (1959). Motivation reconsidered: the concept of competence. *Psychological Review, 66,* 297–333.

Wile, D. B. (1984). Kohut, Kernberg, and accusatory interpretations. *Psychotherapy, 22,* 793–802.

Windholz, M. J., & Silberschatz, G. (1988). Vanderbilt Psychotherapy Process Scale: A replication with adult outpatients. *Journal of Consulting and Clinical Psychology, 56,* 56–60.

Winnicott, D. W. (1960). The theory of the parent-infant relationship. In *The maturational process and the facilitating environment* (pp. 37–55). New York: International Universities Press.

Winnicott, D. W. (1963/1965). From dependence toward independence in the development of the individual. In *The maturational process and the facilitating environment* (pp. 83–92). New York: International Universities Press.

Winnicott, D. W. (1965). *The maturational process and the facilitating environment.* New York: International Universities Press.

Winnicott, D. W. (1971). *Playing and reality.* London: Tavistock.

Winokur, M., & Dasberg, H. (1983). Teaching and learning short-term dynamic psychotherapy. *Bulletin of the Menninger Clinic, 47,* 36–52.

Winokur, M., Messer, S. B., & Schacht, T. E. (1981). Contributions to the theory and practice of short-term dynamic psychotherapy. *Bulletin of the Menninger Clinic, 45,* 125–142.

Winston, A., Laikin, M., Pollack, J., Samstag, L. W., McCullough, L., & Muran, J. C. (1994). Short-term dynamic psychotherapy of personality disorders. *American Journal of Psychiatry, 15,* 190–194.

Winston, A., McCullough, L., & Laikin, M. (1993). Clinical and research implications of patient-therapy interaction in brief psychotherapy. *American Journal of Psychotherapy, 47,* 527–539.

Winston, A., Pollack, J., McCullough, L., Flegenheimer, W., Kestenbaum, R., & Trujillo, M. (1991). Brief psychotherapy of personality disorders. *Journal of Nervous and Mental Disease, 179,* 188–193.

Wiseman, H., Shefler, G., Caneti, L., & Ronen, Y. (1993). A systematic comparison of two cases in Mann's time-limited psychotherapy: An events approach. *Psychotherapy Research, 3,* 227–244.

Wolberg, L. R. (1980). *Handbook of short-term psychotherapy.* New York: Thieme–Stratton.

Woody, G., Luborsky, L., McClellan, A.T., O'Brien, C., Beck, A. T., Blaine, J., Herman, I., & Hole, A.V. (1983). Psychotherapy for opiate addicts: Does it help? *Archives of General Psychiatry, 40,* 639–645.

Zetzel, E. R. (1956). Current concepts of transference. *International Journal of Psycho-Analysis, 37,* 369–378.

Zimet, C. N. (1989). The mental health care revolution: Will psychology survive? *American Psychologist, 44,* 703–708.

Zinberg, N. E. (1965). Special problems of gerontological psychiatry. In M. A. Berezin & S. H. Cath (Eds.), *Geriatric psychiatry: Grief, loss and emotional disorders in the aging process* (pp. 147–159). New York: International Universities Press.

Author Index

Note: Italics indicate reference listing.

359

Subject Index